FETAL WOUND HEALING

FETAL WOUND HEALING

N. Scott Adzick, MD
Michael T. Longaker, MD

Department of Surgery
University of California at San Francisco
School of Medicine
San Francisco, California

Elsevier
New York • Amsterdam • London • Tokyo

No responsibility is assumed by the Publisher for any injury and/or damage to persons or property as a matter of products liability, negligence or otherwise, or from any use or operation of any methods, products, instructions, or ideas contained in the material herein. No suggested test or procedure should be carried out unless, in the reader's judgment, its risk is justified. Because of rapid advances in the medical sciences, we recommend that independent verification of diagnoses and drug dosages should be made. Discussions, views, and recommendations as to medical procedures, choice of drugs, and drug dosages are the responsibility of the authors.

Elsevier Science Publishing Co., Inc.
655 Avenue of the Americas, New York, New York 10010

Distributors outside the United States and Canada:
Elsevier Science Publishers B.V.
P.O. Box 211, 1000 AE Amsterdam, The Netherlands

This book is printed on acid-free paper.

Fetal wound healing / [edited by] N. Scott Adzick, Michael T. Longaker.
p. cm.
Includes index.
ISBN 0-444-01621-X (hard cover : alk. paper)
1. Fetus – Physiology. 2. Wound healing. I. Adzick, N. Scott.
II. Longaker, Michael T.
[DNLM: 1. Fetus – physiology. 2. Wound Healing – physiology.
WO 185 F419]
RG613.F49 1991
618.3'2—dc20
DNLM/DLC 91-34387
for Library of Congress CIP

Current printing (last digit):
10 9 8 7 6 5 4 3 2 1

Manufactured in the United States of America

To our fathers—outstanding teachers and role models.

Contents

Preface

Wound healing in the fetus is fundamentally different from wound healing in the adult. Fetal skin wound healing occurs rapidly and in the absence of scar formation. This phenomenon was first observed clinically during the fetal surgery experience, and now it has extensive experimental confirmation. However, we are just beginning to unravel the underlying mechanisms of fetal tissue repair. Scientists and clinicians from diverse backgrounds have become interested in the remarkable fetal tissue repair process, and we are pleased that many of them have had a hand in this book.

Fetal skin wounds heal without a scar, but SO WHAT? A reply to this question may provide an epiphany for fetal wound healing research. The basic scientist's response to this question is that fetal wound healing studies may provide insights into regeneration and fetal development, as tissue repair, regeneration, and development share many common features: cell proliferation, cell movement, cell differentiation, and the important role of the extracellular matrix. The clinician's response to the SO WHAT question is that fetal wound healing represents a paradigm of ideal tissue repair that we would like to emulate in children and adults. As scarring and fibrosis dominate some diseases in every area of medicine, an understanding of fetal wound healing should help develop therapeutic strategies to avert the devastating consequences of excessive scar formation.

The nidus for this book began in the Fetal Surgery Laboratory at the University of California, San Francisco, and then spread to other investigators who lent their expertise to this project. We recognize here our debt to our UCSF colleagues, particularly the enthusiastic intellectual and moral support of Michael Harrison, and the indefatigable effort of Vilma Zarate in helping us along. We are grateful to all of the authors for their cogent contributions that help elucidate the fetal wound healing process. Several years from now, it is likely that we will poke fun at our initial concepts about fetal tissue repair, but it's a place to start.

N. Scott Adzick, MD
Michael T. Longaker, MD
San Francisco, California
November, 1991

Contributors

N. Scott Adzick, MD
Associate Professor of Surgery and Pediatrics, UCSF School of Medicine, Room 585-HSE, San Francisco, California 94143-0570

Mark N. Ahrendt, MD
Research Fellow, Department of Surgery, University of Minnesota, Minneapolis, Minnesota 55455

Steven Berg, BSc
Technician, Oral and Maxillofacial Surgery Research Laboratory, Department of Oral and Maxillofacial Surgery, UCLA School of Dentistry, Los Angeles, California 90024

Charles N. Bertolami, DDS, DMedSc
Professor and Chairman, Section of Oral and Maxillofacial Surgery, Chief, Dental Service, UCLA Medical Center, Los Angeles, California 90024-1668

Rajendra Bhatnagar, PhD
Professor, Division of Oral Biology, UCSF School of Dentistry, Room C628J, Third and Parnassus Avenues, San Francisco, California 94143-0650

Lawrence F. Brown, PhD
Instructor, Department of Pathology, Beth Israel Hospital, Boston, Massachusetts 02215; Instructor, Department of Pathology, Harvard Medical School, Cambridge, Massachusetts 02115

D. Andrew R. Burd, MD
Department of Plastic & Reconstructive Surgery, Rayne Institute, University College Hospital, London WC1E 6JJ, England

Michael D. Caldwell, MD, PhD
Professor, Department of Surgery, University of Minnesota Hospital and Clinics, Minneapolis, Minnesota 55455

Joseph C. Cheng, MD
Department of Orthopedic Surgery, UCSF School of Medicine, San Francisco, California 94143

Brian W. Duncan, MD
Research Fellow, Fetal Treatment Laboratory, Department of Surgery, UCSF School of Medicine, Room 585-HSE, San Francisco, California 94143-0570

H. Paul Ehrlich, PhD
Shriners Burns Institute, 51 Blossom Street, Boston, Massachusetts 02114

Mark W. J. Ferguson, BSc, BDS, PhD, FFD
Professor and Department Head, Department of Cell and Structural Biology, University of Manchester, Coupland 3 Building, Manchester M13 9PL, England

Charles ffrench-Constant, MRCP, PhD
Wellcome Senior Research Fellow, Wellcome/CRC Institute, Tennis Court Road, Cambridge University, Cambridge CB2 1QR, England

Earl G. Freymiller, DMD, MD
Program Director, Section of Oral and Maxillofacial Surgery, UCLA School of Dentistry, Los Angeles, California 90024-1668

Hari Garg, PhD
Shriners Burns Institute, 51 Blossom Street, Boston, Massachusetts 02114

Michael R. Harrison, MD
Professor of Surgery and Pediatrics, Chief, Division of Pediatric Surgery, Co-Director, Fetal Transplant Program, UCSF School of Medicine, Room 585-HSE, San Francisco, California 94143-0570

Georgina Howarth
Research Fellow, Department of Cell and Structural Biology, University of Manchester, Coupland 3 Building, Manchester M13 9PL, England

Thomas K. Hunt, MD
Professor, Department of Surgery, UCSF School of Medicine, Room 839-HSE, San Francisco, California 94143

Russell W. Jennings, MD
Research Fellow, Fetal Treatment Laboratory, Department of Surgery, UCSF School of Medicine, Room 585-HSE, San Francisco, California 94143-0570

Leonard B. Kaban, DMD, MD
Professor and Chairman, Department of Oral and Maxillofacial Surgery, UCSF School of Medicine, San Francisco, California 94143-0440

Thomas M. Krummel, MD
Professor of Surgery and Pediatrics, Chief, Division of Pediatric Surgery, Department of Surgery, The Milton S. Hershey Medical Center, College of Medicine of The Pennsylvania State University, P.O. Box 850, Hershey, Pennsylvania 17033

Julian H. Lewis, DPhil
Senior Scientist, Developmental Biology Unit, Imperial Cancer Research Fund, Department of Zoology, Oxford University, South Parks Road, Oxford OX1 3PS, England

Michael T. Longaker, MD
Research Fellow, Fetal Treatment Laboratory, Department of Surgery, UCSF School of Medicine, Room 585-HSE, San Francisco, California 94143-0570

Xuan Liu, DDS
Postdoctoral Scholar, UCSF School of Dentistry, San Francisco, California 94143

H. Peter Lorenz, MD
Research Fellow, Fetal Treatment Laboratory, Department of Surgery, UCSF School of Medicine, Room 585-HSE, San Francisco, California 94143

Paul Martin, DPhil
Departmental Demonstrator, Department of Human Anatomy, Oxford University, South Parks Road, Oxford OX1 3QX, England

Bruce A. Mast, MD
The Wound Healing Center, Box 117, MCV Station, Richmond, Virginia 23298-0117

Brent R. W. Moelleken, MD
Research Fellow, Division of Plastic and Reconstructive Surgery, Department of Surgery, UCSF School of Medicine, Room 585-HSE, San Francisco, California 94143-0570

Jing Qian, DDS
Postdoctoral Scholar, UCSF School of Dentistry, San Francisco, California 94143

John W. Siebert, MD
Assistant Professor of Surgery and Director of Microsurgery, New York University Medical Center, 550 First Avenue, New York, New York 10016; Chief, Plastic Surgery and Director of Microsurgery, Bellevue Hospital, First Avenue and 27th Street, New York, New York 10016

David Simmons, PhD
Professor, Division of Orthopedic Surgery, University of Texas, Galveston, Texas 77550-2774

Michael Stern, DMD
Department of Pathology, UCSF School of Medicine, Box 0550, San Francisco, California 94143-0550

Robert Stern, MD
Professor, Department of Pathology, UCSF School of Medicine, Room 551-HSE, Third and Parnassus Avenues, San Francisco, California 94143-0506

Livingston Van De Water, PhD
Assistant Professor, Department of Pathology, Beth Israel Hospital, Boston, Massachusetts 02215; Assistant Professor, Department of Pathology, Harvard Medical School, Cambridge, Massachusetts 02115

David J. Whitby, MBBS, FRCS
Senior Registrar, Department of Plastic Reconstructive Surgery, St. James University Hospital, Leeds, England; Honorary Research Fellow, Department of Cell and Structural Biology, School of Biological Sciences, University of Manchester, Coupland 3 Building, Manchester M13 9PL, England

CHAPTER 1

The Fetal Surgery Experience

N. Scott Adzick
Michael R. Harrison

Prenatal diagnosis has undergone an explosion of growth in the past decade. The primary impetus for this rapid expansion has come from the widespread use of prenatal ultrasonography. After the first reports of in utero ultrasonographic diagnosis of congenital anomalies in the 1970s, increasingly sophisticated equipment and experience in interpretation have led to the accurate prenatal diagnosis of a growing number of surgical lesions.[1]

Antenatal diagnosis and serial sonographic study of fetuses with anatomic lesions now makes it possible to define the natural history of these abnormalities, determine the pathophysiologic features that affect clinical outcome, and formulate management based on prognosis. Prenatal diagnosis has defined a "hidden mortality" for some lesions such as congenital diaphragmatic hernia, bilateral hydronephrosis, sacrococcygeal teratoma, and cystic adenomatoid malformation of the lung. These lesions, when first evaluated and treated postnatally, demonstrate a favorable selection bias. The most severely affected fetuses often die in utero or immediately after birth.[2]

Routine obstetrical sonography has changed the surgical management of many congenital anomalies. Most correctable malformations that can be diagnosed in utero are best managed by appropriate medical and surgical therapy after maternal transport and planned delivery at term. Prenatal diagnosis may influence the timing (Table 1.1) or the mode (Table 1.2) of delivery. In rare cases, various forms of in utero therapy may be possible either currently or in the future (Table 1.3). For instance, hematopoietic stem cell and hepatic enzyme deficiencies may be treated by in utero stem cell and hepatocyte transplantation in the near future.[64] The possibility of open fetal surgical intervention, although a formidable undertaking, may be the only solution for some fetal problems. Fetal surgery is only justifiable, however, if: The natural history and pathophysiology of the disease is well understood; the prenatal diagnosis is accurate, capable of excluding other anomalies, and is able to predict which fetuses have a sufficiently bad prognosis to justify in utero intervention; if in utero correction is shown to be efficacious in animal models; and if maternal risk is proven to be acceptably low.

Over the past decade, we have investigated the rationale and feasibility of in utero repair for a number of fetal anomalies, including congenital hydronephrosis, congenital diaphragmatic hernia, sacrococcygeal teratoma, cystic adenomatoid malformation, chylothorax, simple types of congenital heart disease, and cranio-

TABLE 1.1 Defects That May Lead to Induced Preterm Delivery For Early Correction Ex Utero

Obstructive hydronephrosis
Gastroschisis or ruptured omphalocele
Intestinal ischemia and necrosis secondary to volvulus, meconium ileus, etc.
Amniotic band malformation complex

facial defects. The observation was made from this work that the fetus appears to heal without scar formation.[3–5] The biology of scarless fetal skin healing is the focus of this book. This chapter will review our experimental and clinical experience with open fetal surgery for prenatally diagnosed life-threatening anatomic anomalies.

MANAGEMENT OF THE FETUS WITH CONGENITAL HYDRONEPHROSIS

Unrelieved urinary tract obstruction interferes with fetal development. The severity of damage at birth depends on the type, degree, and duration of the obstruction.[6,7] Although children born with partial bilateral obstruction may have only mild hydronephrosis that is reversible with decompression after birth, children born at term with high-grade obstruction may already have advanced hydronephrosis and renal dysplasia that is incompatible with life. In addition, oligohydramnios secondary to decreased fetal urine output produces pulmonary hypoplasia, which is often fatal at birth.

It is possible that the life-threatening problems of respiratory and renal insufficiency may be ameliorated if the obstruction is relieved early enough in gestation to allow normal development to proceed. Optimal clinical management of both patients, mother and fetus, depends on a thorough understanding of the pathophysiology of fetal obstructive uropathy and its sequelae on the developing fetus.

The approach to fetal hydronephrosis developed over the last decade is a paradigm for fetal treatment in general. In this short period, the management of fetal hydronephrosis has advanced dramatically due to multiple studies defining the natural history and pathophysiology of fetal urinary tract obstruction, and to an intensive search for ways to assess fetal renal function and improve selection for treatment. From this large body of experimental and clinical work, for any individual case, the family can now be counseled about the prognosis and options in management, ranging from termination of a hopeless pregnancy to prenatal intervention for those few fetuses whose renal and pulmonary development is threatened.

TABLE 1.2 Defects That May Lead to Cesarean Delivery

Giant omphalocele
Large sacrococcygeal teratoma, cervical hygroma, cervical teratoma
Malformations requiring preterm delivery in the presence of inadequate labor or fetal distress

TABLE 1.3 Defects That May Require In Utero Treatment

Malformation	Effect on Development	In Utero Treatment
Urethral Obstruction	Hydronephrosis, lung hypoplasia → Renal, respiratory failure	Vesicostomy
Congenital Diaphragmatic Hernia	Pulmonary hypoplasia → Respiratory failure	CDH closure
Fetal Chylothorax	Pulmonary hypoplasia → Respiratory failure	Thoraco-amniotic shunt
Sacrococcygeal Teratoma	Massive arteriovenous shunting → placentomegaly, hydrops	Excision
Cystic Adenomatoid Malformation of the Lung	Pulmonary hypoplasia, hydrops	Resection

Developing the Fetal Lamb Model

To study the pathophysiology of fetal urethral obstruction and the efficacy and feasibility of correction in utero, it was necessary first to develop an animal model. Studies using fetal lambs evaluated the effect of urethral obstruction and its subsequent correction on pulmonary and renal development.[8,9] We produced an accurate model of severe bilateral hydronephrosis in the fetal lamb by ligating the urachus and occluding the urethra with an ameroid constrictor or a ligature at 95–105 days gestation (term = 145 days). We then decompressed some of the obstructed fetuses by performing a suprapubic cystostomy at a second fetal operation about three weeks later and compared obstructed, decompressed, and control lambs at birth (Figure 1.1). Uncorrected lambs did poorly; half were still-

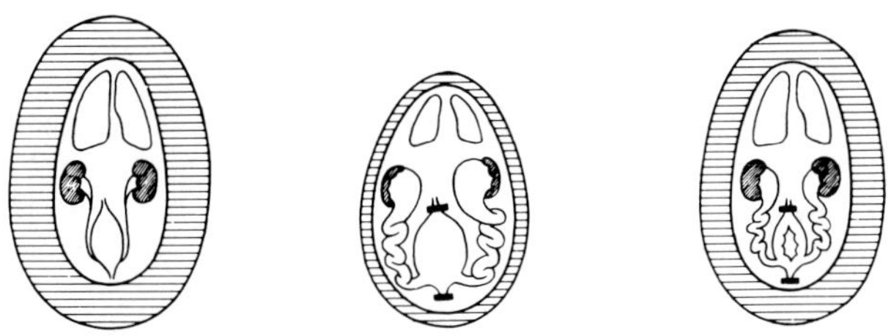

	Controls (n = 8)	Obstructed (n = 8)	Obstructed, decompressed (cystostomy) (n = 9)
Viability	8/8	1/4 (w/resp. distress)	7/7 (w/resp. distress)
(Stillborn)	0	4	2
Urinary tract dilatation	none	2+ to 4+	1+ to 2+
Lung wt./body wt. % ± S.D.	3.03 ± 0.90	1.85 ± 0.46	2.61 ± 0.48
Air cap./body wt. % ± S.D.	5.64 ± 2.07	2.59 ± 0.76	4.34 ± 1.26

Figure 1.1 Summary of data. Obstructed lambs had a high mortality, small lungs, and grossly dilated urinary tracts. Decompression in utero significantly improved survival, lung size, and urinary tract dilation. Four obstructed lambs and two decompressed lambs delivered vaginally prior to planned cesarean delivery, so viability could not be assessed. (Reprinted with permission.[9])

born. Liveborn obstructed lambs had severe respiratory insufficiency, and only one survived the newborn period. The lungs were significantly hypoplastic by weight and volume compared to corrected animals. The bladder, ureters, and renal pelves were severely dilated, mimicking the morphologic disease in human neonates. In contrast, the corrected lambs fared much better. Seven of nine lambs diverted in utero were liveborn, with resolution of the urinary tract dilatation and with far less respiratory difficulty. Relatively late obstruction in the fetal lamb (100 days), however, did not produce the typical cystic and dysplastic changes seen in human urinary tract malformations. To address the relationship between obstruction and renal dysplasia, an earlier gestational model was developed.

To test whether obstruction earlier in fetal life leads to renal dysplasia, we produced complete unilateral ureteral obstruction in fetal lambs at the beginning of the second trimester (55–65 days gestation). We documented that the kidney obstructed at this early stage was both hydronephrotic with ureteral and calyceal dilation proximal to the ligation, and dysplastic when examined at term.[10] This model was then used to determine whether renal dysplasia associated with fetal urinary tract obstruction was preventable by in utero decompression.

Following early second trimester unilateral ureteral ligation in 25 fetal lambs, the fetuses underwent reoperation and ureterostomy of the obstructed ureter after three predetermined time intervals (three, six, or nine weeks). The fetus was returned to the uterus and subsequently delivered at term by cesarean section. Each newborn had the function and morphology of the previously obstructed kidney compared to the contralateral control kidney. This study demonstrated that ureteral obstruction in the early mid-trimester with subsequent decompression prior to term prevents renal dysplasia. Urinary tract decompression reversed the obstructive changes, and the degree of pathologic and functional impairment seen in the obstructed kidney was proportional to the length of time the obstruction existed. Other studies in fetal lambs have shown that the oligohydramnios-induced pulmonary hypoplasia associated with obstructive uropathy is similar to that seen in human fetuses and that decompression of the obstructed urinary tract permits restoration of amniotic fluid volume and compensatory lung growth.[12,13]

There are several lines of evidence which suggest that pulmonary hypoplasia is the result of simple compression of the fetal lung.[14–16] In cases of congenital hydronephrosis, the massively distended urinary tract elevates the diaphragm, and the oligohydramnios results in a small intrauterine cavity that compresses the fetal thorax. If the lung changes are secondary to compression and are not due to a primary pulmonary malformation, restoration of normal amniotic fluid volume by fetal urinary tract decompression would reverse the constraint on normal lung growth. The lamb studies support this hypothesis. Lambs born after correction of urinary tract obstruction in utero fared much better, and the improvement correlated roughly with larger lungs. In addition, we have demonstrated in a fetal rabbit model that decompressing the lungs by restoration of amniotic fluid volume or by reducing pressure on the diaphragm allows the lungs to grow.[17] Further studies in the same experimental preparation suggested that the loss of the internal stenting force of fetal lung fluid is an important etiologic factor.[18]

The Problem of Selection: Assessment of Fetal Renal Function

A major problem in management of the fetus with hydronephrosis is how to select out of a large number of fetuses with dilated urinary tracts only those with obstruction severe enough to compromise renal and pulmonary function at birth,

TABLE 1.4 Prognostic Criteria for the Fetus with Bilateral Obstructive Uropathy

	Fetal Urine Composition and Volume			
Predicted Function	**Sodium (mEq/ml)**	**Chloride (mEq/ml)**	**Osmolarity mosmol**	**Output (ml/hr)**
Poor	>100	>90	>210	<2
Good	<100	<90	<210	>2

yet not so severe that renal function cannot be salvaged even with in utero decompression. The fetus with a dilated low-pressure system who continues to have good urine output and adequate amniotic fluid volume requires no intervention. At the other end of the spectrum, the fetus with severe renal dysplasia that is not reversible even with decompression clearly should not be treated. The fetus with unilateral disease of any type with a normally functioning contralateral kidney can be managed conservatively because the disease is not life-threatening. But the fetus with bilateral hydronephrosis and unknown renal functional potential who might be a candidate for intervention requires methods to assess renal function.

The presence of oligohydramnios is a critical determinant of mortality.[19] Fetuses identified with oligohydramnios in the early second trimester have a mortality in excess of 90%.[20,21] We have attempted to define criteria predicting which of these fetuses would be salvageable. To be a candidate for fetal intervention, the affected fetus must have good residual renal function at the time of diagnosis, despite oligohydramnios. The ultrasound appearance of the fetal kidneys provides valuable prognostic information if the renal parenchyma shows increased echogenicity or cystic changes, but is less predictive in their absence.[22]

We reviewed our experience with 20 fetuses with congenital bilateral hydronephrosis referred for treatment to determine the prognostic value of various criteria used to assess renal functional potential.[23] Based on these results, six prognostic criteria to identify the fetus with "good function" and "poor function" were generated (Table 1.4). Although these results are based on a retrospective analysis, the utility of these parameters have been confirmed in recent prospective and retrospective studies.[20,21] The development of prognostic criteria that predict the potential for recovery has greatly simplified counseling of the families and selection of appropriate management. The prognostic criteria (urine Na < 100 mEq/L, Cl < 90 mEq/L, Osm < 210 mosm, and normal fetal kidneys by ultrasound) have proven to reliably predict neonatal and long-term outcome after in utero urinary tract decompression, and the urine studies can be obtained by a single bladder aspiration under ultrasound guidance.

An Algorithm for Management

From our cumulative clinical and laboratory experience, we have derived the following general guidelines for management of the fetus with hydronephrosis (Figure 1.2). Initial evaluation should begin with an ultrasound to confirm the diagnosis, the anatomic level of obstruction, the status of the amniotic fluid, and the presence of associated anomalies. If an associated life-threatening anomaly is present, the family should be counseled and allowed to choose expectant management or termination of the pregnancy. If hydronephrosis appears to be an isolated defect and the amniotic fluid volume is adequate, the mother should be

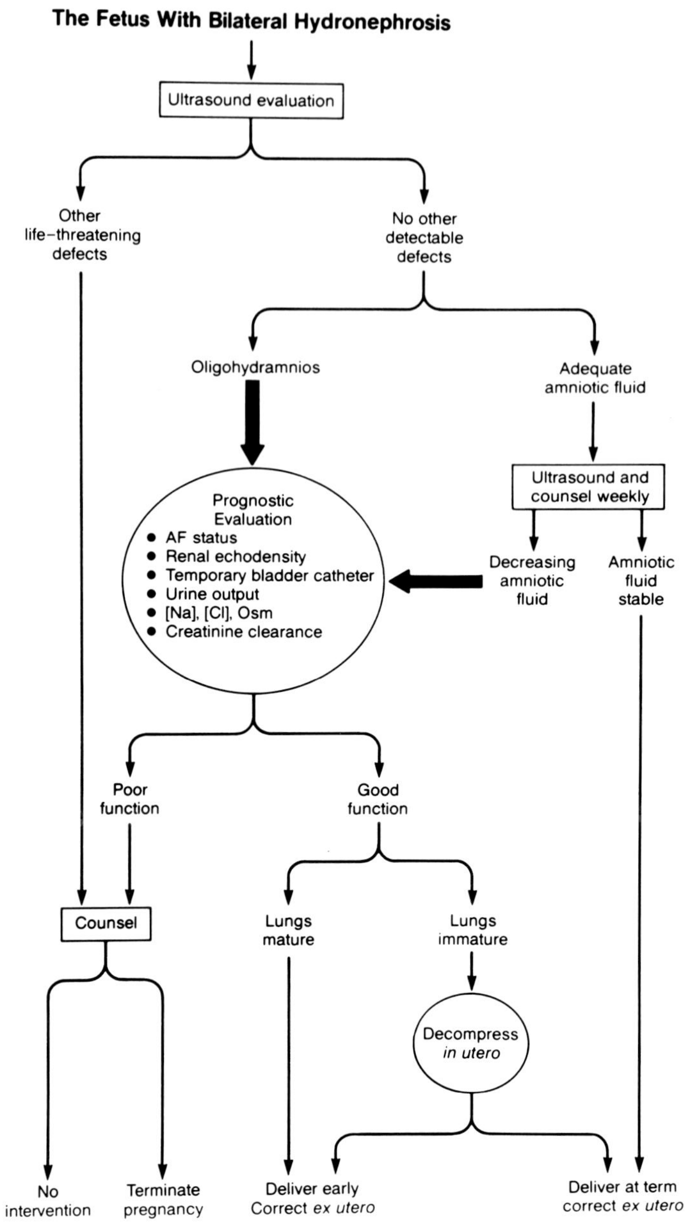

Figure 1.2 Management scheme for the fetus with bilateral hydronephrosis. (Reprinted with permission.[23])

followed by serial ultrasound. If amniotic fluid volume remains adequate, then the mother should receive routine obstetrical care, and the fetus can be treated postnatally. If moderate to severe oligohydramnios develops, then the fetus should undergo a complete prognostic evaluation to determine the fetus' potential for normal renal and pulmonary function at birth. For the fetus with predicted renal dysplasia, aggressive obstetrical care or in utero decompression is not indicated. For the fetus with predicted preserved renal function, there are two management options depending on fetal lung maturity. For the fetus with mature lungs, immediate delivery and ex utero decompression is indicated, and for the fetus with immature lungs, in utero decompression is recommended. For open fetal surgery, the gestational age at diagnosis should be less than 28 weeks, as successful decompression can occasionally be performed after this time with a percutaneously placed fetal bladder catheter. Prior to 28 weeks gestation, fetal catheter placement has been unsuccessful due to frequent obstruction and dislodgement.[24]

The Evolution of Open Fetal Surgery for Hydronephrosis

The criteria for attempting open fetal surgery were satisfied by our group in the early 1980s. The first open case for hydronephrosis was performed in 1981,[25] and six others have been performed since then. It is important to remember that only seven out of more than 200 cases of bilateral hydronephrosis referred for management over the last decade were deemed appropriate for open surgery.[24,26] The first fetus had bilateral ureterostomies and the subsequent six had marsupialization of the bladder at 18–24 weeks gestation. The first five pregnancies proceeded to cesarean delivery at 32 to 35 weeks gestation. The sixth fetus never drained urine well after vesicostomy and was removed at re-exploration by the parent's request because of a severe cloacal anomaly. The seventh fetus underwent successful urinary tract decompression, but subsequently died two weeks later from pulmonary hypoplasia. This baby was delivered prematurely as a result of the mother's discontinuing her oral tocolytic therapy.

Three fetuses had prolonged return of normal amniotic fluid dynamics and all three had adequate pulmonary function at birth, suggesting that fatal pulmonary hypoplasia associated with early severe oligohydramnios had been reversed. Two other neonates died at birth with pulmonary hypoplasia. One had no amniotic fluid even after decompression due to our inability to predict fetal renal function early in our experience. The other had some amniotic fluid after decompression but a tiny chest cavity due to a long period of severe oligohydramnios before decompression. Of the three surviving infants, one had normal renal function when she died of unrelated causes at nine months of age. One has normal renal function at age three. The third developed failing renal function by three years, has grown and developed normally, and subsequently received a successful kidney transplant. Our current selection criteria would now accurately exclude from treatment the two fetuses who died of pulmonary hypoplasia.

Throughout this initial period of performing fetal surgery, our selection criteria have been evolving. Improvements in selection now make it possible to avoid intervention in hopeless cases. This small series of human cases confirms that the development of fatal pulmonary hypoplasia can be prevented if amniotic fluid dynamics can be restored by decompression of the obstructed urinary tract. It is still unclear if in utero intervention arrested or reversed cystic dysplastic changes caused by obstructive uropathy, since it is possible that the dysplastic changes initiated in utero will compromise renal function progressively as functional demand increases with growth. We believe, however, that relief of obstruction during the most active phase of nephrogenesis, between 20 and 30 weeks gestation, may obviate further damage and allow nephrogenesis to proceed normally.[23] Further experience and long-term follow-up are necessary to determine the effectiveness of in utero decompression in reversing or arresting renal damage caused by obstruction.

MANAGEMENT OF THE FETUS WITH CONGENITAL DIAPHRAGMATIC HERNIA

Congenital diaphragmatic hernia (CDH) is an anatomically simple defect easily correctable by removing the herniated viscera from the chest and closing the diaphragm.[27] However, many infants with CDH die of pulmonary insufficiency despite optimal postnatal care because their lungs are too hypoplastic to support extrauterine life. The pulmonary hypoplasia seen with CDH has been well documented clinically and experimentally; it appears to be caused by compression of the developing fetal lung by herniated bowel. In this section, the evolution of in utero therapy for CDH will be described. As was the case for bilateral hydronephrosis, 10 years of experimental and clinical work that supports the pathophysiologic rationale for correction of CDH in utero will be reviewed.

The Fetal Lamb Model

To study the pulmonary hypoplasia that accompanies CDH and the possibility of reversing these changes by correcting the CDH in utero, a model was developed in which a conical, silicone-rubber balloon was progressively inflated in the left hemithorax of fetal lambs over the last trimester to simulate compression of the growing fetal lung by abdominal viscera.[28] Lambs born with inflated intrathoracic balloons deteriorated rapidly and died of respiratory insufficiency despite maximal resuscitation and ventilatory support. Deflation of the balloon midway through the third trimester (simulated "correction") allowed sufficient lung growth to alleviate respiratory insufficiency and to assure survival in five of five lambs delivered by cesarean section.[29] Simulated correction produced a significant increase in lung weight, air capacity, compliance, and area of the pulmonary vascular bed (Figure 1.3).

Although the balloon model established the efficacy of in utero repair, it could not be used to study the feasibility of correction or to develop the surgical techniques necessary for actual successful fetal surgical repair. For this purpose we had to create and then attempt to surgically repair actual fetal diaphragmatic

	CONTROLS (n=6)	SIMULATED CDH BALLOON INFLATED (n=7)	"CORRECTED" CDH BALLOON DEFLATED AT 120 DAYS (n=8)

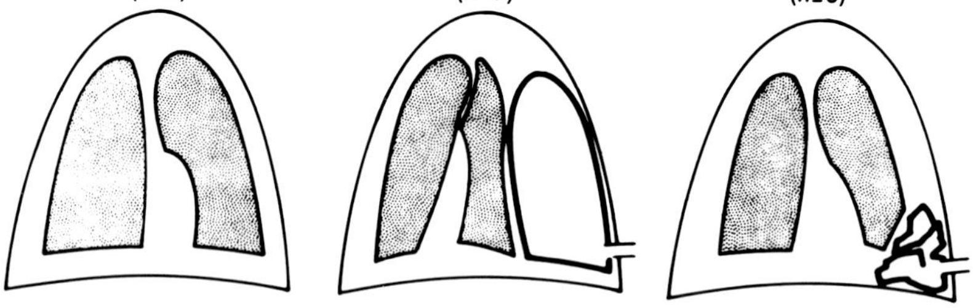

VIABILITY	6/6 LIVED	6/6 DIED	5/5 LIVED (with resp. distress)
Lung Weight	123.2±25.4	49.6±6.6	79.1±6.0
Lung Wt./Body Wt.	3.42±0.30	1.71±.03	2.26±.14
Air Capacity	222.5±47.9	58.8±7.6	151±10.0
Air Cap./Body Wt.	6.24±0.84	2.37±0.12	4.55±0.32

Figure 1.3 Summary of data for lambs with simulated CDH. (Reprinted with permission.[29])

hernias. We created diaphragmatic hernias in fetal lambs by making a hole in the left diaphragm and demonstrated that herniated viscera produced pulmonary hypoplasia comparable to that produced by the balloon. We then tried to repair the CDH surgically at a second operation.[29]

The first attempts at repair were unsuccessful because increased intra-abdominal pressure secondary to replacement of the viscera into the abdomen resulted in severely compromised umbilical venous blood flow. It became clear that the abdominal cavity would need to be enlarged to prevent increased intra-abdominal pressure after fetal CDH repair. Incorporating a piece of silastic into the abdominal wall proved to be a satisfactory solution allowing the abdominal contents to be accommodated without increased pressure. When we used these techniques for repair of fetal CDH, the lambs survived at term and at sacrifice the lungs were well expanded, histologically mature, and much larger than those of uncorrected animals.[30] These findings have been confirmed by others using a similar fetal lamb model.[31] Subsequent pulmonary morphometric studies have shown that an early gestational CDH lamb model simulates the morphologic features that correlate with fatal outcome for human neonates with CDH and persistent fetal circulation, and that fetal surgical repair ameliorates these vascular changes and permits compensatory lung growth and development.[32]

The Natural History of Congenital Diaphragmatic Hernia

Survey data derived from neonatal centers underestimate the incidence and mortality of CDH because the more severely affected infants often die before the anomaly is recognized. Minimum incidence figures derived from various sources range from one in 2400 to one in 5000 live births; the true incidence including stillborns is probably around one in 2200 births.[2,33–35] Paradoxically, the mortality of infants with CDH reported from major neonatal centers has not improved with the recent improvements in neonatal transport and intensive care. Earlier reported series quoted mortality rates around 50% for postnatally detected CDH, but included only the most favorable cases—those that survived to be transferred to the major referral center. The most severely affected infants died before they came to the attention of the referral center, accounting for a significant "hidden mortality,"[2] a situation directly analogous to that seen with prenatally diagnosed bilateral hydronephrosis. With improved neonatal transport and respiratory support, some of these desperately ill infants now survive long enough to be treated. Because mortality is extremely high in this group, recent series from highly capable centers often show dismal results.[36]

Management of the fetus with prenatally diagnosed CDH is dependent on an understanding of the natural history, pathophysiology, and prognostic factors affecting outcome. It would seem that antenatal diagnosis of CDH would result in immediate postnatal repair and survival. However, our initial reported experience with fetal CDH was very disappointing—no survivors out of seven fetuses prospectively diagnosed before birth.[37] This led to a multicenter survey that documented the natural history and clinical outcome of fetal CDH in 94 cases.[38] This study demonstrated that the prenatal sonographic diagnosis is accurate, the mortality is high (80%), and polyhydramnios is a prenatal predictor of poor clinical outcome. A subsequent study of 38 prenatally diagnosed cases from a single medical center permitted a detailed assessment of prognostic factors and evaluation of the impact of extracorporeal membrane oxygenation (ECMO) on outcome.[39]

This study found that survival was poor despite optimal postnatal therapy including ECMO, and that both polyhydramnios and an early gestational diagnosis were associated with a dismal outcome. Thus the severity of a fetal CDH can be judged by the timing of herniation, the degree of pulmonary compression (lung to thorax ratio at the level of a four-chamber view of the heart), and the presence of polyhydramnios.

Initial Experience with Repair In Utero

We obtained the approval of the Committee on Human Research in 1983 for open fetal surgery for CDH. Only eight cases in seven years have met our stringent selection criteria. In addition, it has been imperative that the families understand the risks of fetal surgery and are willing to travel to San Francisco. Finances were a major stumbling block as insurance companies refused to cover any expenses associated with this experimental procedure. Although there were no professional fees, the cost of the procedures and hospitalization were considerable and had to be borne by the investigating institution. Although we were contacted by telephone about a large number of fetuses with CDH, only a fraction (less than 1 in ten) was even a candidate to come to San Francisco for further evaluation. Of the potential candidates, at least half were excluded by social and financial considerations.

After extensive experimental work demonstrated the efficacy, feasibility, and safety of repair in utero, we attempted to salvage eight highly selected fetuses with severe CDH by open fetal surgery.[40,66] The experience with these very severe cases was initially discouraging, but each of these cases contributed to invaluable knowledge and experience that eventually led to the first clinical success. The first three fetuses died at operation because attempts to reduce the friable incarcerated liver from the fetal chest were unsuccessful. In the fourth case, a Gore-Tex diaphragm was constructed around the liver, but lung decompression was ineffective and the baby died at birth. The last four fetuses were successfully repaired, and the technical problem with the herniated liver proved to be surmountable. All four demonstrated rapid growth of the lung in utero, and had surprisingly good lung function after birth. Two subsequently died of non-pulmonary problems (an unrelated nursery accident in one and intestinal complications in the other), but the last two babies have done well.[66]

An Algorithm for Prenatal Management of CDH

Figure 1.4 shows our proposed algorithm for management. Once a diaphragmatic hernia is diagnosed by ultrasound, the patient should be referred for chromosomal analysis by amniocentesis (results in about 2 weeks) or percutaneous umbilical blood sampling (results in about 2 days), screening for other anatomic abnormalities by an experienced obstetrical sonographer, and evaluation for cardiac abnormalities by fetal echocardiography. When associated serious anomalies are discovered, the family may choose to terminate the pregnancy.

There is a wide spectrum of severity in CDH. Some mildly affected fetuses will be detected later in gestation, develop polyhydramnios later or not at all, and have a smaller volume of viscera in the chest. These fetuses should be followed by sonogram and delivered at an appropriate tertiary perinatal center after the lungs are mature. Unfortunately, the majority of fetuses will be on the severe end of the spectrum and will not survive even with optimal conventional pre- and postnatal management. In general, these fetuses will be detected earlier, develop

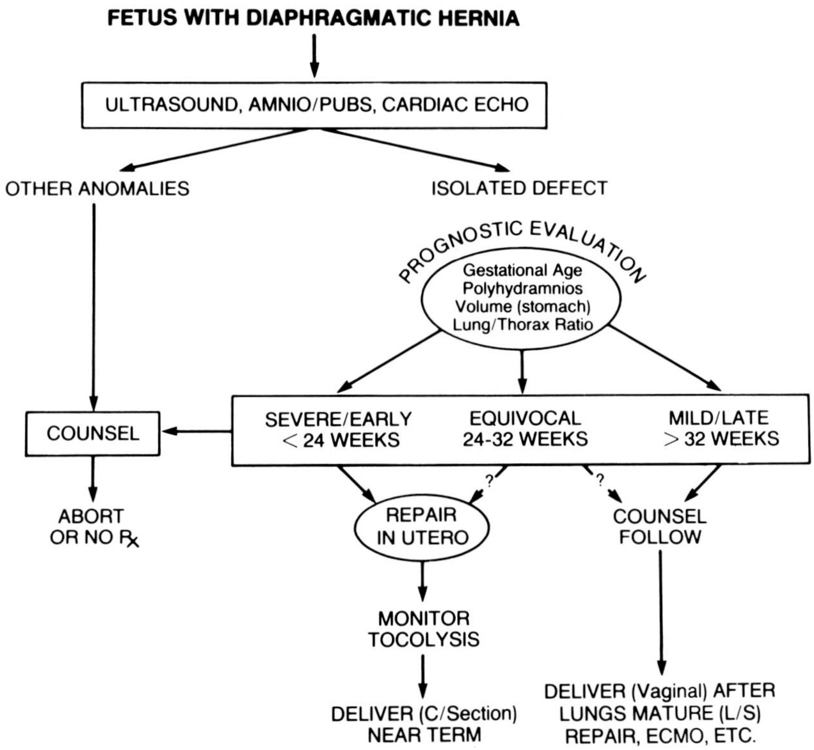

Figure 1.4 Algorithm for management of the fetus with CDH. (Reprinted with permission.[40])

polyhydramnios earlier, and have a larger volume of viscera in the chest (dilated stomach, impressive mediastinal shift, little lung visible in either thorax). Every effort should be made to determine if the liver is herniated into the chest as this affects prognosis and the technical difficulty of repair before birth. Between 20 and 30 weeks, the family can choose between conventional management or fetal repair depending on assessment and their personal attitude. After 30 weeks, the only option is conventional management aimed at maximizing postnatal care. Although fetal repair is theoretically possible until 32 weeks, it is probably best performed before 30 weeks for two reasons. First, the longer the decompressed lung has to grow before it is required to support life at birth, the better (and preterm labor associated with hysterotomy may shorten the remaining gestation). Second, it is our impression that the risk of inducing preterm labor is greater when the procedure is performed later in gestation. Although it would seem technically advantageous to operate on a larger fetus with more mature tissues, surgical procedures have proven feasible in fetuses as young as 18 weeks. At present, we will consider fetuses between 20 and 30 weeks gestation for in utero repair.

MANAGEMENT OF FETAL CHYLOTHORAX

Congenital pleural effusions are often due to fetal chylothorax (FCT), and can be diagnosed as early as 16 weeks gestation.[41] Small effusions may be harmless, while large effusions may result in pulmonary compression, pulmonary hypoplasia, and hydrops.

We recently reported a series of 32 cases.[42] The overall mortality was 53%.

Polyhydramnios was present in 22 cases and was not associated with a higher mortality. Early diagnosis (less than 32 weeks gestation) and hydrops were associated with a higher mortality. Pleural fluid was available in 12 patients, all of which had more than 80% lymphocytes on cell count, which confirmed the diagnosis of FCT.

Small effusions diagnosed late in gestation often have a satisfactory outcome without prenatal treatment, and some resolve spontaneously. In these cases, serial ultrasounds should be performed, with appropriate postnatal follow-up. For large effusions causing hydrops, in utero decompression may offer the only hope for survival. Although success with repeated percutaneous thoracenteses in utero has been reported, we have recently used a thoraco-amniotic shunt to successfully decompress the FCT after multiple attempts at aspiration failed to permanently drain the fetal chest. Rodeck reported the successful placement of a thoraco-amniotic shunt in eight fetuses with massive FCT.[43] Six of these infants survived, five without respiratory difficulty postnatally. Lung re-expansion was seen in all of the survivors, but not in the two who died.

MANAGEMENT OF FETAL TUMORS

Sacrococcygeal Teratoma

The majority of babies with sacrococcygeal teratoma (SCT) are diagnosed as newborns when the malignant potential is low and the prognosis is good. However, prenatal diagnosis has identified cases of SCT that die in utero. The gestational age has important prognostic significance. We reported a series where six out of eight cases survived when the diagnosis was made after 30 weeks gestation, but only one of 14 cases survived when the diagnosis was made before 30 weeks gestation.[44] When diagnosed prior to 30 weeks gestation, invariably there has been development of massive tumor enlargement, fetal hydrops, and placentomegaly. In each of six cases diagnosed at 14–23 weeks gestation, the mothers developed "mirror syndrome" with vomiting, hypertension, edema, and proteinuria; two of the six affected mothers required treatment in the intensive care unit for pulmonary edema.

We have recently demonstrated by Doppler ultrasound that the tumor in these severe cases behaves as a large arteriovenous fistula with markedly increased distal aortic blood flow and shunting of blood away from the placenta.[45] Fetal demise presumably occurs because of high-output cardiac failure with the development of hydrops.

These findings have important implications for management. Fetuses with lesions greater than 5 centimeters should be delivered by cesarean section to avoid dystocia, tumor rupture, or hemorrhage into the tumor which may occur with vaginal delivery.[44] Cases with hydrops diagnosed after 30 weeks gestation should be delivered when pulmonary maturity is attained. Lesions diagnosed prior to 30 weeks gestation usually have a poor outcome and may require fetal surgical excision.

Congenital Cystic Adenomatoid Malformation (CCAM)

CCAM can present itself as a fatal lesion in a fetus or neonate, or as a relatively mild lesion causing respiratory difficulty or recurrent infections in an infant or child. CCAM represents a spectrum of disease characterized by cystic lesions of the lung. The macrocystic type has cysts that grow to several centimeters in diameter. Microcystic disease has multiple cystic lesions less than 5 millimeters in diameter. Prenatal ultrasound can generally distinguish individual cysts in macrocystic disease while microcystic lesions usually have the appearance of an echogenic, solid lung mass.[46]

Differences in survival rate of patients with CCAM have been previously ascribed to the histologic type of the lesion, but our experience and that of others demonstrates that an unfavorable outcome is most closely associated with hydrops. Hydrops is probably secondary to vena cava obstruction or cardiac compression from the extreme mediastinal shift caused by these lesions, and hydrops has been associated with other space-occupying thoracic lesions.[47] The invariably fatal outcome seen with large CCAM lesions is related to several factors including development of hydrops, hypoplasia of normal lung tissue secondary to prolonged compression in utero, and lack of early diagnosis and immediate postnatal surgery. Macrocystic lesions may resolve spontaneously when followed by serial ultrasound throughout the course of pregnancy.[48]

It is now clear that in utero surgical decompression or removal of the CCAM will reverse the hydrops and allow sufficient lung growth to permit survival in these severe cases.[67] We have demonstrated experimentally that in utero pulmonary resection is feasible and that compensatory lung growth of the opposite lung occurs.[49] Thoracentesis of macrocystic lesions in utero does not provide lasting decompression of normal lung tissue.[46] However, percutaneous placement of a double pigtail catheter shunt between a large lung cyst and the amniotic space in a 20 week gestation fetus with CCAM resulted in sustained cyst decompression, and resolution of hydrops with delivery 17 weeks later and successful postnatal surgery.[50]

Maternal Mirror Syndrome: An Unsolved Problem after Resection of Fetal Tumors

Large fetal tumors may result in placentomegaly, hydrops, and fetal death. The "maternal mirror syndrome" (MMS) is a hyperdynamic state in which the maternal physiology "mirrors" that of the hydropic fetus with hypertension, peripheral and pulmonary edema, and gastrointestinal and renal dysfunction. Maternal mirror syndrome is associated with severe Rh disease and other fetal conditions that cause placentomegaly and complicates control of preterm labor.[51] We have encountered this syndrome twice after resection of large tumors in hydropic moribund fetuses.

The first case was a 21 week gestation fetus referred with a huge sacrococcygeal teratoma, placentomegaly, and hydrops due to massive arteriovenous shunting through the tumor.[45] Successful complete resection of the tumor in utero led to marked improvement in the fetal hydrops. The second case was a 27 week gestation fetus referred with a giant congenital cystic adenomatoid malformation with massive mediastinal shift, hydrops, and placentomegaly. A thoracoamniotic shunt was not possible since the lung lesion was microcystic. The mass was successfully resected in utero by right middle lobectomy with consequent improvement in the fetal pathophysiology.[67] In both cases, placentomegaly persisted postoperatively, and the mothers developed progressive MMS that prevented adequate tocolysis despite fetal improvement. A cesarean section was performed for maternal safety

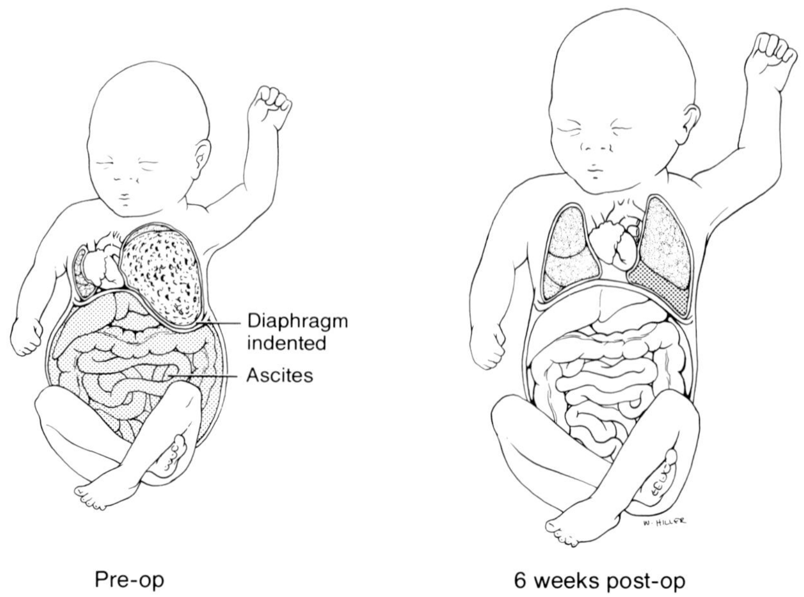

Figure 1.5 Schematic drawing of fetal anatomy preoperatively (A) and six weeks after fetal surgery for cystic adenomatoid malformation (B). Postoperatively, the fetal ascites resolved, the mediastinum returned to the midline, and the remaining left upper lobe and right lung showed remarkable growth. (Reprinted with permission.[67])

in case one after 12 days and case two after 6 days, and the MMS quickly resolved. The premature infants soon died from respiratory insufficiency.

Although fetal tumor excision is technically feasible, reversal of the fetal pathophysiology did not rapidly correct the placentomegaly or resolve the MMS. MMS may be caused by placental release of vasoactive compounds resulting in a severe pre-eclamptic state. Until the MMS riddle is solved, earlier intervention before the onset of placentomegaly and hydrops may be the only approach to salvage these doomed fetuses.

Recently, successful in utero resection of a huge CCAM was performed in a 23 week fetus with ascites but no placentomegaly. The ascites resolved, and good lung growth occurred in utero (Figure 1.5). That child is currently thriving at 14 months of age.[67] In that case, the early diagnosis, the large size of the tumor, and the early onset of hydrops indicated a dismal prognosis, which led us to consider prenatal intervention as the only hope for a successful outcome. We can now add appropriately selected cases of CCAM to the list of congenital lesions that are amenable to fetal surgical therapy. An algorithm for management of the fetus with CCAM is shown in Figure 1.6.

CONGENITAL HEART DISEASE

Many types of congenital cardiac disease can now be readily diagnosed in utero with a high degree of accuracy.[52] Prenatally diagnosed complete heart block (CHB) can occur without associated cardiac anomalies, and it is often refractory to attempts to increase heart rate and cardiac output by medical therapy and results in fetal demise.[53] We have developed a model of CHB in fetal lambs and have demonstrated the feasibility of epicardial ventricular or atrioventricular pac-

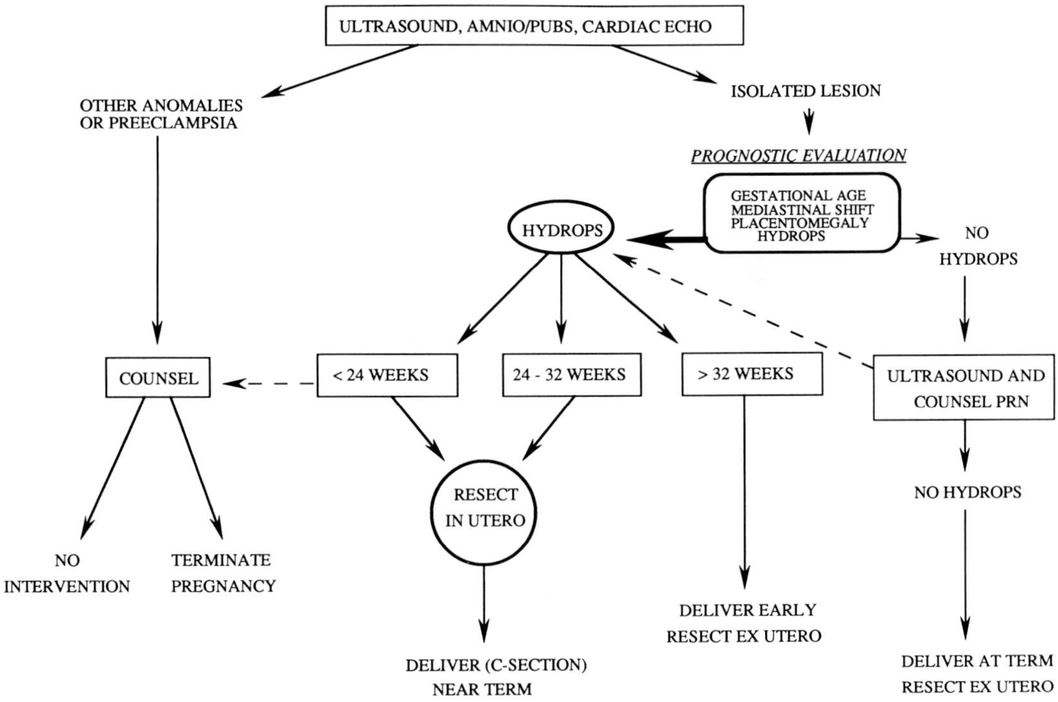

Figure 1.6 Algorithm for management of the fetus with a CCAM.

ing to increase cardiac output. The model may facilitate the development of new clinical therapies to salvage refractory cases of fetal CDH.[54] Another group of investigators has attempted percutaneous transthoracic pacing in a hydropic fetus with CHB, but this effort failed for technical reasons.[55]

Although the in utero pathophysiology of congenital cardiac lesions is not completely understood, it appears that decreased blood flow during fetal life can result in secondary hypoplasia of vessels or cardiac chambers.[56] Experimental intrauterine repair of pulmonary artery stenosis is feasible without cardiac bypass,[57,58] percutaneous angioplasty balloon dilatation for critical fetal aortic stenosis has been attempted in a human fetus, and hypothermia or bypass techniques may make open fetal cardiac surgery a possibility in the future.[59]

MATERNAL MANAGEMENT AND RISK

Maternal safety is the paramount consideration in fetal surgery. A series of 102 fetal operations in 94 monkeys permitted us to develop anesthetic, surgical, and tocolytic regimens for fetal surgery and demonstrate satisfactory maternal safety.[60–62]

Clinical Experience: Operative Technique

Perioperative clinical management principles have their basis directly from the experimental nonhuman primate work. Maternal preparation begins with a 100 mg suppository of indomethacin preoperatively and placement of an epidural catheter for postoperative analgesia. Intraoperatively, halothane is used for uterine

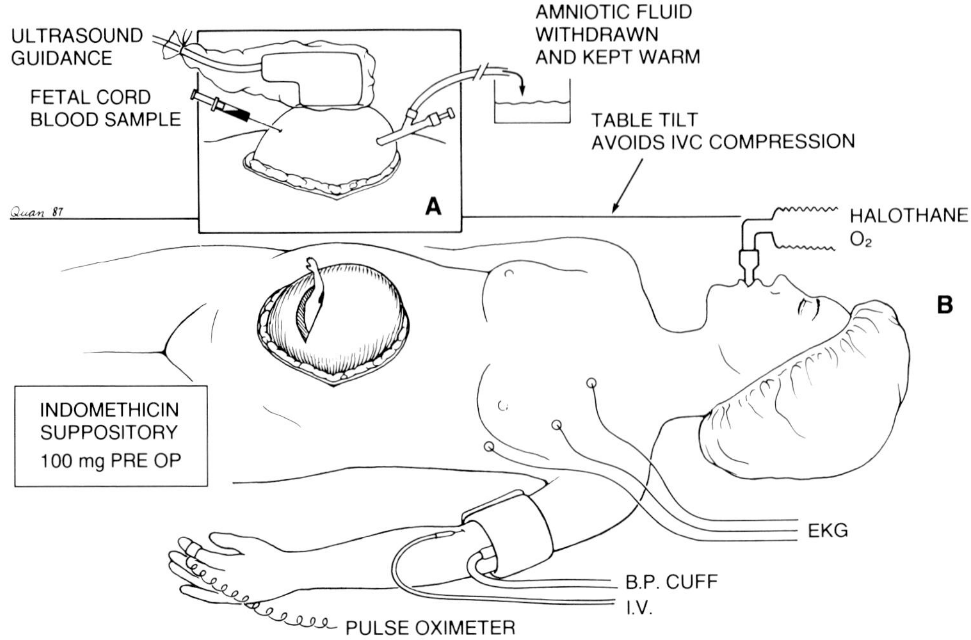

Figure 1.7 Drawing of maternal positioning and monitoring for open fetal surgery. (Reprinted with permission.[68])

relaxation and for fetal and maternal anesthesia. Postoperatively, ritodrine, magnesium sulfate and indomethacin are used for tocolysis. Maternal intraoperative monitoring includes a blood pressure cuff, large bore intravenous catheters, a bladder catheter, EKG leads, and a transcutaneous pulse oximeter (Figure 1.7).

The mother is positioned supine with towels placed under her right side to lift her uterus off of the inferior cava to avoid compromise of venous return. The uterus is exposed through a low transverse abdominal incision and delivered into the operative field. A large abdominal ring retractor is utilized to maintain exposure. Sterile intraoperative ultrasound is used to confirm the fetal position and placental location. The position and orientation of the hysterotomy is planned to stay as far away from the placenta as possible and still allow exposure of the appropriate part of the fetus. Excess amniotic fluid is aspirated with a trocar and kept warm. The hysterotomy can be performed with an absorbable stapler that

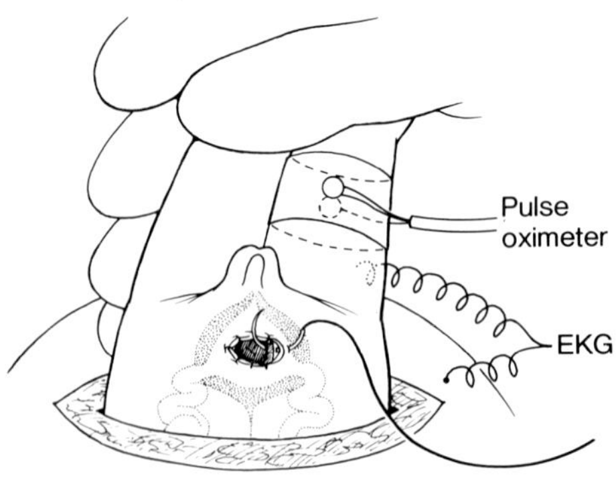

Figure 1.8 Diagram of intraoperative appearance of bladder marsupialization to the fetal abdominal wall to create a vesico-amniotic fistula. (Reprinted with permission.[24])

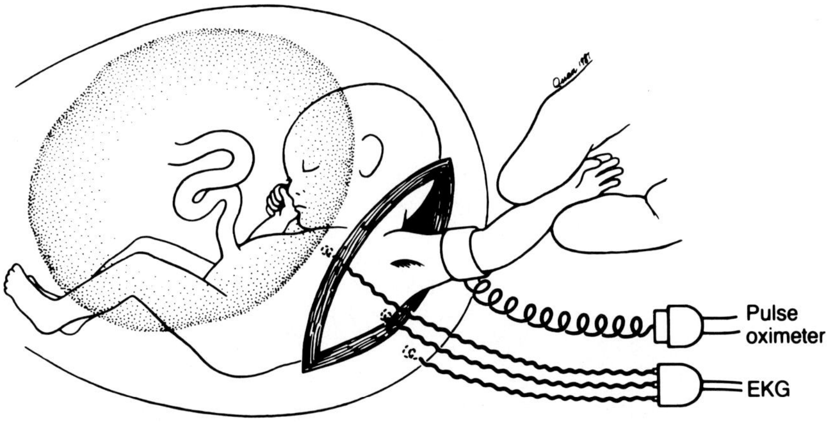

Figure 1.9 Left arm and chest exteriorized and monitors placed with subcostal incision shown. (Reprinted with permission.[40])

is fast and hemostatic.[63] An alternative method to minimize blood loss during hysterotomy is by manual compression on either side of the proposed hysterotomy; the uterine incision is then made between the assistant's hands using electrocautery. Immediately, specially designed compression clamps are placed around the edge of the uterine incision to prevent bleeding.

For urinary tract decompression,[24–26] the lower extremities of the fetus are exteriorized and a transcutaneous pulse oximeter is placed around the fetal thigh. A midline suprapubic incision is made through the fetal abdominal wall exposing the thick-walled and distended bladder. The bladder is then opened and marsupialized to the abdominal wall using interrupted 4-O silk sutures (Figure 1.8).

For diaphragmatic hernia,[40,66] the left arm of the fetus is exteriorized for monitoring, and the left side of the chest and upper abdomen is stabilized by placing a Babcock clamp onto the costal margin (Figure 1.9). The diaphragm is repaired with a Gore-Tex patch through a subcostal incision and the abdomen is enlarged to accommodate the viscera using another synthetic patch (Figures 1.10 and 1.11).

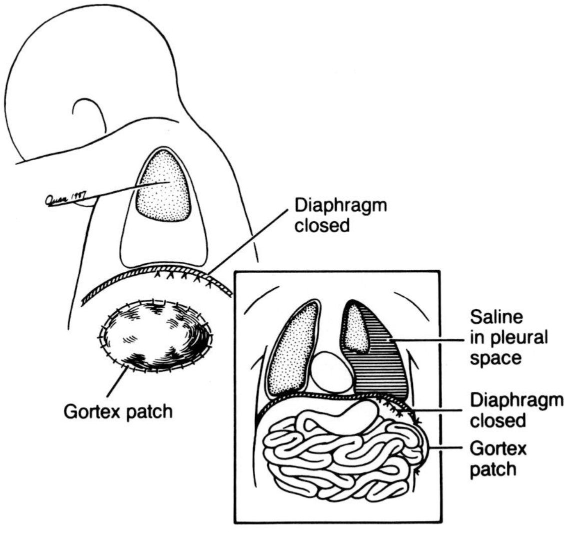

Figure 1.10 Diaphragm closed. Abdomen enlarged with patch to accommodate viscera without increasing intra-abdominal pressure. (Reprinted with permission.[40])

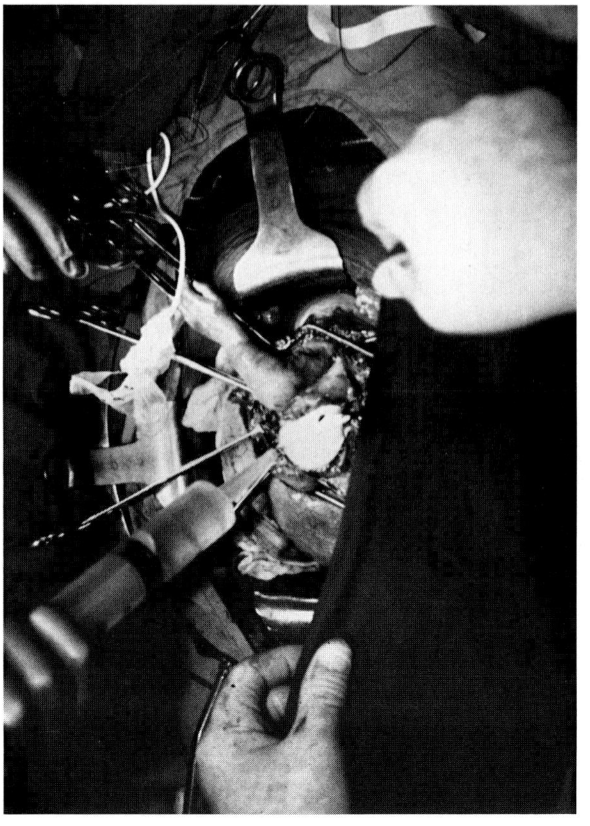

Figure 1.11 Intraoperative photograph of 25 week gestation human fetus at the end of CDH repair. The GoreTex patch abdominoplasty is shown just below the left arm. The large syringe is replacing amniotic fluid.

The fetus is returned to the uterine cavity and the amniotic fluid is restored with either warm normal saline or warm amniotic fluid containing 500 mg nafcillin. The uterus is closed with three layers of absorbable sutures and fibrin glue. The low transverse abdominal incision is closed in layers using running O-prolene suture and the skin is closed with a subcuticular suture. Beyond these technical points, we have learned that, as a general principle, fetal surgery should be "all or none", i.e., the fetal repair should be complete and adequate to ensure a good chance for fetal survival, or else the otherwise doomed fetus should be removed. A partial or inadequate repair presents an ongoing threat to the mother for little potential benefit.

Postoperative Management

Premature labor remains the largest obstacle to a successful outcome in the postoperative course. Postoperatively, uterine contractions and fetal heart rate are monitored and tocolytic therapy with betamimetics, magnesium sulfate, and prostaglandin synthetase inhibitors is adjusted accordingly. Once the initial period of uterine contractions has subsided (usually within 5 days), oral tocolytics are gradually substituted for intravenous drugs and are then continued throughout the remainder of the pregnancy. Preoperative antibiotics, generally a cephalosporin, are continued for 3 days postoperatively. The patient is kept at bedrest for at least 3 days following surgery and then begins a progressive ambulation program. A postoperative adynamic ileus is common for 2–3 days, and oral intake resumes with the return of bowel function. Generally, the patient is discharged on only oral tocolytic therapy within ten days of the procedure.

Maternal Outcome

Between 1981 and 1990, 18 women have undergone open fetal surgery in the Fetal Treatment Program at UCSF. The operations were performed for four indications: bladder outlet obstruction, congenital diaphragmatic hernia, sacrococcygeal teratoma, and congenital cystic adenomatoid malformation. Of these procedures, 15 were technically successful resulting in a viable fetus postoperatively. In three cases, the fetal anatomic problem proved to be irreparable at the time and the fetus was removed. Women with continuing pregnancies are committed to cesarean section at the time of delivery.

Obviously, maternal safety is the first priority in all cases. There have been no maternal deaths, and few maternal complications. There was one case of mild antibiotic-associated pseudomembranous colitis that responded to oral vancomycin. One patient developed a small amniotic fluid leak from the hysterotomy site causing abdominal pain several weeks after she returned home. This was easily stopped during reoperation with a single suture and has not happened again since we changed our method of hysterotomy closure to three layers. The maternal mirror syndrome developed in two mothers after resection of fetal tumors as previously described. This complication made control of preterm labor difficult, and ultimately necessitated cesarean delivery. Finally, poor patient compliance occurred in one case—the mother stopped her oral tocolytics and promptly went into premature labor and delivered vaginally.

Effect on Reproductive Potential

One of the principal concerns following fetal surgery is the ability of the mother to carry subsequent pregnancies. We first evaluated the potential for future reproduction after fetal surgery in a large series of nonhuman primates.[62] Computerized medical records are maintained for each primate at the California Primate Research Center, Davis, California. This database provided reliable information regarding subsequent breeding and contraception and permitted comparison of our experimental fetal surgery group with the normal breeding colony. We found that in animals that had uterine closure with absorbable sutures, fetal surgery did not interfere with subsequent fertility.[62] However, animals that had metal staple hysterotomy closure had a markedly decreased fertility rate. It is now clear that metal staples migrate through the uterine wall, and we speculate that exposure of the endometrial cavity to permanent foreign body hinders fertility. Based on this experience, we no longer use the metal stapler for uterine closure, and we have subsequently developed a stapler for hysterotomy that uses absorbable staples.[63]

Uterine rupture is a dreaded complication during labor following previous cesarean section, and it occurs more commonly after a classic cesarean section than after a lower uterine segment incision. The hysterotomy used for fetal surgery is invariably in the upper segment of the uterine corpus and this is comparable to a classic cesarean section. In our nonhuman primate series there were five cases of uterine rupture, while 62 other primates labored and delivered vaginally without complication during the fetal surgery pregnancy. Based on this experience, cesarean section delivery should be mandatory after fetal surgery in order to avoid rupture of the relatively fresh uterine wound.

In follow-up of our 18 patients, six have had subsequent pregnancies, and all deliveries were by repeat cesarean section with good outcome. The first patient has had two normal pregnancies. The remaining women are too close to their operative date to assess for subsequent fertility after fetal surgery.

From our experience in animals and in our initial clinical experience with open fetal surgery, we conclude that the anesthetic regimen first developed in the nonhuman primate model has been successfully employed in humans, with an acceptable perioperative risk. We believe that the paucity of complications in the first 18 patients with open fetal procedures is a direct result of our extensive preparation in experimental fetal animals, which should be a prerequisite for anyone contemplating these inherently dangerous procedures. We know of only one other human open fetal surgical case that was performed at a medical center where the investigators chose not to do preparatory work in nonhuman primates, and that procedure failed.

The uterine irritability induced by hysterotomy can be successfully suppressed intraoperatively with halothane anesthesia and postoperatively with intravenous and oral tocolytic agents, but premature labor remains a serious and frequent problem with fetal surgery, requiring early confinement in most cases. The morbidity associated with management of preterm labor will be reduced with further experience. Finally, the clinical and experimental evidence suggests that a midgestation hysterotomy, closed with absorbable sutures, does not adversely affect future fertility.

Our ability to diagnose fetal birth defects has achieved considerable sophistication and offers new hope for improved management of the fetus with a life-threatening defect. However, the more invasive diagnostic and therapeutic procedures involve significant risks for both fetus and mother, raising difficult ethical questions about risks versus benefits and about the rights of the fetus and the mother. It is imperative that all who consider embarking on this type of treatment be committed to continuously developing the enterprise through ongoing research and responsible reporting of all clinical experience.

Fetal treatment, particularly fetal surgery, is at a crossroads. There is sufficient evidence from experimental models and clinical experience to suggest that in a few carefully selected conditions (e.g., some cases of diaphragmatic hernia and bilateral hydronephrosis), intervention before birth can ameliorate the pathophysiologic features and can be accomplished with reasonable safety. However, we do not know (and may never know without proper trials) how effective the new intervention is in treating the fetal disease or how cost effective it is in managing a given fetal condition. With feasibility established but efficacy unknown, now is the time to put fetal surgery to the test of a prospective controlled trial, performed in a way that minimizes the ethical and emotional problems of assigning or withholding a potentially life-saving fetal treatment.

REFERENCES

1. Harrison MR, Golbus MS, Filly RA: The Unborn Patient, 2d ed. WB Saunders, Philadelphia, 1990.
2. Harrison MR, Bjordal RI, Landmark F, et al.: Congenital diaphragmatic hernia: The hidden mortality. J Pediatr Surg 1979;13:227–231.
3. Adzick NS, Harrison MR, Glick PL, et al.: Comparison of fetal, newborn, and adult wound healing by histologic, enzyme-histochemical, and hydroxyproline determination. J Pediatr Surg 1985; 20:315–319.
4. Krummel TM, Nelson JM, Diegelmann RF, et al.: Fetal response to injury in the rabbit. J Pediatr Surg 1987;22:640–644.
5. Longaker MT, Chiu ES, Harrison MR, et al.: Studies in fetal wound healing. IV: Hyaluronic acid stimulating activity distinguishes fetal wound fluid from adult wound fluid. Ann Surg 1989;210:667–672.
6. Harrison MR, Filly RA, Parer JRT, et al.: Management of the fetus with a urinary tract malformation. JAMA 1981;246:635–639.
7. Harrison MR, Golbus MS, Filly RA: Management of the fetus with a correctable congenital defect. JAMA 1981;246:774–777.
8. Harrison MR, Ross NA, Noall R, et al.: Correction of congenital hydronephrosis in utero. I. The model: Fetal urethral obstruction produces hydronephrosis and pulmonary hypoplasia in fetal lambs. J Pediatr Surg 1983;18:247–256.
9. Harrison MR, Nakayama DK, Noall R, et al.: Correction of congenital hydronephrosis in utero. II. Decompression reverses the effects of obstruction on the fetal lung and urinary tract. J Pediatr Surg 1982;17:965–974.
10. Glick PL, Harrison MR, Noall R, et al.: Correction of congenital hydronephrosis in utero. III. Early mid-trimester urethral obstruction produces renal dysplasia. J Pediatr Surg 1983;18:681–687.
11. Glick PL, Harrison MR, Adzick NS, et al.: Correction of congenital hydronephrosis in utero. IV. In utero decompression prevents renal dysplasia. J Pediatr Surg 1984;19:649–657.
12. Adzick NS, Harrison MR, Hu L, et al.: Pulmonary hypoplasia and renal dysplasia in a fetal lamb urinary tract obstruction model. Surg Forum 1987;38:666–668.
13. Docimo SG, Luetic T, Crone RK, et al.: Pulmonary development in the fetal lamb with severe bladder outlet obstruction and oligohydramnios: A morphometric study. J Urol 1989;142:657–660.
14. Wigglesworth JS, Desai R, Guenini P: Fetal lung hypoplasia: Biochemical and structural variations and their possible significance. Arch Dis Child 1981;56:606–610.
15. Inselman LS, Mellins RB: Growth and development of the lung. J Pediatr 1981;98:1–7.
16. Reid L: The lung: Its growth and remodeling in health and disease. Am J Roentgenol 1977;129:777.
17. Nakayama DK, Glick PL, Villa RL, et al.: Experimental pulmonary hypoplasia due to oligohydramnios and its reversal by relieving thoracic compression. J Pediatr Surg 1983;18:347–353.
18. Adzick NS, Harrison MR, Glick PL, et al.: Experimental pulmonary hypoplasia and oligohydramnios: Relative contribution of lung fluid and fetal breathing movements. J Pediatr Surg 1984; 19:658–663.
19. Harrison MR, Filly RA, Golbus MS, et al.: Fetal treatment 1982. N Engl J Med 1982;307:1651–1652.
20. Muller F, Dumez Y, Dommergues M, et al.: Can fetal urinary biochemistry predict postnatal renal function? Fetal Therapy (in press).
21. Crombleholme TM, Harrison MR, Golbus MS, et al.: Fetal intervention in obstructive uropathy: Prognostic indicators and efficacy of intervention. Am J Ob Gyn 1990;162:1239–1244.
22. Mahoney BS, Filly RA, Callen PW, et al.: Sonographic evaluation of fetal renal dysplasia. Radiology 1984;152:143–146.
23. Glick PL, Harrison MR, Adzick NS, et al.: Management of the fetus with congenital hydronephrosis. II. Prognostic criteria and selection for treatment. J Pediatr Surg 1985;20:376–387.
24. Crombleholme TM, Harrison MR, Langer JC, et al.: Early experience with open fetal surgery for congenital hydronephrosis. J Pediatr Surg 1988;23:1114–1116.
25. Harrison MR, Golbus MS, Filly RA, et al.: Fetal surgery for congenital hydronephrosis. N Engl J Med 1982;306:591–593.
26. Harrison MR, Golbus MS, Filly RA, et al.: Management of the fetus with congenital hydronephrosis. J Pediatr Surg 1982;17:728–742.
27. Harrison MR, deLorimier AA: Congenital diaphragmatic hernia. Surg Clin North America 1981; 61:1023–1028.

28. Harrison MR, Jester JA, Ross NA: Correction of congenital diaphragmatic hernia in utero. I. The model: Intrathoracic balloon produces fatal pulmonary hypoplasia. Surgery 1980;88:174–182.
29. Harrison MR, Bressack MA, Churg AM: Correction of congenital diaphragmatic hernia in utero. II. Simulated correction permits fetal lung growth with survival at birth. Surgery 1980;88:260–268.
30. Harrison MR, Ross NA, deLorimier AA: Correction of congenital diaphragmatic hernia in utero. III. Development of a successful surgical technique using abdominoplasty to avoid compromise of umbilical blood flow. J Pediatr Surg 1981;16:934–942.
31. Soper RT, Pringle KC, Scofield JC: Creation and repair of diaphragmatic hernia in the fetal lamb: Technique and survival. J Pediatr Surg 1984;19:33–37.
32. Adzick NS, Outwater KM, Harrison MR, et al.: Correction of congenital diaphragmatic hernia in utero IV. An early gestational model for pulmonary vascular morphometric analysis. J Pediatr Surg 1985;20:673–680.
33. Fitzgerald RJ: Congenital diaphragmatic hernia as a cause of perinatal mortality. Ir J Med Sci 1979;146:280–284.
34. Butler N, Claireaux AE: Congenital diaphragmatic hernia as a cause of perinatal mortality. Lancet 1962;1:659–665.
35. Puri P, Gorman F: Lethal nonpulmonary anomalies associated with congenital diaphragmatic hernia: Implications for early intrauterine surgery. J Pediatr Surg 1984;19:29–35.
36. O'Rourke PP, Vacanti JP, Crone RK, et al.: Use of the postductal PaO_2 as a predictor of pulmonary vascular hypoplasia in infants with congenital diaphragmatic hernia. J Pediatr Surg 1989;23:904–907.
37. Nakayama DK, Harrison MR, Chinn DH, et al.: Prenatal diagnosis and management of the fetus with a congenital diaphragmatic hernia: Initial clinical experience. J Pediatr Surg 1985;20:118–122.
38. Adzick NS, Harrison MR, Glick PL, et al.: Diaphragmatic hernia in the fetus: Prenatal diagnosis and outcome in 94 cases. J Pediatr Surg 1985;20:357–361.
39. Adzick NS, Vacanti JP, Lillehei CW, et al.: Fetal diaphragmatic hernia: Ultrasound diagnosis and clinical outcome in 38 cases from a single medical center. J Pediatr Surg 1989;24:654–658.
40. Harrison MR, Langer JC, Adzick NS, et al.: Correction of congenital diaphragmatic hernia in utero V. Initial clinical experience. J Pediatr Surg 1990;25:47–57.
41. Benacerraf BR, Frigoletto FD, Wilson M: Successful midtrimester thoracentesis with analysis of the lymphocyte population in the pleural effusion. Am J Ob Gyn 1986;155:398–399.
42. Longaker MT, Laberge JM, Dansereau J, et al.: Primary fetal hydrothorax: Natural history and management. J Pediatr Surg 1989;24:573–576.
43. Rodeck CH, Fisk NM, Fraser DI, et al.: Long-term in utero drainage of fetal hydrothorax. N Engl J Med 1988;319:1135–1138.
44. Flake AW, Harrison MR, Adzick NS, et al.: Fetal sacrococcygeal teratoma. J Pediatr Surg 1986; 21:563–566.
45. Langer JC, Harrison MR, Schmidt KG, et al.: Fetal hydrops and demise from sacrococcygeal teratoma: Rationale for fetal surgery. Am J Ob Gyn 1989;160:1145–1150.
46. Adzick NS, Harrison MR, Glick PL, et al.: Fetal cystic adenomatoid malformation: Prenatal diagnosis and natural history. J Pediatr Surg 1985;20:483–488.
47. Golladay ES, Mollitt DL: Surgically correctable fetal hydrops. J Pediatr Surg 1984;19:59–64.
48. Saltzman DH, Adzick NS, Benacerraf BR: Fetal cystic adenomatoid malformation of the lung: Apparent improvement in utero. Obstet Gynecol 1988;71:1000–1003.
49. Adzick NS, Harrison MR, Hu LM, et al.: Compensatory lung growth after pneumonectomy in fetal lambs: A morphometric study. Surg Forum 1986;37:309–314.
50. Clark SL, Vitale DJ, Minton SD, et al.: Successful fetal therapy for cystic adenomatoid malformation associated with second trimester hydrops. Am J Ob Gyn 1987;157:294.
51. Nicolay KS, Gainey HL: Pseudotoxemic state associated with severe Rh-isoimmunization. Am J Ob Gyn 1964;89:41–43.
52. Kleinman CS, Hobbins JC, Jaffe CC, et al.: Echocardiographic studies of the human fetus: Prenatal diagnosis of congenital heart disease and cardiac dysrhythmias. Pediatrics 1980;65:1059–1066.
53. Taylor PV, Scott JS, Garlis LM, et al.: Maternal antibodies against fetal cardiac antigens in congenital complete heart block. N Engl J Med 1986;315:667–772.
54. Crombleholme TM, Longaker MT, Langer JC, et al.: Complete heart block and AV-sequential pacing in fetal lambs: The atrial contribution to cardiac output in the fetus. Surg Forum 1989; 40:268–270.

55. Carpenter RJ, Strasburger JF, Garson A, et al.: Fetal ventricular pacing for hydrops secondary to complete atrioventricular block. J Am Coll Cardiol 1986;8:1434–1436.
56. Fishman NH, Hof RB, Rudolph AM, et al.: Models of congenital heart disease in fetal lambs. Circulation 1978;58:354–364.
57. Becal O, Gallix P, Toussaint M, et al.: Intrauterine creation and repair of pulmonary artery stenosis in the fetal lamb. J Thorac Cardiovasc Surg 1987;93:761–766.
58. Slate RK, Stevens MB, Verrier ED, et al.: Intrauterine repair of pulmonary stenosis in fetal sheep. Surg Forum 1985;36:246–248.
59. Adzick NS, Harrison MR, Slate RK, et al.: Surface cooling and rewarming the fetus: a technique for experimental fetal cardiac surgery. Surg Forum 1984;35:313–316.
60. Harrison MR, Anderson J, Rosen M, et al.: Fetal surgery in the primate. I. Anesthetic, surgical, and tocolytic management to maximize fetal-neonatal survival. J Pediatr Surg 1982;17:115–122.
61. Nakayama DK, Harrison MR, Seron-Ferre M, et al.: Fetal surgery in the primate. II. Uterine electromyographic response to operative procedures and pharmacologic agents. J Pediatr Surg 1984;19:333–339.
62. Adzick NS, Harrison MR, Anderson JV, et al.: Fetal surgery in the primate. III. Maternal outcome after fetal surgery. J Pediatr Surg 1986;21:477–480.
63. Adzick NS, Harrison MR, Flake AW, et al.: Automatic uterine stapling devices in fetal surgery: Experience in a primate model. Surg Forum 1985;36:479–480.
64. Flake AW, Harrison MR, Adzick NS, et al.: Transplantation of fetal hematopoietic stem cells in utero: The creation of hematopoietic chimeras. Science 1986;233:766–778.
65. Richter RC, Slate RK, Rudolph AM, et al.: Fetal blood flow during hypothermic cardiopulmonary bypass in utero. J Cardiovasc Surg 1985;26:86.
66. Harrison MR, Adzick NS, Longaker MT, et al.: Successful repair in utero of a fetal diaphragmatic hernia after removal of herniated viscera from the left thorax. N Engl J Med 1990;322:1582–1584.
67. Harrison MR, Adzick NS, Jennings RW, et al.: Antenatal intervention for congenital cystic adenomatoid malformation. Lancet 1990;336:965–967.
68. Longaker MT, Golbus MS, Filly RA, et al.: Maternal outcome after open fetal surgery. JAMA 1991;265:737–741.

CHAPTER 2

Overview of Postnatal Wound Healing

Russell W. Jennings
Thomas K. Hunt

INTRODUCTION

Only a century ago, complicated and incomplete healing after injury or surgery was the rule rather than the exception. The close observation of healing wounds and subsequent evolution of wound care and antisepsis in the 18th and 19th centuries improved surgery dramatically. Nevertheless, poor healing, infection, and excessive scarring remained frequent consequences of injury and operation.

The 20th century has seen investigation of wound healing on a more fundamental level. Knowledge about the basic mechanisms of tissue repair has grown rapidly, and surgeons who have a detailed knowledge of these mechanisms have learned to influence healing. Surgeons now anticipate and often prevent problems of infection and inadequate or excessive tissue repair. Recent insights into the basic molecular events involved in the repair process hold even greater promise (Figure 2.1).

Tissue loss or damage results in either regeneration, repair by scar tissue, or a combination of both. Some amphibians can regenerate amputated appendages.[1] Lower mammals such as neonatal mice and opossums have some capacity to regenerate digits,[2] but higher mammals have almost no regenerative capability except for the liver.[3] Repair by scar, the postnatal mammalian response to injury, occurs as a sequential cascade of overlapping processes. Tissue injury initiates bleeding, coagulation, inflammation, cell replication, angiogenesis, epithelization, and matrix synthesis.

Injured vessels rapidly constrict. Coagulation then limits loss of blood and generates biologically active substances that begin the early and late inflammatory phases of tissue repair. Coagulation also releases biologically active products that convert fibroblasts and endothelial cells into their reparative mode, forming local tissue and capillary tube forming cells.

The next phase of healing—inflammation—begins with activation of complement and initiation of the classical molecular cascade, which leads to infiltration of the wound by granulocytes. These cells consume contaminating bacteria and debris and are largely replaced by monocytes in the next few days. Monocytes differentiate into tissue macrophages after entering the wound site and subsequently are important regulators of repair.

Tissue macrophages continue the debridement process begun by granulocytes, but they also secrete biologically active substances that initiate the development

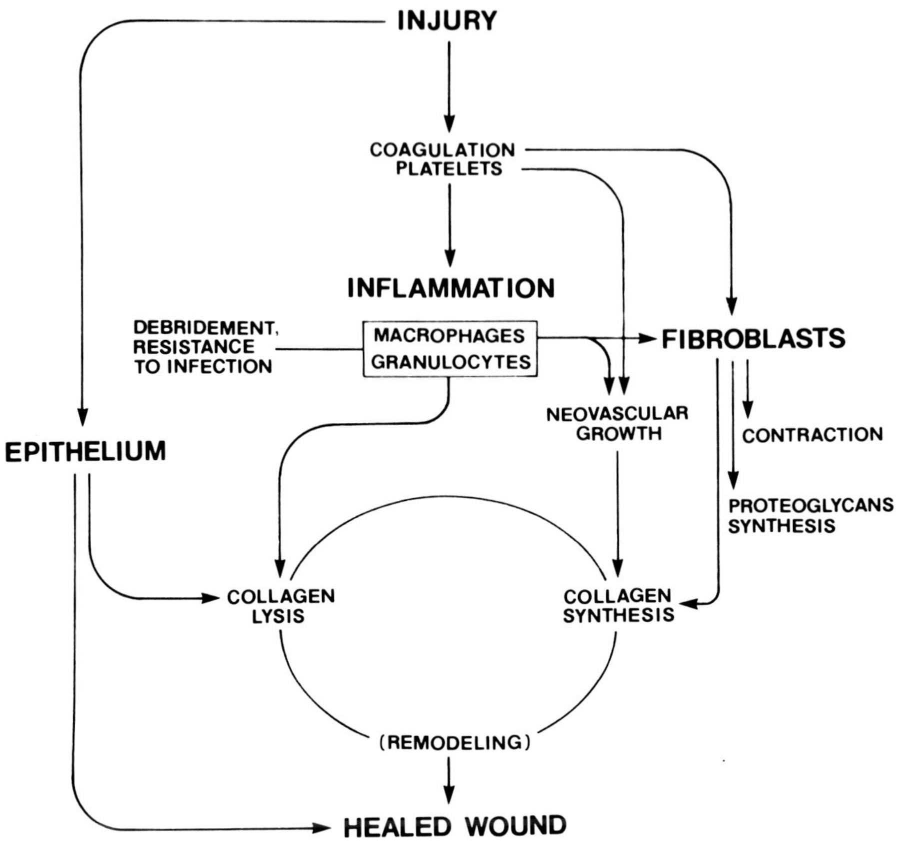

Figure 2.1 The complex interactions of the many cell types to achieve repair of an injury.

of granulation tissue, composed of fibroblasts and new vessels, in the next phase of wound repair. If wound conditions warrant, macrophages recruit additional inflammatory cells. Lymphocytes contribute in much the same manner but probably to a lesser degree.

Wound fibroblasts derive from cells surrounding the wound that change their differentiated phenotype(s) and become mobile during the process of replication. As they migrate into the wound in the process of fibroplasia, they proliferate and secrete extracellular matrix.

Growth and migration of cells requires angiogenesis. The directed growth of vascular endothelial cells occurs simultaneously with fibroplasia during granulation tissue formation, stimulated in much the same manner as fibroblasts, namely by platelet and activated macrophage products. Angiogenesis gives granulation tissue its deep red color due to its rich microvasculature. Granulation tissue is a loose matrix that appears in open wounds and is composed of collagen, fibronectin, and hyaluronic acid with dense infiltration by macrophages, fibroblasts, and capillary endothelial cells. The new tissue that unites simple closed or coapted wounds is not quite the same as granulation tissue although it is composed of the same tissue elements.

In wounds exposed to the external environment, re-epithelization begins within minutes after injury. Epithelial cells surrounding the defect become mobile and move into the defect. Within one to two days, epithelial cells at the wound edge begin proliferating, and the new cells migrate either along an undisrupted basement membrane or across a provisional matrix of fibrin and fibronectin, which is then replaced with basement membrane. Necrotic tissue or foreign bodies are gradually separated from the wound as the epithelial cells migrate under them. Once epithelial integrity is completed, the cells reform hemidesmosomes and attach to the new basement membrane, thus reforming a barrier to further contamination and moisture loss.

Repair is not complete for some time after coverage and tensile integrity are accomplished. Remodeling requires months for completion and is concerned with the removal of loose extracellular matrix materials such as fibronectin, and slow deposition of type I collagen in fibrils. During remodeling, the tissue becomes stronger and more flexible.

The end result is scar formation. This scar lacks some components of normal tissue and is therefore less functional than the surrounding uninjured tissue. The major benefit of repair by scar is the rapid reformation of tissue integrity.

TISSUE INJURY

The type of injury has a great deal of influence over the wound healing process. Minor wounds need little debridement and incite little inflammation. A very mild tissue injury may remove only the epithelial cell layer, leaving the basement membrane intact. Healing then occurs rapidly by simple re-epithelization and little scar. On the other hand, a severe tissue injury involving damage to large amounts of tissue at all depths with heavy bacterial contamination requires all phases of tissue repair and often leaves a disfiguring and dysfunctional scar.

Uncontaminated incisional wounds with clean coapted wound edges need little repair since bleeding is minimal, little tissue needs debridement, and contamination is light, so the early granulocyte inflammatory phase is limited to one or two days. The wound edges are apposed, minimizing the need for new tissue deposition and epithelization. The net effect is rapid healing with minimal scar formation.

If there is severe tissue injury that needs debridement or there is heavy bacterial contamination with infection, the acute inflammatory phase with granulocyte infiltration is exaggerated and prolonged. Microvessels continue to thrombose for several days. Some of the products secreted by granulocytes are toxic to surrounding tissue, and progressive tissue injury follows.

Understanding these concepts allows therapeutic modulation of the healing process. The conversion of a heavily injured or grossly contaminated wound, with its resulting poor tissue repair, into a clean incisional wound with coapted edges can help achieve acceptable tissue repair with less morbidity and improved function. For instance, healing of deep burns can be accelerated and cosmetic results improved by early excision and grafting. The simplest repair usually heals the most rapidly and with the most return of function. Even when healing is complex, however, the most rapid repair is almost always the most functional.[4]

COAGULATION

Tissue injury severe enough to injure blood vessels leads to plasma, platelet, and cellular extravasation. This initiates the coagulation cascade that culminates in formation of a fibrin (and fibronectin) clot that limits further bleeding by trapping platelets, blood borne cells, and plasma proteins. This clot is often the initial step in wound healing, the step that initiates the subsequent events. The clot acts as an attractant and temporary matrix for inflammatory cells and fibroblasts. In addition, it provides a growth medium for reparative cells. If the clot is exposed to air it will dry, forming a scab as a temporary wound cover.

Any mechanism of vessel injury including inflammation, direct vessel injury, and even histamine release, causes blood vessels around the wounded area to dilate and leak between separated endothelial cells from the small venules into the injured tissue.[5,6] The extravascular fibrin forms a hygroscopic gel that is partly responsible for the induration seen around wounds. The resulting fibrin clot in the interstitial tissue then facilitates inflammatory cell migration.[7]

All three mechanisms of coagulation—the extrinsic and intrinsic coagulation cascades, and platelet activation—contribute to subsequent repair. The ultimate function of each is the activation of prothrombin to thrombin which then converts fibrinogen to fibrin which then is polymerized into a stable clot.

The extrinsic coagulation cascade is primarily responsible for coagulation and hemostasis. It is initiated by tissue thromboplastin, a lipoprotein expressed by fibroblasts, smooth muscle cells, and endothelial cells in injured tissue.[8,9] Tissue thromboplastin is also expressed at sites of early inflammation by granulocytes and sites of late inflammation by monocytes and tissue macrophages.[10,11] The intrinsic coagulation cascade is primarily responsible for vasodilation by bradykinin, which causes increased permeability and plasma extravasation. The intrinsic coagulation cascade is initiated by activated factor XII (the Hageman factor), prekallikrein, and high molecular weight (HMW) kininogen. Many tissues secrete active tissue kallikrein which then cleaves HMW-kininogen to release bradykinin.[12] Kallikrein also activates plasminogen[13] and complement,[14] and is both chemotactic and stimulatory for granulocytes.[15,16]

Products of the coagulation cascade are regulatory for the cells in the injury area. Intact thrombin functions as a potent growth factor for fibroblasts and endothelial cells.[17,18] Degraded thrombin fragments stimulate monocytes and platelets.[19–21] Both fibrinogen and thrombin contain growth-promoting peptide sequences and some fibrinopeptides are chemoattractant to monocytes.[22] The clot also induces angiogenesis with directed capillary endothelial cell ingrowth.[23] This complex pattern of interactions is easier to understand when one realizes that many growth-promoting peptides involved in wound healing are contributed by several sources.[24] The combination of the processes influences the next series of events: an increase in vascular permeability,[25] and an increase in chemotaxis toward the fibrin clot.[26]

Platelets

Platelet activation by tissue injury or thrombosis augments coagulation and the formation of kinins. Platelets also provide an appropriate surface for the vitamin K dependent factors (factors VII, IX, X, and prothrombin) to bind to calcium dependent sites on the platelet membrane.[27] Platelet-endothelial cell interaction requires factor VIII which circulates as a complex with von Willebrand factor.[28,29]

Platelets are activated by thrombin and factors XI and XIa.[30,31] This leads to platelet aggregation that limits bleeding, and platelet degranulation with release of clotting factors and inflammatory mediators.[32] One effect is mast cell degranulation, which leads to increased plasma extravasation.[33] The release of platelet

ADP, fibrinogen, fibronectin, and thrombospondin acts to bind platelets together forming a more stable clot.

Platelets also release a number of cytokines into the injury area from their storage granules. These include transforming growth factor beta (TGF-β), insulin-like growth factor-1 (IGF-1), platelet factor 4, platelet derived growth factor (PDGF), and other less well-characterized substances. The functions of the cytokines are not always clear. For example, platelet factor 4 inhibits growth factor stimulated endothelial cell proliferation, while other platelet derived growth factors are stimulatory for endothelial cells.[34] Others, like TGFβ, are chemoattractants. The net effect of platelet activation is the attraction and activation of fibroblasts, endothelial cells, and macrophages. As wound healing progresses to later stages, most of these platelet derived cytokines will be secreted by other cells.

Fibrin

Coagulation activates fibrinogen to fibrin, which then crosslinks to form a fibrin plug or clot. Factor XIIIa covalently links the fibrin monomers together to stabilize the clot. Fibroblasts are attracted to many agents involved in the clot including lymphokines, complement, collagen, and fibronectin.[35]

The fibrin gel forms a variably conducive environment for cellular movement. The concentration of thrombin, for instance, influences the ability of cells to migrate through it. Macrophages express fibrinogen and fibrin receptors and migrate into the clot during the early wound stages when the fibrin levels are low.[36,37] Later the fibrin levels increase and inhibit macrophage migration, keeping them in the wound.

Fibrin clots are gradually lysed and converted into a collagen matrix to complete tissue repair. Tissues contain tissue plasminogen activator, which converts plasminogen to plasmin. This activates the fibrinolysis cascade. Tissue plasminogen activator can be found in most wound cells, including damaged endothelial cells,[38] and activated granulocytes and macrophages.[39,40]

The provisional fibrin gel matrix allows macrophages, fibroblasts, and capillaries to infiltrate and form granulation tissue.[41] The fibrin gel is then degraded in about three weeks.[42,43] Fibronectin is laid down early, then decreases in concentration. Endothelial cells are attracted to the soluble fibronectin. Collagens type I and III are then laid down, initially deposited in association with the fibrin strands.[44] Epithelial cells lay down laminin and type IV collagen as part of their basement membrane as they penetrate the clot.

THE EARLY INFLAMMATORY PHASE

The reader should refer to Chapter 15 for a complete discussion of inflammation in fetal and adult wound healing.

Granulocytes infiltrate into wounds within the first 24 hours. Their primary function is to debride necrotic cellular debris and foreign material, including bacteria. Healing may progress normally in the absence of granulocytes in a clean wound.[45]

Upon exposure to chemoattractants the granulocytes alter their adherence characteristics and tend to adhere locally to endothelial cells in post capillary venules. This process depends upon granulocytes expressing integrins such as

CD18 β-chain receptors Mac-1, LFA-1, and p150,95.[46] Adhesion can be made even more efficient if endothelial cells express attachment molecules in response to IL-1, tumor necrosis factor (TNF), or bacterial LPS.[47,48]

After they attach, granulocytes emigrate by diapedesis between endothelial cells into the extravascular space.[49,50] They normally express specific laminin receptors, and when these receptors are blocked by antibodies their migration through the basement membrane is impeded.[51] Once a cell has produced a defect in the vessel wall other leukocytes and red blood cells follow the same path.[52]

Granulocytes move to the injury area predominantly by chemotaxis, which is the directed movement of a cell up a concentration gradient of a soluble chemoattractant. They also demonstrate contact guidance by following the three-dimensional shape of the matrix.[53] There is no requirement for proteolytic degradation of the collagen matrix during granulocyte infiltration, though some degradation does occur.[54]

The many granulocyte chemoattractants include products such as C5a from complement activation, formyl-methionyl peptide products from bacteria, and thrombin and other fibrinopeptides from clot formation.[55] Granulocytes are also attracted to matrix degradation products from elastin,[56] collagen,[57] and plasma fibronectin.[58] Chemoattractants may also increase the oxidative metabolism of the granulocyte, and may induce exocytosis of lysosomal enzymes and oxygen radicals.[59]

Granulocytes provide the major, though temporary, line of defense against infection by ingesting and killing invading microorganisms. Phagocytosis induces a respiratory burst that produces toxic oxygen metabolites. These toxic products include hypohalides (such as hypochlorite anion OCl^-)[60], superoxide anion (O_2^-)[61], and the hydroxyl radical ($^\cdot OH$).[62] They also can generate chloramines as the toxic products of the reaction of hypochlorite with ammonia or amines.[63] Although granulocytes produce some of these toxic metabolites as part of a normal mechanism that destroys invading microorganisms, they may also release them into the surrounding tissues causing further tissue damage.[64,65]

In addition, granulocytes produce a 75 kDa interstitial collagenase that is relatively specific for type I collagen in solution instead of fibrillar collagen, and that probably participates in wound debridement.[66]

Granulocytes add little to the normal healing process; their role is limited to the prevention of infection and debridement of wounds. If wounds become infected, however, the accumulation of activated granulocytes to fight the infection can lead to extensive tissue injury and more severe scarring.

THE LATE INFLAMMATORY PHASE

Macrophages are the critical controlling cells in wound healing. Depletion of monocytes and macrophages causes a severe alteration in wound healing with poor debridement, delayed fibroblast proliferation, inadequate angiogenesis, and poor fibrosis.[67] Macrophages secrete growth factors in response to a number of stimuli including foreign bodies, fibrin, and the local hypoxic and/or high lactate conditions in the wound. These growth factors stimulate proliferation and matrix production by fibroblasts, proliferation of smooth muscle cells, and proliferation of endothelial cells resulting in angiogenesis.

Tissue macrophages can proliferate locally.[68] However, during inflammatory conditions such as that found after injury, circulating blood monocytes are actively recruited into the tissues where they are converted into tissue macrophages.[69]

Macrophages are attracted by a variety of chemoattractants including complement, clotting components, IgG fragments, and breakdown products of the extracellular matrix including collagen, fibronectin, and elastin fragments. Macrophages also respond to secreted cytokines such as leukotriene B4 and platelet factor 4, and they localize at sites of bacterial accumulation where they are attracted by bacterial peptides.[70]

Cytokines

PDGF: Platelet Derived Growth Factors

Coagulation releases platelet granule contents, which in turn attract granulocytes and macrophages. PDGF is contained in the α-granules of the platelets and is released in response to thrombin or fibrillar collagen.[71–73] A similar molecule is secreted by activated, but not resting, monocytes and alveolar macrophages in response to a variety of stimuli.[74,75] PDGF exists in two equally active forms, PDGF I and II in a 1:2.5 ratio in the platelet and is composed of two chains, an α and a β chain, although small amounts of each homodimer exist.[76–78]

PDGF is the most potent mitogen for fibroblasts, glial cells, and smooth muscle cells.[79–81] Mesenchymal cells have a high-affinity membrane receptor that works through tyrosine kinase.[82] There are no PDGF receptors on epithelial cells or endothelial cells. Nevertheless, PDGF seems to initiate angiogenesis.

PDGF is a potent chemoattractant for inflammatory cells.[83] High concentrations can activate granulocytes.[84] Smooth muscle cells and fibroblasts are attracted to low concentrations of PDGF, which also induces them to proliferate.[85,86] PDGF also increases the amount of fibroblast secreted collagenase, indicating a role in tissue remodeling. In the serum it binds to α_2-macroglobulin, which is then cleared by the liver.[87]

EGF: Epidermal Growth Factor

Epidermal growth factor is the same protein as urogastrone, a hormone found in human urine that inhibits gastric acid secretion.[88–90] It is a single chain polypeptide 53 amino acids long, and circulates bound to a specific "carrier protein" from which it is easily cleaved by proteolytic enzymes.[91,92] EGF is found in many tissues but is in particularly high concentrations in milk, the maxillary glands of male mice,[93] and the Brunner's glands in the small intestine.[94]

EGF acts via a cell membrane receptor mechanism.[95–97] Other proteins, such as TGFα, also bind to the EGF receptor and cause similar alterations in cellular physiology. TGFα may act as EGF in the fetus.[98]

The putative EGF receptor is found on all cells but is most dense on epithelial cells and fibroblasts.[99–102] The receptor acts through tyrosine kinase autophosphorylation and causes an elevation in intracellular calcium.[103,104] Stimulation of the EGF receptor causes the cells to become less differentiated and to divide and grow rapidly. Fibroblasts may stop making collagen while in this less differentiated state. The end result, however, is an increased number of differentiated cells.

The major effect of EGF is to encourage cells to continue through the cell cycle. In wounds, it has this effect on epithelial cells,[105] fibroblasts,[106] and endothelial cells.[107] EGF is also chemotactic for epithelial cells and increases the secretion of collagenases by fibroblasts, which is an important step in tissue remodeling.[108,109]

FGF: Fibroblast Growth Factors

Fibroblast growth factor has both an acidic form and a basic form.[110] Basic FGF is about 10 times as potent as acidic FGF, but has identical effects since it binds to the same FGF receptor. Fibroblast growth factor, and a number of similar growth factors, are found in a wide variety of tissues and share the common property of binding to heparin. Most differ only in the length of their N-terminus peptides.[111] The source of FGF in wounds is unclear, but it is thought to be present in tissues bound to heparan sulfate in the extracellular matrix.[112] Injury is thought to induce the breakdown of the matrix with release of the stored FGF.

FGF is angiogenic in rabbit corneas and chick chorioallantoic membranes.[113–115] Its angiogenic activity can be increased by the addition of heparin, possibly indicating that it interacts with endothelial cell surface heparan sulfate.[116] It is a mitogen for mesodermally derived cells such as fibroblasts and endothelial cells, causing them to dedifferentiate, become more mobile, and proliferate.[117] FGF added to tissue culture induces synthesis of the extracellular matrix with secretion of fibronectin and collagen.[118]

FGF also promotes neovascularization and re-epithelization in wounds.[119] FGF impregnated PVA sponges have increased levels of cellular infiltration without inflammation, and demonstrate increased collagen deposition as well as elevated DNA and protein synthesis. Application of FGF improves wound healing by increasing granulation tissue and neovascularization.[120,121]

TGF-β: Type β Transforming Growth Factors

TGFβ is a 25000 kDa homodimer composed of two 112 amino acid peptides. The term TGFβ actually refers to a small family of peptide hormones including types 1 through 3 found in humans and type 4 and 5 found in the chick.[122–125] All appear to act through a membrane receptor mechanism.[126,127] TGFβ is distinct from TGFα, which is related to EGF, binds the EGF receptor, and elicits EGF-like responses.[128–130]

TGFβ is found in high concentrations in platelet α-granules associated with its binding protein and is released by platelet degranulation.[131–133] Other inflammatory cells also secrete TGFβ, including activated T-lymphocytes.[134] Many cells secrete TGFβ in a latent form associated with a binding protein, which makes the TGFβ biologically inactive.[135,136] This inactive, or latent, form may be a storage form of the cytokine until it is activated by macrophages or local conditions.

In tissue culture, TGFβ may either increase or decrease cell proliferation.[137–139] Wound cylinder studies using the Hunt-Schilling chamber have demonstrated the presence of TGFβ in wounds,[140] and both an elevation in fibroblast infiltration and increased collagen deposition has been documented when exogenous TGFβ is applied.[141,142] There is an increased wound healing effect by combining TGFβ with PDGF and EGF after adriamycin has been given to impair wound healing.[143] The subcutaneous injection of TGFβ induces angiogenesis, mucopolysaccharide synthesis,[144] and collagen deposition resulting in fibrosis in newborn mice,[145] but much of this evidence appears to be indirect. In cell culture, fibroblasts respond to the addition of TGFβ by secreting more collagen, elastin, and fibronectin, indicating an induction of extracellular matrix synthesis.[146,147]

The addition of TGFβ also decreases collagenase and stromelysin production, further enhancing overall extracellular matrix synthesis. TGFβ also causes secretion of more TGFβ, a positive feedback cycle that may account for its prolonged activity after a single administration.[48] The normal role of TGFβ in wound healing is far from clear.

IGFs: Insulin-like Growth Factors

The insulin-like growth factors, or somatomedins, are a family of proteins with approximately 50% amino acid homology to proinsulin. They function on two levels: as classical hormones bound to specific binding proteins and distributed to the target tissues via the blood, and also as autocrine and paracrine proteins with local actions. Secretion of IGF-I is under control of growth hormone, and is largely responsible for the growth-promoting action of growth hormone.

There are two classes of IGF: types I and II. They share 60%–70% homology in the critical binding regions. The genes that encode for these proteins are complex with each having both three introns and four exons.[149,150] Both genes transcribe several forms of mRNA. The IGF-II gene has at least three promoters, one of which encodes for a fetal specific transcript, which is produced during development.[151] Postnatally this promoter is inactivated and is associated with a 20-fold decrease in blood IGF-II concentrations. Developmental control of IGF-II has been studied in rats where fetal fibroblasts secreted increased amounts in response to human placental lactogen, but postnatal fibroblasts did not.[152]

Fibroblasts secrete a pro-IGF-I that is similar to IGF-I and is biologically active.[153] PDGF stimulates secretion of IGFs by many cell types.[154] This effect is distinct from the factors that increase plasma levels of IGFs, such as growth hormone. A multimodal form of IGF control has been proposed in which: 1) the local microenvironment stimulates cell type specific secretion, 2) regional paracrine regulation may modify processes such as wound healing, and 3) systemic growth is maintained by blood IGFs.[155] This is supported by the finding of increased IGF-I mRNA and protein in smooth muscle cells after injury to the aorta.[156] IGFs apparently arrive in wounds by both blood delivery and local cellular production.

Some growth factors are either competence or progression factors depending on where they act in the cell cycle. Competence factors move the cell from the resting state into the cell cycle and may involve alterations in gene expression and cytoplasmic calcium and pH changes. Progression factors stimulate mitogenesis with DNA synthesis.[157] The IGFs function synergistically with competence growth factors such as PDGF or FGF to facilitate DNA synthesis.[158] The IGFs cannot recruit quiescent cells, but once the cells are recruited into the cell cycle by a competence factor, IGFs function as progression factors. The combination of IGF-I and PDGF, with PDGF acting as the competence factor, causes maximal rates of cell division and re-epithelization in rat wounds.[159]

PARENCHYMAL CELL MIGRATION INTO WOUNDS

Healing requires migration of mesenchymal cells into the wounded region. The types of cells, the number, and the distance that they infiltrate depends on the tissue injured and the type of injury. Infiltration requires cellular guidance. Directed cell migration is a common feature of several processes that also include growth, development, and tumor metastasis.[160–162] Directed cell motion requires cells to polarize and form both a leading edge that attaches to the matrix and a trailing edge that is pulled along.

There are four types of directed cell motility: chemotaxis, haptotaxis, contact guidance, and the free edge effect. Chemotaxis involves movement up a concentration gradient of a soluble chemoattractant and has been most extensively studied in inflammatory cells. Parenchymal cells can also respond to chemotactic signals but are usually prevented from moving by their adherence to the matrix and surrounding cells.

Haptotaxis involves movement up a concentration gradient of substrate bound adhesion elements by extension of lamellipodia. As the cell moves, it pulls its trailing edge along, and new membrane is inserted into the leading edge.[163]

Contact guidance occurs as the cell is forced to move along paths of least resistance through the extracellular matrix. It results in the cell aligning along the matrix. When two groups of cells are placed at opposite edges of a plasma clot they move toward each other. This is thought to be the effect of cellular contraction acting on the plasma clot to cause the fibrin strands to stretch out between the two groups, thus providing the path of least resistance between the strands. This may also account for the orientation of fibroblasts in granulation tissue.[164]

The free-edge effect occurs in epithelial cells and will be discussed with epithelial cells.

ANGIOGENESIS

Angiogenesis is the process of formation of new blood vessels by directed endothelial cell migration and growth. This is a widespread process occurring in embryos,[165] developing tissue,[166] physical conditioning, and wound healing.[167] Wound healing provides a paradigm for multicellular production of a variety of angiogenic factors that culminates in a well-regulated healing process. At present, all we know is that some factors that can induce angiogenesis are present in the area of healing, although they actually may not do so.

Platelets arrive very early in the process of wound healing and are involved in the angiogenic cascade. Among the many products secreted at the wound site is TGF-β, which is an indirect angiogenic factor and a macrophage chemoattractant.[168,169] Platelets also secrete PDGF, which attracts macrophages and granulocytes.[170]

In addition, platelets release an enzyme that degrades the heparin and heparan sulfate components of basement membrane and endothelial cell surface.[171] Basement membrane is thought to be a storage depot for FGF, which is released upon degradation of the heparin components of basement membrane.[172,173] Other stores of FGF include the intracellular spaces of endothelial cells, smooth muscle cells, and fibroblasts that may be released upon cell damage or when the cell becomes ischemic. Release of FGF from any of the stores may lead to endothelial cell activation and stimulation of angiogenesis. Activation of endothelial cells leads to both migration and proliferation via FGF surface receptors. Endothelial cell activation also results in secretion of collagenases and other hydrolytic enzymes that further degrade the basement membranes and may release more FGF. It has been suggested that this process results in new capillary ingrowth into the relatively hypovascular wound area.[174]

Macrophages play a key role in angiogenesis when activated to produce angiogenic substances by a number of factors including accumulation of lactate (which macrophages produce in large quantities even in aerobic conditions) and/ or by local hypoxia.[175] Once activated, they release several factors involved in angiogenesis including TNF-α, basic FGF, and other unidentified factors that increase endothelial cell migration.[176–178]

Both the intrinsic lactate production and oxidation-reduction potential of the cell influence angiogenesis. Local hypoxia causes a further shift to anaerobic glycolysis with even greater lactate production, a resultant decrease in oxidized nicotinamide-adenine-dinucleotide (NAD^+), and activation of both angiogenesis and collagen synthesis.[179] This hypothesis is attractive because it implies that wounds use a process that is also prominent in growth and development.

Once new blood vessels form they acquire a layer of pericytes and their basement membrane composition changes. Pericytes inhibit growth of adjacent endothelial cells, thus directing angiogenesis toward the site of attraction.[180] With maturation, fewer platelets release their granules, and endothelial cells begin to deposit heparin-like compounds in their basement membranes that bind FGF. As the blood vessels mature they carry more oxygen to the healing area. One consequence of this might be that the normalized oxygen and lactate levels then decrease macrophage angiogenic factor production and allow healing to stop at an appropriate point.

RE-EPITHELIZATION

Loss of epidermis breaks the natural separation between the organism and the environment allowing body fluids to escape and some environmental elements to penetrate into the skin. Fluids that accumulate at the injury site form a clot that acts as a temporary cover for the wound and allows migration of epithelial elements under the scab. Epithelial migration and proliferation are often the first signs that wound repair is underway.

In deep wounds the migrating epithelium arises only from the cells at the wound edge, while in more superficial wounds epithelium may also arise from dermal appendages such as hair follicles.[181,182] Epithelium moves across the defect as an advancing front, called the free edge effect, where the cells facing a defect in a sheet of cells move out to cover the defect. The free edge effect varies with the epithelial tissue involved. Stratified epithelium, such as epidermis, multiplies near the leading edge. Cells from this point migrate across a defect with nearby cells moving over the newly anchored leading edge cells, similar to the game "leap frog."[183] Simple epithelium and endothelium migrate across defects in serial fashion, where the leading edge cells advance and the others follow.[184]

Epithelial cells are attached to their substratum by hemidesmosomes.[185] Cell-cell attachments include zonulae occludens (occluding junctions, tight junctions), which seal cells together to prevent leakage through the epithelial sheet, zonulae adherens (anchoring junctions) and macula adherens (desmosomes), which attach cells to their matrix and neighboring cells, and nexi (gap junctions, communicating junctions), which permit chemical or electrical communication between cells. In order to move, the epithelial cells must overcome their attachments. The marginal cells at the edge of a defect in an epithelial sheet alter their phenotype to become mobile by breaking their desmosomal and hemidesmosomal contacts, and by extending lamellopodia.[186] The peripheral cells surrounding the epithelial defect are involved in movement across the defect, while the cells close to the area of injury are actively dividing to provide new cells.[187]

The leading edge cells also become phagocytic, allowing them to clear debris and plasma clot from their path.[188] The rate of epithelial coverage is increased if the wound does not need debridement, if the basal lamina is left intact,[189] or if the wound is kept moist.[190] Once epithelial continuity is achieved, the entire epithelium alters its phenotype back to normal with rapid reformation of desmosomes, hemidesmosomes, and basement membrane.[191]

Postnatal epithelization, in contrast to fetal, must often overcome a dried clot (eschar). To migrate under the eschar, the leading cells must enzymatically cleave the eschar off the wound bed. Epithelization is faster when a moist environment prevents eschar formation.

MATRIX FORMATION AND REMODELING

Fibronectin

See Chapter 19 for a complete discussion of fibronectins.

Fibronectins are prominent matrix molecules involved in wound contraction, cell migration, collagen matrix deposition, and re-epithelization. Fibronectins are found predominantly in the tissue stroma and in the basal lamina, where they are produced normally by fibroblasts, epithelial cells, and macrophages.[192] They are among the first proteins to be laid down in a wound, and thus form part of the preliminary matrix.[193,194] The molecule is a complex glycoprotein made up of two subunits, each of which has specific collagen binding sites.[195] The differences between soluble plasma fibronectin and stromal fibronectin, as well as the differences between its two subunits, are due to post-translational modification of a single fibronectin gene product.[196]

Fibronectin has the ability to bind a wide variety of molecules involved in wound healing including collagen types I–IV,[197] actin,[198] fibrin,[199] hyaluronic acid,[200] dermatan sulfates and heparan sulfates,[201] fibronectin itself,[202] and cell surface receptors on fibroblasts.[203] Fibronectin seems to function as a linkage between the collagen matrix and the cell's cytoskeleton through specific receptors.[204] These cell surface receptors recognize a specific amino acid sequence, arginyl-glycyl-aspartyl-serine (RGDS using the single letter amino acid code), with the RGD sequence critical for receptor binding and the fourth amino acid modulating the receptor binding.[205,206] Many other matrix receptors also recognize the RGD sequence, and it appears that the region surrounding the RGD sequence determines the binding specificity.[207]

During wound healing fibronectin is supplied by local cells such as fibroblasts and endothelial cells,[208] after the deposition of soluble fibronectin from the plasma.[209] Plasma fibronectin is produced by hepatocytes and appears early in wounds during the coagulation phase.[210] Plasma fibronectin is crosslinked to the fibrin clot, and facilitates fibroblast attachment.[211] In addition, soluble fibronectin fragments are chemotactic for fibroblasts and monocytes.[212] Fibroblasts that infiltrate the wound secrete fibronectin in two stages. Initially fibronectin provides cell attachments for the fibroblasts[213]; later it is secreted as part of the three-dimensional matrix in close association with collagen,[214] decreasing as the wound matures and type I collagen replaces type III.[215,216]

Fibronectin is important for the deposition of the collagen matrix. Granulation tissue fibroblasts are coated with a layer of fibronectin matrix,[217] and myofibroblasts are covered with fibronectin that forms part of the fibronexus attachment with the stress fibers in the wound.[218] This fibronectin acts as the scaffold for collagen deposition. Blocking formation of the fibronectin matrix suppresses collagen deposition to a large degree.[212]

Proteoglycans and Hyaluronic Acid

Proteoglycans are a large and varied group of structural core proteins that are covalently linked to glycosaminoglycans, a type of polysaccharide. Hyaluronic acid consists of repeating sequences of disaccharides of a broad range of molecular weights without a protein core. The variations in protein cores and types of sugar moities provides for tremendous variability in structure, but their polyanionic charge, which influences all interactions with them, is a constant feature.

Four major types of mucopolysaccharide participate in tissue structure and repair: chondroitin sulfate, heparan sulfate, keratan sulfate, and hyaluronic acid. Chondroitin sulfates consist of a large varied group of proteoglycans that contain N-acetylglucosamine as the hexosamine component and glucuronic acid as the uronic acid component. The polysaccharide moities are linked to a core protein via serine residues in the protein. Smooth muscle cells, fibroblasts, and chondrocytes all are capable of producing hyaluronic acid-binding chondroitin sulfates.[219] Cartilage contains large amounts of a complex chondroitin sulfate, which is composed of a large core protein with hyaluronic acid and large numbers of attached chondroitin sulfates that ensure the physical properties necessary for function.[220] Skin contains interstitial proteoglycans, called dermatan sulfates, which are involved in collagen formation and may be important in wound repair.[221,222] Chondroitin sulfates impair the adhesion of cells to fibronectin and collagen, possibly promoting cell mobility.[223–225]

Heparan sulfates are composed of a glucosamine and uronic acid backbone linked to the serine residues of a protein core in a similar fashion to chondroitin sulfates. Their unique feature is the presence of N-sulfated hexosamine groups. Heparins are a subtype with anticoagulant activity. Heparan sulfates, produced by most cells,[226] adhere to the cell surface and basement membranes,[227–230] and may be involved with cell adhesion.[231]

Keratan sulfates consist of sulfated galactose and glucosamine moities attached to a core protein and are limited to the cornea, sclera, and cartilage. Their role in wound healing is unknown.

Hyaluronic acid, often a massive molecule but without either sulfated groups or a core protein, is composed solely of glucuronic acid and N-acetylglucosamine. It is ubiquitous in connective tissue and is present in particularly high concentrations in the umbilical cord and vitreous humor. Its hydrophilic nature may facilitate cell mobility. Cellular migration during wound repair occurs through hyaluronic acid-rich areas (see Chapters 12–14).

The role of proteoglycans during wound repair is poorly understood. They appear to create a charged, hydrated environment that facilitates cell mobility. This function may involve alterations of the cellular adhesion complexes.[232] Eventually, their complexity and hydrophilic properties provide the visco-elastic properties of normal connective tissues.

Collagens

The collagens are a large group of triple helix structural matrix proteins which in general give connective tissues their strength. Type I collagen is the major structural component of bones, skin and tendons. Type II is found predominantly in cartilage. Type III is found in association with type I, although the ratio varies in different tissues. Type IV collagen is found in basement membranes in association with mucopolysaccharides and laminin, while type V is found in the cornea in association with type III and is important in maintaining transparency.[233] Other types of collagen (up to type XII) are found in small amounts in many tissues and serve unknown functions.

Collagens are a key component of all phases of wound repair. Immediately after injury the exposure of fibrillar collagen to blood promotes platelet aggregation and activation and the release of chemotactic factors that initiate healing. Collagen fragments released by leukocytic collagenases attract fibroblasts to the injured area.[234]

Later collagen becomes the foundation of the new extracellular matrix. Normal dermis contains about 80% type I collagen and 20% type III collagen.[235] The amount of type III collagen in healing wounds in the postnatal period is elevated for three to four days before the levels of type I collagen increase.[236] Invading fibroblasts synthesize and secrete type I and III collagen to form the neomatrix as early as 24 hours after injury.[237,238] Granulation tissue has higher levels of type III collagen than most normal tissues, although type I is still the major component.[239,240]

Collagens in general are synthesized like most proteins. Several steps are unusual, however. For instance, although extracellular collagen contains significant amounts of hydroxyproline—the only major protein to do so—its genes code only for proline. As the growing alpha chain leaves the ribosomal network, it is inserted into the endoplasmic reticulum where it is glycosylated and about 40% of its prolines, but only about 14% of its lysines, are hydroxylated by three dioxygenases called prolyl 4-hydroxylase, prolyl 3-hydroxylase, and lysyl hydroxylase.[241] The 4-hydroxyprolines are critical for triple helix formation and thermal stability.[242] If insufficient prolines are 4-hydroxylated the collagen alpha chains cannot assume a stable triple helix at body temperature, the collagen cannot be exported, and the unassociated alpha chains are broken down. The function of 3-hydroxyproline is not known, but it is present in high proportions (7% of hydroxyprolines) only in type IV collagen.[243] Hydroxylysine residues serve two functions: as the attachment sites for carbohydrates,[244] and as the essential interchain cross-links that stabilize extracellular collagen.[245]

The substrates and cofactors for these essential steps include iron (Fe^{2+}), 2-oxoglutarate, ascorbate, and oxygen, the latter three all being consumed. The K_m of prolyl 4-hydroxylase and lysyl hydroxylase for oxygen is about 20 mm Hg for biologic substrates.[246,247] Thus the reaction is pO_2 dependent in the range from zero to about 200 mm Hg—far beyond the zone in which hypoxia might interfere with energy and ATP production. Since both ascorbic acid and oxygen are essential to this reaction, hypoxia and scurvy have identical effects on collagen synthesis, and both interfere profoundly with deposition of collagen into the extracellular matrix.

Once triple helical procollagen molecules are exported, their telopeptides, the ends of the molecules that prevent polymerization, are cleaved and the remaining molecules are polymerized by several types of chemical bonds among which lysines are oxidized and condensed to lysyl-lysine bonds. This last step is catalyzed by extracellular lysyl oxidase. Again pO_2 is important since the lysyl oxidase K_m for oxygen is also quite high. Without these lysyl-lysine bonds, or if lysyl oxidase is deficient, collagen fibers fail to gain structural stability.

The control of collagen synthesis—what starts it and what stops it—remains one of the major mysteries of wound healing. Many signals influence collagen synthesis including growth factors, nutritional elements, the partial pressure of oxygen, and lactate concentration.[248,249] Fibroblasts exposed to hypoxia or high lactate concentrations, conditions found in the wound microenvironment, increase their rate of collagen synthesis when oxygen levels are raised.[250–252]

The traditional assumption that collagen synthesis is a constitutive property of fibroblasts appears untrue. This means collagen synthesis is not necessarily proportional to the number of fibroblasts. Thus, the cytokine growth factors that increase cell number are only a beginning to collagen deposition. TGFβ is the one known growth factor that appears to influence collagen synthesis independent of cell number.[253]

More primitive metabolic stimuli seem to control collagen synthesis as well as TGFβ. Accumulation of lactate in injured tissue, due to damaged microvasculature and constitutive production by macrophages, elicits both TGFβ secretion from macrophages and collagen synthesis by fibroblasts by increasing transcription of collagen genes, and derepressing controls on posttranslational processing. This control mechanism seems to involve several steps. Lactate (and hypoxia) reduce the NAD^+ pool by converting NAD^+ to NADH. This reduces the amount of the only other metabolite of NAD^+ (NADH does not contribute), ADP-ribose (ADPR), which is merely NAD^+ with its nicotinamide removed. The polymerized form of ADPR (PADPR) normally appears to down-regulate collagen gene transcription in the resting state. Prolyl hydroxylase is also inhibited by ADPR. Thus, ADPR removal, by decreasing levels of NAD^+, "activates" both the gene and the critical enzyme. Lactate therefore increases both the genetic expression of unhydroxylated procollagen gene transcripts in the cell nucleus and the cytoplasmic hydroxylation of these peptides. Under normal circumstances, collagen synthesis is limited mainly by the prolyl hydroxylase substrates, ascorbate and oxygen (Figure 2.2).

Though the mechanisms are unclear, lactate also appears to induce both macrophages and fibroblasts to release TGFβ. Thus, the cytokines increase cell number, and macrophages produce lactate and TGFβ, which amplify each other to induce production of collagen peptides whose rate of production then depends on ascorbate and pO_2. This creates a peculiar circumstance in which increased lactate incites a reaction that proceeds faster in hyperoxia. Since macrophage lactate production continues despite hyperoxia, this circumstance does actually exist and has been measured.

This postnatal circumstance stands in fairly sharp contrast to fetal wound collagen production, which proceeds far faster than adult despite very low oxygen tension. Even so, the ADPR reaction seems to play a role, though a somewhat different one, in fetal healing as well (see Chapter 20).

Provision of oxygen and ascorbate allows collagen biosynthesis and deposition to proceed at higher rates. As angiogenesis proceeds, these metabolites are delivered in increasing amounts and permit acceleration of collagen matrix synthesis. When the vascular system develops to the point that lactate no longer accumulates, the impetus for collagen synthesis apparently diminishes to normal levels.

Accumulation of collagen in the wound area is dependent on the ratio of col-

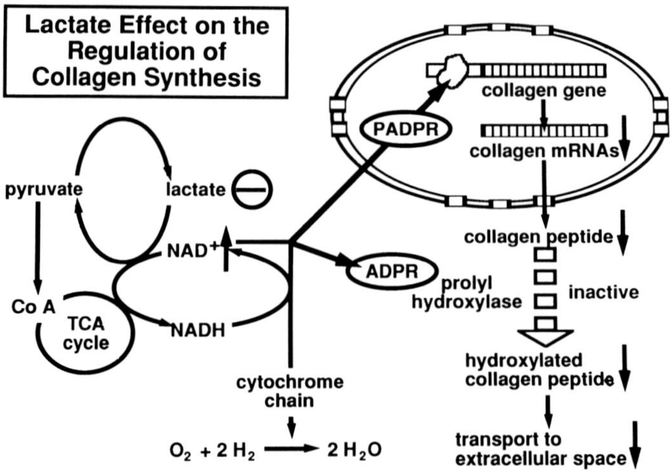

Figure 2.2 Lactate effect on collagen synthesis. PADPR normally inhibits collagen gene transcription and ADPR normally suppresses prolyl hydroxylase activity. Lactate lowers PADPR and ADPR, releases these inhibitions, and permits increased collagen gene transcription and prolyl hydroxylase activity.

lagen synthesis to collagen degradation by local enzymes. Early in the wound healing phase the amount of collagen degradation is low, but it increases as the wound matures.[254] Interstitial collagenases are the principal degradative enzymes, and they cleave all three chains of the collagen type I and III triple helix at one specific bond. The fragments are susceptible to other proteinases. Interstitial collagenases are secreted by granulocytes, macrophages, fibroblasts and epithelial cells as inactive zymogens that are activated by proteases.[255] Local inhibition of collagenase can occur with protease inhibitors like α_2-macroglobulin.[256]

Control of collagen synthesis, secretion, crosslinking, and degradation is incompletely understood but the subject of much wound healing research. Collagen is obviously an important factor in all phases of wound healing and is critical for return of tissue integrity and strength.

WOUND CONTRACTION

See Chapter 9 for a complete discussion of fetal wound contraction.

During healing of open injuries, especially wounds in loose skin, the tissue edges are slowly brought closer to each other by the process of wound contraction. Though slow, contraction in some wounds accounts for the majority of coverage. In postnatal animals wound contraction is a double edged sword. On the one hand, it reduces the size of the tissue defect, but on the other, if allowed to continue too far, it can inhibit function and cause disfigurement and excessive scarring.[257] There is some evidence that the cell responsible for wound contraction is the myofibroblast, a fibroblast with contractile properties.[258] More recent data suggest that fibroblasts without contractile fibers easily contract collagen gels, probably by membrane wrinkling, as a locomotive force, and subsequently by chemical bonding.[259–261]

Myofibroblasts contain an actin-myosin contractile system similar to the actin microfilaments found in smooth muscle cells. These microfilaments, also called stress fibers, are contractile fibers containing actin,[262] myosin,[263] tropomyosin,[264] filamin,[265] and α-actinin.[266] The microfilaments are arranged along the long axis of the fibroblasts and are associated with dense bodies for attachment to the surrounding extracellular matrix.[267] It is attractive to ascribe contraction to cells that have obvious contractile properties, but all fibroblasts also have well-developed systems of microtubules and microfilaments, which are cytoskeletal components found in most cells. Thus, all fibroblasts have mechanical strength. The microtubules run parallel to the long axis of the myofibroblasts with the microfilaments.[268] Myofibroblasts show other characteristics of smooth muscle cells. Gap junctions connect granulation tissue myofibroblasts but are not found in normal tissue fibroblasts.[269] Myofibroblasts are generally covered in a layer of material similar to basement membrane found around smooth muscle cells and endothelial cells.[270] Myofibroblasts also possess a unique attachment entity connecting the cytoskeleton to the extracellular matrix called the fibronexus. It is essentially a connection across the cell membrane of intracellular microfilaments and extracellular fibronectin.[271,272] Finally, granulation tissue expands and contracts in response to drugs that similarly affect smooth muscle tone.[273]

In short, there are two competing, or perhaps complementary, hypotheses to explain wound contraction. The unresolved issue is whether myofibroblasts are important, necessary, or irrelevant to the process of wound contraction.

SUMMARY

The repair of injured tissue in the postnatal individual is a complex event that culminates in return of tissue integrity and exclusion of the external environment. In contrast to fetal wound healing, it does so at the not trivial expense of scar tissue formation with some loss of function.

The earliest response to wounding in postnatal animals must, by necessity, be concerned with control of blood loss. Perhaps for this reason, early healing is dominated by coagulation phenomena, fibrin, thrombin, and factors released from platelets. Postnatal wounds often require disposal of devitalized tissue and control of infection. Therefore, inflammation is perpetuated, perhaps more than is necessary in the fetus. Once macrophages arrive in the wound, they dominate the subsequent inflammatory events perhaps to the detriment of regeneration.

Invasion of the wound by fibroblasts, secretion of a neomatrix, and re-epithelization culminate in return of tissue integrity. The new tissue then continues to remodel for a considerable period of time by altering the types, amounts, and geometry of the extracellular and cellular elements. The resulting scar is a region of dense collagen with some loss of normal tissue architecture and function.

Wound healing is an injured organism's response to a life-threatening event. An unhealed wound provides a distinct survival disadvantage. In the postnatal animal, the cellular response to achieve tissue integrity by scar formation after injury overrides the potential for perfect regeneration and return of all function, placing importance on early recovery free of infection. Perhaps the ability to regenerate tissue is not lost, but is subdued by the necessity for survival. We offer this analysis in the spirit that the study of fetal wound healing may allow us someday to make possible in adults that which is now possible only in the unborn.

REFERENCES

1. Goss RJ: The Physiology of Growth. New York, Academic Press, 1978.
2. Borgens RB: Mice regrow the tips of their foretoes. Science 217:74, 1982.
3. McMinn RMH: Tissue Repair. New York, Academic Press, 1969.

4. Deitch EA: The management of burns. N Engl J Med 323:1249–1253, 1990.
5. Majno G, Shea SM, Leventhal M: Endothelial contraction induced by histamine type mediators: An electron microscopic study. J Cell Biol 42:647–672, 1969.
6. Peacock EE Jr, van Winkle W Jr: Wound Repair. Philadelphia, WB Saunders, 1976.
7. Dvorak HF, Senger DR, Dvorak AM, et al.: Regulation of extravascular coagulation by microvascular permeability. Science 227:1059–1061, 1985.
8. Nemersaon Y, Zur M, Bach R, et al.: The mechanisms of action of tissue factor: A provisional model, in: The Regulation of Coagulation, KG Mann and FB Taylor, eds., pp. 193–203, Elsevier/North-Holland, New York, 1980.
9. Smariga PE and Maynard JR: Platelet effects on tissue factor and fibrinolytic inhibition of cultured human fibroblasts and vascular cells. Blood 60:140–147, 1982.
10. Niemetz J: Coagulant activity of leukocytes. Tissue factor activity. J Clin Invest 5:307–313, 1972.
11. Edwards RL and Rickes FR: The role of human T cells (and T cell products) for monocyte tissue factor generation. J Immunol 125:606–609, 1980.
12. Thompsen RE, Mandle R, and Kaplan AP: Characterization of human HMW-kininogen. Procoagulant activity associated with the light chain of kinin-free HMW kininogen. J Exp Med 147:488–499, 1978.
13. Mandle RJ, and Kaplan AP: Hageman factor substrates: Human prekallikrein. Mechanism of fibrinolysis. J Biol Chem 252:6097–6104, 1977.
14. DiScipio, RG: The activation of the alternative pathway C3 convertase by human plasma kallikrein. Immunology 45:587–595, 1982.
15. Kaplan AP, Kay AP, and Austen KF: A prealbumin activator of kallikrein. III. Appearance of chemotactic activity in human neutrophils by the conversion of human prekallikrein to kallikrein. J Exp Med 135:81–97, 1972.
16. Wachtfogel YT, Kucich U, James UL, et al.: Human plasma kallikrein releases neutrophil elastase during blood coagulation. J Clin Invest 72:1672–1677, 1983.
17. Chen LB, Buchanan JM: Mitogenic activity of blood components. I. Thrombin and prothrombin. Proc Natl Acad Sci USA 72:131–135, 1975.
18. Wesler BB, Ley CW, Jaffe EA: Stimulation of endothelial cell prostacycline production by thrombin, trypsin, and ionophore A23187. J Clin Invest 62:923–930, 1978.
19. Bar-Shivat R, Wilner GD: Biologic activities of nonenzymatic thrombin: Elucidation of a macrophage interactive domain. Sem Throm Hem 12:244–249, 1986.
20. Bar-Shivat R, Kahn AJ, Mann KG, et al.: Identification of a thrombin sequence with growth factor activity on macrophages. Proc Natl Acad Sci USA 83:976–980, 1986.
21. Lyons RM, Stanford NM, Majerus PW: Thrombin-induced protein phosphorylation in human platelets. J Clin Invest 56:924–936, 1975.
22. Gray AJ, Reeves JT, Harrison NK, et al.: Growth factors for human fibroblasts in the solute remaining after clot formation. J Cell Sci 96:271–274, 1990.
23. Dvorak HF, Harvey VS, Estrella P, et al.: Fibrin containing gels induce angiogenesis: Implications for tumor stroma generation and wound healing. Lab Invest 57:673–686, 1987.
24. Jones FS, Burgoon MP, Hoffman S, et al.: A cDNA clone for cytotactin contains sequences similar to epidermal growth factor-like repeats and segments of fibronectin and fibrinogen. Proc Natl Acad Sci USA 85:2186–2190, 1988.
25. Gerdin B and Saldeen T: Effect of fibrin degradation products on microvascular permeability. Thromb Res 13:995–1006, 1978.
26. Richardson DL, Pepper DS, and Kay AB: Chemotaxis for human monocytes by fibrinogen-derived peptides. Br J Haematol 32:507–513, 1976.
27. Esmon CT, Suttie JW and Jackson CM: The functional significance of vitamin K action. Difference in phospholipid binding between normal and abnormal prothrombin. J Biol Chem 250:4095–4099, 1975.
28. Fujimoto T, O'hara S, and Hawiger J: Thrombin-induced exposure and prostacyclin inhibition of the receptor for Factor VIII/Von Willebrand Factor on human platelets. J Clin Invest 69:1212–1222, 1982.
29. Schullek J, Jordan J, and Montgomery RR: Interaction of Von Willebrand Factor with human platelets in the plasma milieu. J Clin Invest 73:421–428, 1984.
30. Greengard JS, Heeb MJ, Ersdal E, et al.: Binding of Factor XI to washed human platelets. Biochemistry 25:3884–3890, 1986.
31. Sinha D, Seaman FS, Koshy A, et al.: Blood coagulation Factor XIa binds specifically to a site on activated platelets distinct from that for Factor XI. J Clin Invest 73:1550–1556, 1984.
32. Marr J, Barboriak JJ, and Johnson SA: Relationship of appearance of adenosine diphosphate,

fibrin formation, and platelet aggregation in the haemostatic plug in vivo. Nature (Lond.) 205:259–262, 1985.
33. Weiss HJ: Platelet physiology and abnormalities of platelet function (first of two parts). N Engl J Med 293:531–541, 1975.
34. Maione TE, Gray GS, Petro J, et al.: Inhibition of angiogenesis by recombinant human platelet factor-4 and related peptides. Science 247:77–79, 1990.
35. Clark RAF: Fibronectin in the skin. J Invest Dermatol 81:475–479, 1983.
36. Gonda SR, and Shainoff JR: Adsorptive endocytosis of fibrin monomer by macrophages: Evidence of a receptor for the amino terminus of the fibrin alpha-chain. Proc Natl Acad Sci USA 79:4565–4569, 1982.
37. Ciano P, Colvin R, Dvorak A, et al.: Macrophage migration in fibrin gel matrices. Lab Invest 54:62–129, 1986.
38. Allen RA and Pepper DC: Isolation and properties of human vascular plasminogen activator. Thromb Haemost 45:43–50, 1981.
39. Granelli-Piprro P, Vassailli JD and Reich E: Secretion of plasminogen activation by human polymorphonuclear leukocytes: Modulation by glucocorticoids and other effectors. J Exp Med 146:1693–1706, 1977.
40. Vasalli JD, Hamilton J, and Reich E: Macrophage plasminogen activator modulation of enzyme production by anti-inflammatory steroids, mitotic inhibitors, and cyclic nucleotides. Cell 8:271–281, 1976.
41. Hunt TK, ed: Wound Healing and Wound Infection. Appleton-Century-Crofts, New York 1980.
42. Clark RAF, Lanigan JM, DellaPelle P, et al.: Fibronectin and fibrin provide a provisional matrix for epidermal cell migration during wound re-epithelialization. J Invest Dermatol 79:264–269, 1982.
43. Kurkinen M, Vaheri A, Roberts PJ, et al.: Sequential appearance of fibronectin and collagen in experimental granulation tissue. Lab Invest 43:47–51, 1980.
44. Harris N, Dvorak A, Smith J, et al.: Fibrin deposits in Hodgkin's disease. Am J Pathol 108:119–129, 1982.
45. Simpson DM and Ross R: The neutrophil leucocyte in wound repair: A study with antineutrophil serum. J Clin Invest 51:2009–2020, 1972.
46. Sanchez-Madrid F, Nagy JA, Robbins E, et al.: A human leukocyte differentation antigen family with distinct alpha subunits and a common beta subunit: The lymphocyte function-associated antigen (LFA-1), the C3bi complement receptor (OKM1/Mac-1) and the p150,95 molecule. J Exp Med 158:1785–1803, 1983.
47. Bevilacqua MP, Pober JS, Wheeler ME, et al.: Interleukin-1 acts on cultured human vascular endothelium to increase the adhesion of polymorphonuclear leukocytes, monocytes, and related leukocyte cell lines. J Clin Invest 76:2003–2011, 1985.
48. Gamble JR, Harlan JM, Klebanoff SJ, et al.: Stimulation of the adherence of neutrophils to umbilical vein endothelium by human recombinant tumor necrosis factor. Proc Natl Acad Sci USA 82:8667–8671, 1985.
49. Wilkinson PC: Chemotaxis and Inflammation, 2d ed. Churchill Livingstone, New York, 1982.
50. Snyderman R and Goetzl EJ: Molecular and cellular mechanisms of leukocyte chemotaxis. Science 213:830–837, 1981.
51. Terranova VP, DiFlorio R, Hujanen ES, et al.: Laminin promotes rabbit neutrophil motility and attachment. J Clin Invest 77:1180–1186, 1986.
52. Johnston DE: Wound healing in skin. Veterinary Clinics of North America 20:1–25, 1990.
53. Wilkinson PC and Lackie JM: The influence of contact guidance on chemotaxis of human neutrophil leukocytes. Exp Cell Res 45:255–264, 1983.
54. Brown AF: Neutrophil granulocytes: Adhesion and locomotion on collagen substrata and in collagen matrices. J Cell Sci 58:445–467, 1982.
55. Bar-Shivat R, Kahn A, Fenton JW, et al.: Chemotactic response of monocytes to thrombin. J Cell Biol 96:282–285, 1983.
56. Senior RM, Griffin GL and Mecham RP: Chemotactic activity of elastin-derived peptides. J Clin Invest 66:859–862, 1980.
57. Postlethwaite AE and Kang AH: Collagen and collagen peptide-induced chemotaxis of human blood monocytes. J Exp Med 143:1299–1307, 1976.
58. Norris DA, Clark RAF, Swigart LM, et al.: Fibronectin fragment(s) are chemotactic for human peripheral blood monocytes. J Immunol 129:1612–1618, 1982.
59. Roos D, Goldstein IM, Kaplan HB, et al.: Dissociation of phagocytosis, metabolic stimulation and lysosomal enzyme release in human leukocytes. Agents Actions 6:256–259, 1976.

60. Klebanoff SJ, Hamon CB: Role of myeloperoxidase-mediated antimicrobial systems in intact leukocytes. J Reticuloendothel Soc 12:170–196, 1972.
61. Babior BM, Kipnes RS, Curnutte JT: Biological defense mechanisms: The production by leukocytes of superoxide, a potential bactericidal agent. J Clin Invest 52:741–744, 1973.
62. Weiss SJ, King GW, LoBuglio AF: Evidence for hydroxyl radical generation by human monocytes. J Clin Invest 60:370–373, 1977.
63. Thomas EL: Myeloperoxidase, hydrogen peroxide, chloride antimicrobial system: Nitrogen-chlorine derivatives of bacterial components in bactericidal action against Escherichia coli. Infect Immun 23:522–531, 1979.
64. Johnston RB and Lehmeyer JE: Elaboration of toxic oxygen by-products by neutrophils in a model of immune complex disease. J Clin Invest 57:836–841, 1976.
65. Henson PM and Johnston RB: Tissue injury in inflammation: Oxidants, proteinases, and cationic proteins. J Clin Invest 79:669–674, 1987.
66. Hasty KA, Hibbs MS, Kang AH, et al.: Secreted forms of human neutrophil collagenase. J Biol Chem 261:5645–5648, 1986.
67. Leibovich SJ and Ross R: The role of the macrophage in wound repair. A study with hydrocortisone and antimacrophage serum. Am J Pathol 78:71–100, 1975.
68. vanFurth R, Diesselhoff-den Dulk MMC, et al.: New perspectives on the kinetics of mononuclear phagocytes, in Mononuclear Phagocytes: Characteristics, Physiology, and Function. R. van Furth, ed.; pp 201–208, Martinus Nijhoff, Dordrecht, Holland, 1985.
69. van Furth R, Diesselhoff-den Dulk MMC, Mattie H: Quantitative study on the production and kinetics of mononuclear phagocytes during an acute inflammatory reaction. J Exp Med 138:1314–1330, 1973.
70. Riches DW: The multiple roles of macrophages in wound healing, in The Molecular and Cellular Biology of Wound Healing. RAF Clark and PM Henson, eds.; pp 218, Plenum Press, New York, 1988.
71. Witte LD, Kaplan KL, Nossel HL, et al.: Studies of the release from human platelets of the growth factor for cultured human arterial smooth muscle cells. Circ Res 42:402–409, 1978.
72. Kaplan DR, Chao FC, Stiles CD, et al.: Platelet-alpha granules contain a growth factor for fibroblasts. Blood 53:1043–1052, 1979.
73. Kaplan KL, Broekman MJ, Chernoff A, et al.: Platelet-alpha granule proteins: Studies on release and subcellular localization. Blood 53:604–616, 1979.
74. Martinet Y, Bitterman PB, Mornex JF, et al.: Activated human monocytes express the c-sis protooncogene and release a mediator showing PDGF-like activity. Nature (Lond.) 319:158–160, 1986.
75. Mornex JF, Martinet Y, Yamauchik K, et al.: Spontaneous expression of the c-sis gene and release of a platelet-derived growth factor-like molecule by human alveolar macrophage. J Clin Invest 78:61–66, 1986.
76. Antonaides HN: Human platelet-derived growth factor (PDGF): Purification of PDGF-I and PDGF-II and separation of their reduced subunits. Proc Natl Acad Sci USA 78:7314–7317, 1981.
77. Deuel TF, Senior RM, Chang D, et al.: Platelet factor 4 is chemotactic for neutrophils and monocytes. Proc Natl Acad Sci USA 78:4584–4587, 1981.
78. Rains EW and Ross R: Platelet-derived growth factor I. High yield purification and evidence for multiple forms. J Biol Chem 257:5154–5160, 1982.
79. Deuel TF and Huang JS: Platelet-derived growth factor: Structure, function, and roles in normal and transformed cells. J Clin Invest 74:669–676, 1984.
80. Deuel TF and Huang JS: Platelet-derived growth factor: Purification, properties, and biological activities. Prog Hematol 13:201–221, 1983.
81. Heldin CH and Westermark B: Growth Factors: Mechanism of action and relation to oncogenes. Cell 37:9–20, 1984.
82. Daniel TO, Tremble PM, Frankelton ARJ, et al.: Purification of the platelet-derived growth factor receptor by using an anti-phosphotyrosine antibody. Proc Natl Acad Sci USA 82:2684–2687, 1985.
83. Deuel TF, Senior RM, Huang JS, et al.: Chemotaxis of monocytes and neutrophils to platelet-derived growth factor. J Clin Invest 69:1046–1049, 1982.
84. Tzeng DY, Deuel TF, Huang JS, et al.: Platelet-derived growth factor promotes polymorphonuclear leukocyte activation. Blood 64:1123–1128, 1984.
85. Grotendorst GR, Chang T, Seppa HEJ, et al.: Platelet-derived growth factor is a chemoattractant for vascular smooth muscle cells. J Cell Physiol 113:261–266, 1982.

86. Senior RM, Griffin GL, Huang JS, et al.: Chemotactic activity of platelet alpha granule proteins for fibroblasts. J Cell Biol 96:382–385, 1983.
87. Huang JS, Huang SS, Deuel TF: Specific covalent binding of platelet-derived growth factor to human plasma α-2-macroglobulin. Proc Natl Acad Sci USA 81:342–346, 1984.
88. Gray JS, Wieczorowski E, Ivy AC: Inhibition of gastric secretion by extracts of normal male urine. Science 89:489–490, 1939.
89. Gray JS, Culmer CU, Wieczorowski E, et al.: Preparation of a pyrogen-free urogastrone. Proc Soc Exp Biol and Med 43:225–228, 1940.
90. Gregory H: Isolation and structure of urogastrone and its relationship to epidermal growth factor. Nature (Lond.) 257:325–327, 1975.
91. Zapf J, Waldvogel M, and Froesch ER: Binding of nonsuppressible insulin-like activity to human serum: Evidence for a carrier protein. Arch Biochem Biophys 168:638–645, 1975.
92. Hintz RL and Liu F: Demonstration of specific plasma protein binding sites for somatomedin. J Clin Endocrinol Metab 45:988–995, 1977.
93. Jansson L, Karlson FA, Westermark B: Mitogenic activity and epidermal growth factor content in human milk. Acta Paediatr Scand 74:250–253, 1985.
94. Olsen PS, Poulsen SS, Kirkegaard P: Adrenergic effects on secretion of epidermal growth factor from Brunner's glands. Gut 26:920–927, 1985.
95. Wiley HS, VanNostrand W, McKinley DN, et al.: Intracellular processing of epidermal growth factor and its effect on ligand-receptor interactions. Cancer Res 45:1934–1939, 1985.
96. Hunter T: The epidermal growth factor receptor gene and its product. Nature (Lond.) 311:477–480, 1984.
97. Carpenter G: Epidermal growth factor: Biology and receptor metabolism. J Cell Sci 3(Suppl):1–9, 1985.
98. Derynck R, Roberts AB, Winkler ME, et al.: Human transforming growth factor-α: Precursor structure and expression in E. coli. Cell 38:287–297, 1984.
99. Chabot JG, Walker P and Pelletier G: Distribution of epidermal growth factor binding sites in the adult rat liver. Am J Physiol 250:G760, 1986.
100. Toyoda S, Lee PC, and Lebenthal E: Interaction of epidermal growth factor with specific binding sites of enterocytes isolated from rat small intestine during development. Biochem Biophys Acta 886:295–301, 1986.
101. Green MR and Couchman JR: Distribution of epidermal growth factor receptors in rat tissues during embryonic skin development, hair formation, and adult hair growth cycle. J Invest Dermatol 83:118–123, 1984.
102. Lim RW and Hauschka SD: A rapid decrease in epidermal growth factor-binding capacity accompanies the terminal differentiation of mouse myoblasts in vitro. J Cell Biol 98:739–747, 1984.
103. Downward J, Parker P, Waterfield MD: Autophosphorylation sites on the epidermal growth factor receptor. Nature (Lond.) 311:483–485, 1984.
104. Moolenaar WH, Tertoolen LG, de Laat SW: Growth factors immediately raise cytoplasmic free Ca^{2+} in human fibroblasts. J Biol Chem 259:8066–8069, 1984.
105. Grove RI, Pratt RM: Influence of epidermal growth factor and cyclic AMP on growth and differentiation of palatal epithelial cells in culture. Dev Biol 106:427–437, 1984.
106. Stanulis-Praeger BM and Gilchrest BA: Growth factor responsiveness declines during adulthood for human skin-derived cells. Mech Aging Dev 35:185–198, 1986.
107. Nakagawa S, Yoshida S, Hirao Y, et al.: Biological effects of biosynthetic human EGF on the growth of mammalian cells in vitro. Differentiation 29:284–288, 1985.
108. Blay J and Brown KD: Epidermal growth factor promotes the chemotactic migration of cultured rat intestinal epithelial cells. J Cell Physiol 124:107–112, 1985.
109. Chua CC, Geiman DE, Keller GH, et al.: Induction of collagenase secretion in human fibroblast cultures by growth promoting factors. J Biol Chem 260:5213–5216, 1985.
110. Gospodarowicz, D: Localization of a fibroblast growth factor and its effect alone and with hydrocortisone on 3T3 cell growth. Nature (London) 249:123–127, 1974.
111. Li QG, Blacher R, Esch F, et al.: A heparin-binding erythroid cell stimulating factor from fetal bovine serum has the N-terminal sequence of insulin-like growth factor. II. Biochem Biophys Res Commun 166:557–561, 1990.
112. Shing Y, Folkman J, Sullivan R, et al.: Heparin affinity: Purification of a tumor-derived capillary endothelial cell growth factor. Science: 223:1296–1299, 1984.
113. Gospadarowicz, D: Fibroblast and epidermal growth factors: Their uses in vivo and in vitro in studies on cell functions and cell transplantation. Mol Cell Biochem 25:79–110, 1979.

114. Klagsbrun M, Knighton D, and Folkman J: Tumor angiogenesis in cells grown in tissue culture. Cancer Res 36:110–114, 1975.
115. Auerbach R, Kubai L, Knighton D, et al.: A simple procedure for the long-term cultivation of chicken embryos. Dev Biol 41:391–394, 1974.
116. Shing Y, Folkman J, Sullivan R, et al.: Heparin affinity: Purification of a tumor-derived capillary endothelial cell growth factor. Science 223:1296–1299, 1984.
117. Gospodarowicz D and Bialecki H: The effects of epidermal and fibroblast growth factors on the replicative lifespan of cultured bovine granulosa cells. Endocrinology 103:854–858, 1978.
118. Gospodarowicz D: Hormonal Proteins and Peptides. Vol. XII, CH Li, ed.: pp 205–230. Academic, New York, 1984.
119. Fourtanier A, Courty J, Muller E, et al.: Eye-derived growth factor isolated from bovine retina and used for epidermal wound healing in vivo. J Invest Dermatol 87:76–80, 1986.
120. Buntrock P, Jentzsch KD, and Heder G: Stimulation of wound healing, using brain extract with fibroblast growth (FGF) activity. I. Quantitative and biochemical studies into formation of granulation tissue. Exp Pathol 21:46–53, 1982.
121. Buntrock P, Jentzsch KD, and Heder G: Stimulation of wound healing, using brain extract with fibroblast growth factor (FGF) activity. II. Histological and morphometric examination of cells and capillaries. Exp Pathol 21:62–67, 1982.
122. Cate RL, Mattaliano RJ, Hession C, et al.: Isolation of the bovine and human genes for Mullerian Inhibiting Substance and expression of the human gene in animal cells. Cell 45:5312–5316, 1986.
123. Mason AJ, Hayflick JS, Ling N, et al.: Complementary DNA sequences of ovarian follicular fluid inhibin show precursor structure and homology with transforming growth factor-beta. Nature (Lond.) 318:659–663, 1985.
124. Seyedin SM, Thomas TC, Thompson AY, et al.: Purification and characterization of two cartilage-inducing factors from bovine demineralized bone. Proc Natl Acad Sci USA 82:2267–2271, 1985.
125. Seyedin SM, Thompson AY, Bentz H, et al.: Cartilage-inducing factor-A: Apparent identity to transforming growth factor-beta. J Biol Chem 261:5693–5695, 1986.
126. Frolick CA, Wakefield LM, Smith DM, et al.: Characterization of a membrane receptor for transforming growth factor-beta in normal rat kidney fibroblasts. J Biol Chem 259:10995–11000, 1984.
127. Massague J: Subunit structure of a high-affinity receptor for type beta transforming growth factor: Evidence for a disulfide-linked glycosylated receptor complex. J Biol Chem 260:7059–7066, 1985.
128. Nexo E, Hollenberg MD, Figueroa AA, et al.: Detection of epidermal growth factor-urogastrone and its receptor during fetal mouse development. Proc Natl Acad Sci USA 77:2782–2785, 1980.
129. Twardzik DR, Ranchalis JE, and Todaro GJ: Mouse embryonic transforming growth factors related to those isolated from tumor cells. Cancer Res 42:590–593, 1982.
130. Lee DC, Rochfor R, Todaro GJ, et al.: Developmental expression of rat transforming growth factor-alpha mRNA. Mol Cell Biol 5:3644–3646, 1985.
131. Pincher R, Jullien P, and Lawrence DA: Beta-transforming growth factor is stored in human blood platelets as a latent high molecular weight complex. Biochem Biophys Res Commun 136:30–37, 1986.
132. Assoian RK, Komoriya A, Meyers CA, et al.: Transforming growth factor-beta in human platelets: Identification of a major storage site, purification, and characterization. J Biol Chem 258:7155–7160, 1983.
133. Assoian RK and Sporn MB: Anchorage-independent growth of primary rat embryo cells is induced by platelet-derived growth factor and inhibited by type-beta transforming growth factor. J Cell Physiol 126:312–318, 1986.
134. Kehrl JH, Wakefield LM, Roberts AB, et al.: Production of transforming growth factor-beta by human T lymphocytes and its potential role in the regulation of T cell growth. J Exp Med 163:1037–1050, 1986.
135. Pincher R, Lawrence DA, and Jullien P: Latent beta-transforming growth factor in non-transformed and Kirsten sarcoma virus-transformed normal rat kidney cells, clone 49F. Cancer Res 44:5538–5543, 1984.
136. Lawrence WT, Sporn MB, Gorschboth C, et al.: The reversal of an adriamycin induced healing impairment with chemoattractants and growth factors. Ann Surg 203:142–147, 1986.
137. Tucker RF, Shipley GD, Moses HL, et al.: Growth inhibitor from BSC-1 cells closely related to platelet type beta transforming growth factor. Science 226:705–707, 1984.
138. Roberts AB, Anzano MA, Lamb LC, et al.: Type beta transforming growth factor: A bifunctional regulator of cellular growth. Proc Natl Acad Sci USA 83:119–123, 1985.

139. Sporn MB, Roberts AB, Wakefield LM, et al.: Transforming growth factor-beta: Biological function and chemical structure. Science 233:532–534, 1986.
140. Cromack DT, Sporn MB, Roberts AB, et al.: Transforming growth factor β levels in rat wound chambers. J Surg Res 42:622–628, 1987.
141. Lawrence WT, Sporn MB, Gorschboth C, et al.: The reversal of an adriamycin induced healing impairment with chemoattractants and growth factors. Ann Surg 203:142–147, 1986.
142. Sporn MB, Roberts AB, Shull JH, et al.: Polypeptide transforming growth factor isolated from bovine sources and used for wound healing in vivo. Science 219:1329–1331, 1983.
143. Salomon GD, Kasid A, Bernstein E, et al.: Gene expression in normal and doxorubicin-impaired wounds: Importance of transforming growth factor-beta. Surgery 108:318–323, 1990.
144. Ogawa Y, Sawamura SJ, Ksander GA, et al.: Transforming growth factors-b1 and b2 induce synthesis and accumulation of hyaluronate and chondroitin sulfate in vivo. Growth Factors 3, 53–62, 1990.
145. Roberts AB, Sporn MB, Assoian RK, et al.: Transforming growth factor type beta: Rapid induction of fibrosis and angiogenesis in vivo and stimulation of collagen formation in vitro. Proc Natl Acad Sci USA 83:4167–4171, 1986.
146. Roberts CJ, Birkenmeier TM, McQuillan JJ, et al.: Transforming growth factor beta stimulates the expression of fibronectin and of both subunits of the human fibronectin receptor by cultured human lung fibroblasts. J Biol Chem 263:4586–4592, 1988.
147. Ignotz RA, and Massague J: Transforming growth factor-beta stimulates the expression of fibronectin and collagen and their incorporation into the extracellular matrix. J Biol Chem 261:4337–4345, 1986.
148. Quaglino D, Nanney LB, Kennedy R, et al.: Transforming growth factor-β stimulates wound healing and modulates extracellular matrix gene expression in pig skin. I. Excisional wound model. Lab Investigation 63:307–319, 1990.
149. Rotwein P, Pollack KM, Didier DK, et al.: Organization and sequence of the human insulin-like growth factor I gene. J Biol Chem 261:4828, 1986.
150. Pagter-Holthuizen P de, van Schaik FMA, Verdujin GH, van Ommen GJB, Bouma BN, Jansen M, Sussenback JS: Organization of the human genes for insulin-like growth factors I and II. FEBS Letters 195:179–184, 1986.
151. Pagter-Holthuizen P de, Jansen M, Van der Kammen R, et al.: The human insulin-like growth factor II gene contains two development-specific promoters. FEBS Letters 214:259–264, 1987.
152. Adams SO, Nissley SP, Handwerger S, et al.: Developmental patterns of insulin-like growth factor I and II synthesis and regulation in rat fibroblasts. Nature 302:150–153, 1983.
153. Clemmons DR and Shaw DS: Purification and biologic properties of fibroblast somatomedin. J Biol Chem 263:2841–2849, 1986.
154. Clemmons DR: Structural and functional analysis of insulin-like growth factors. Brit Med Bulletin 45:465–480, 1989.
155. Clemmons DR: Multiple hormones stimulate the production of somatomedin by cultured human fibroblasts. J Clin Endocrinol Metab 58:850–856, 1984.
156. Clemmons DR: Structural and functional analysis of insulin-like growth factors. Brit Med Bulletin 45:465–480, 1989.
157. Pledger WJ, Stiles CD, Antonaides HN, et al.: Induction of DNA synthesis in BALB/c3t3 cells by serum components. Re-evaluation of the commitment process. Proc Natl Acad Sci USA 74:4481–4485, 1977.
158. Stiles CD, Capone GT, Scher CD, et al.: Dual control of cell growth by somatomedin and platelet derived growth factor. Proc Natl Acad Sci 76:1279–1283, 1979.
159. Calvin RB, Antonaides HN: Role of platelet-derived growth factor in wound healing: Synergistic effects with other growth factors. Proc Natl Acad Sci USA 84:7696–7700, 1987.
160. Singer SJ and Kupfer A: The directed migration of eukaryotic cells. Annu Rev Cell Biol 2:337–365, 1986.
161. Thiery JP: Mechanisms of cell migration in the vertebrate embryo. Differentiation 15:1–15, 1984.
162. Trinkhaus JP: Cells Into Organs. The Forces that Shape the Embryo. Prentice-Hall, Englewood Cliffs, New Jersey, 1984.
163. Bergmann, Kupfer A, and Singer SJ: Membrane insertion at the leading edge of motile fibroblasts. Proc Natl Acad Sci USA 80:1367–1371, 1983.
164. Bryant WM: Wound healing. CIBA Clin Symp 29:1–36, 1977.
165. Wagner RC: Endothelial cell embryology and growth. Adv Microcirc 9:45–75, 1980.
166. Hudlicka O: Development of microcirculation: Capillary growth and adaptation. In: Handbook

of Physiology-section 2: The Cardiovascular System. Vol IV; Microcirculation, Part 1;165–216, Baltimore, Waverly Press, 1984.
167. Hunt TK: Wound Healing and Wound Infection: Theory and Surgical Practice. New York: Appleton-Century-Crofts, 1980.
168. Knighton DR, Phillips GD, Fiegel VD: Wound healing angiogenesis: Indirect stimulation by basic fibroblast growth factor. J Trauma 30 (12 Suppl):S134–144, 1990.
169. Pepper MS, Belin D, Montesano R, et al.: Transforming growth factor-beta 1 modulates basic fibroblast growth factor-induced proteolytic and angiogenic properties of endothelial cells in vitro. J Cell Biol 111:743–755, 1990.
170. Senior RM, Huang JS, Griffin GL, et al.: Dissociation of the chemotactic and mitogenic activities of platelet-derived growth factor by human neutrophil elastase. J Cell Biol 100:351–356, 1985.
171. Oosta GM, Favreau LV, Beeler DL, et al.: Purification and properties of human platelet heparinase. J Biol Chem 257:11249–11255, 1982.
172. Vlodasky I, Folkman J, Sullivan R, et al.: Endothelial cell-derived basic fibroblast growth factor synthesis and deposition into subendothelial extracellular matrix. Proc Natl Acad Sci USA 84:2292–2296, 1987.
173. Baird A and Ling N: Fibroblast growth factors are present in the extracellular matrix produced by endothelial cells in vitro: Implications for a role of heparinase-like enzymes in the neovascular response. Biochem Biophys Res Commun 142:428–435, 1987.
174. Zetter BR: Angiogenesis: State of the art. Chest 93 (suppl):159S–166S, 1988.
175. Knighton DR, Hunt TK, Scheuenstuhl H, et al.: Oxygen tension regulates the expression of angiogenesis factor by macrophages. Science 221:1283–1285, 1983.
176. Banda MJ, Knighton DR, Hunt TK, et al.: Isolation of a nonmitogenic angiogenesis factor from wound fluid. Proc Natl Acad Sci USA 79:7773–7777, 1982.
177. Hockel M, Beck T, Wissler JH: Neomorphogenesis of blood vessels in rabbit skin produced by a highly purified monocyte-derived polypeptide (monocyto-angiotropin) and associated tissue reactions. Intl J Tiss Reac 6:323–331, 1984.
178. Jensen JA, Hunt TK, Scheuenstuhl H, et al.: Effect of lactate, pyruvate, and pH on secretion of angiogenesis and mitogenesis factors by macrophages. Lab Invest 54:574–578, 1986.
179. Hussain MZ, Ghani QP, Hunt TK: Inhibition of prolyl hydroxylase by poly(ADP-ribose) and phosphoribosyl AMP. Possible role of ADP-ribosylation in intracellular prolyl hydroxylase regulation. J Biol Chem 264:7850–7855, 1989.
180. Orlidge A, D'Amore PA: Inhibition of capillary endothelial cell growth by pericytes and smooth muscle cells. J Cell Biol 105:1455–1462, 1987.
181. Pang SC, Daniels WH, Buck RC: Epidermal migration during the healing of suction blisters in rat skin: A scanning and transmission electron microscopic study. Amer J Anat 153:177–191, 1978.
182. Hinshaw JR and Miller ER: Histology of healing split-thickness, full thickness autogenous skin grafts and donor sites. Arch Surg 91:658–670, 1965.
183. Repsh LA and Oberprillar: Ultrastructural studies on migrating epidermal cells during the wound healing stage of regeneration in the adult newt, Notophthalmus visidescents. Am J Anat 159:187–208, 1980.
184. Mahan JT, and Donaldson DJ: Events in the movement of newt epidermal cells across implanted substrates. J Exp Zool 235:35–44, 1985.
185. Trinkhaus-Randall V, and Gipson IK: Role of calcium and calmodulin in hemidesmosome formation in vitro. J Cell Biol 98:1565–1571, 1984.
186. Andersen L and Fejerskov O: Ultrastructure of initial epithelial cell migration in palatal wounds of guinea pigs. J Ultrastruct Res 48:313–324, 1974.
187. Gipson IK and Kiorpes TC: Epithelial sheet movement: Protein and glycoprotein synthesis. Dev Biol 92:259–262, 1982.
188. Gibbons JR: Epithelial migration in organ culture. A morphological and time-lapse cinematographic analysis of migrating stratified squamous epithelium. Pathology 10:207–218, 1978.
189. Krawczyk WS: A pattern of epidermal cell migration during wound healing. J Cell Biol 49:247–263, 1971.
190. Miller TA: The healing of partial thickness skin injuries, in: Wound Healing and Wound Infection. TK Hunt (ed.): pp 81–96, Appleton-Century-Crofts, New York, 1980.
191. Martinez IR: Fine structural studies of migrating epidermal cells following incisional wound, in Epidermal Wound Healing. Maibach HI and Rovee DT, eds. Year Book, Chicago; pp 323–342, 1972.

192. Alitalo K, Hovi T, Vaheri A: Fibronectin is produced by human macrophages. J Exp Med 151:602–613, 1980.
193. Hynes RO: Fibronectins: Sci Am 254:42–51, 1986.
194. Hynes RO, Yamada KM: Fibronectins: Multifunctional modular glycoproteins. J Cell Biol 95:369–377, 1982.
195. Hynes RO: Molecular biology of fibronectin, in: Annual Review of Cell Biology, vol 1, Palade GE, Alberts BM, Spudich JA, eds., pp 67–90, Annual Reviews, Palo Alto, California, 1985.
196. Tamkun JW, DeSimone DW, Fonda D, et al.: Structure of integrin, a glycoprotein involved in the transmembrane linkage between fibronectin and actin. Cell 46:271–282, 1986.
197. McDonald JA, Kelley DG, Broekelmann TJ: Role of fibronectin in collagen deposition: Fab′ to the gelatin-binding domain of fibronectin inhibits both fibronectin and collagen organization in fibroblast extracellular matrix. J Cell Biol 92:485–492, 1982.
198. Keski-Oja J and Yamada KM: Isolation of an actin-binding fragment of fibronectin. Biochem J 193:615–620, 1981.
199. Garcia-Pardo A, Pearlstein E, Frangione B: Primary structure of human plasma fibronectin. Characterization of a 31,000 dalton fragment from the COOH-terminal region containing a free sulfhydryl group and a fibrin-binding site. J Biol Chem 260:10320–10325, 1985.
200. Yamada KM, Kennedy DW, Kimata K, et al.: Characterization of fibronectin interactions with glycosaminoglycans and identification of active proteolytic fragments. J Biol Chem 255:6055–6063, 1980.
201. Gold LI, Frangione B, Pearlstein E: Biochemical and immunological characterization of three binding sites of human plasma fibronectin with different affinities for heparin. Biochemistry 22:4113–4119, 1983.
202. Homandberg GA and Erickson JW: A model of fibronectin tertiary structure based on studies of interactions between fragments. Biochemistry 25:6917–6925, 1986.
203. Pytela R, Pierschbacher MD, Ruoslahti E: Identification and isolation of a 140 kd cell surface glycoprotein with properties expected of a fibronectin receptor. Cell 40:191–198, 1985.
204. Horwitz A, Duggan K, Buck C, et al.: Interaction of plasma membrane fibronectin receptor with talin-A transmembrane linkage. Nature 320:531–533, 1986.
205. Pierschbacher MD, Ruoslahti E: Cell attachment activity of fibronectin can be duplicated by small synthetic fragments of the molecule. Nature (Lond.) 309:30–33, 1984.
206. Pierschbacher MD, Ruoslahti E: Variants of the cell recognition site of fibronectin that retain attachment-promoting activity. Proc Natl Acad Sci USA 81:5985–5988, 1984.
207. McCarthy JB, Sas DF, Furcht LT: Mechanisms of parenchymal cell migration into wounds, in: The Molecular and Cellular Biology of Wound Repair. Clark RAF and Henson PM, eds., pp 281–319, Plenum Press, New York, 1988.
208. Clark RAF, Colvin RB: Wound repair, in: Plasma Fibronectin: Structure and Function. McDonagh J, ed., pp 197–262, Dekker, New York.
209. Oh E, Pierschbacher M, Ruoslahti E: Deposition of plasma fibronectin in tissues. Proc Natl Acad Sci USA 78:3218–3221, 1981.
210. Sekiguchi K, Klos AM, Kurachi K, et al.: Human liver fibronectin complementary DNAs-Identification of 2 different messenger RNAs possibly encoding the alpha-subunit and beta-subunit of plasma fibronectin. Biochemistry 25:4436–4441, 1986.
211. Mosher DF and Johnson RB: Specificity of fibronectin-fibrin cross-linking. Ann NY Acad Sci 408:583–594, 1983.
212. Postlethwaite A, Keski-Oja J, Balian G, et al.: Induction of fibroblast chemotaxis by fibronectin. Localization of the chemotactic region to a 140,000 molecular weight non-gelatin-binding fragment. J Exp Med 153:494–499, 1981.
213. Grinnell F, Feld MK: Initial adhesion of human fibroblasts in serum-free medium: Possible role of secreted fibronectin. Cell 17:117–129, 1979.
214. Irish PS, Hasty DL: Immunocytochemical localization of fibronectin in human fibroblast cultures using a cell surface replica technique. J Histochem Cytochem 31:69–77, 1983.
215. Williams IF, McCullagh KG, Silver IA: The distribution of types I and III collagen and fibronectin in the healing equine tendon. Connect Tissue Res 12:211–227, 1984.
216. Grinnell F and Bennett MH: Fibroblast adhesion on collagen substrata in the presence and absence of plasma fibronectin. J Cell Sci 48:19–34, 1981.
217. Repesh LA, Fitzgerald TJ, Furcht LT: Fibronectin involvement in granulation tissue and wound healing in rabbits. J Histochem Cytochem 30:351–358, 1982.
218. Singer II, Kazais DM, Kawka DW: Localization of the fibronexus at the surface of granulation

tissue myofibroblasts using double-label immunogold electron microscopy on ultrathin frozen sections. Eur J Cell Biol 38:94–101, 1985.

219. Heinegard D, Franzen A, Hedbom E, et al.: Common structures of the core proteins of interstitial proteoglycans, in: Functions of the Proteoglycans, Ciba Foundation Symposium 124, Evered D, Whelen J, eds.; pp 65–88, Wiley, New York, 1986.

220. Hassell JR, Kimura JH, Hascall VC: Proteoglycan core protein families. Annu Rev Biochem 55:539–567, 1986.

221. Scott JE, Orford CR: Dermatan sulfate-rich proteoglycan associated with rat tail-tendon cartilage at the d band in the gap region. Biochem 197:213–216, 1981.

222. Gallagher JT, Gasiunas N, Schor SL: Specific association of iduronic acid-rich dermatan sulfate with the extracellular matrix of human skin fibroblasts cultured on collagen gels. Biochem J 215:107–116, 1983.

223. Brennan MJ, Oldberg A, Hayman EG, et al.: Effect of a proteoglycan produced by rat tumor cells on their adhesion to fibronectin-collagen substrata. Cancer Res 43:4302–4307, 1983.

224. Funderburg FM and Markwald RR: Conditioning of native substrates by chondroitin sulfate proteoglycan during cardiac mesenchymal cell migration. J Cell Biol 103:2475–2487, 1986.

225. Laterra J, Ansbacher R, Culp LA: Glycosaminoglycans that bind cold-insoluble globulin in cell-substratum adhesion sites of murine fibroblasts. Proc Natl Acad Sci USA 77:6662–6666, 1980.

226. Marcum JA, Rosenberg RD: Anticoagulantly active heparin-like molecules from vascular tissue. Biochemistry 23:1730–1737, 1984.

227. Kjellen L, Pettersson I, Hook M: Cell-surface heparan sulfate: An intercalated membrane proteoglycan. Proc Natl Acad Sci USA 78:5371–5375, 1981.

228. Jalkanen M, Nguyen H, Rapraeger A, et al.: Heparin sulfate proteoglycan from mouse mammary epithelial cells: Localization on the cell surface with a monoclonal antibody. J Cell Biol 101:976–984, 1985.

229. Parthasathy N, Spiro RG: Isolation and characterization of the heparin sulfate proteoglycan of the bovine glomerular basement membrane. J Biol Chem 259:12749–12755, 1984.

230. Kanwar YS, Farquhar MG: Isolation of glycosaminoglycans (heparin sulfate) from glomerular basement membranes. Proc Natl Acad Sci USA 76:4493–4497, 1979.

231. Woods A, Hook M, Kjellen L, et al.: Relationship of heparin sulfate proteoglycans to the cytoskeleton and extracellular matrix of cultured fibroblasts. J Cell Biol 99:1743–1753, 1984.

232. Lembach KJ: Enhanced synthesis and extracellular accumulation of hyaluronic acid during stimulation of quiescent human fibroblasts by mouse epidermal growth factor. J Cell Physiol 89:277–288, 1976.

233. McLaughlin JS, Linsenmayer TF, Birk DE: Type V collagen synthesis and deposition by chicken embryo corneal fibroblasts in vitro. J Cell Science 94:371–379, 1989.

234. Postlethwaite EE, Seyer JM, Kang AH: Chemotactic attraction of human fibroblasts to type I, II, and III collagens and collagen derived peptides. Proc Natl Acad Sci USA 75:871–875, 1978.

235. Miller EJ: Biochemical characteristics and biological significance of genetically distinct collagens. Molec Cell Biochem 13:165–189, 1976.

236. Gay S, Viljanto J, Raekallio J, et al.: Collagen types in early phases of wound healing in children. Acta Chir Scand 144:205–211, 1978.

237. Heughan C, Hunt T: Some aspects of wound healing research: A review. Can J Surg 18:118–126, 1975.

238. Cohen IK, Moore CD, Diegelmann RF: Onset and localization of collagen synthesis during wound healing in open rat skin wounds. Proc Soc Exp Biol Med 160:458–462, 1979.

239. Bailey AJ, Sims TJ, LeLous M, et al.: Collagen polymorphism in experimental granulation tissue. Biochem Biophys Res Commun 66:1160–1165, 1975.

240. Clore JN, Cohen IK, Diegelman RF: Quantitation of collagen types I and III during wound healing in rat skin. Proc Soc Exp Biol Med 161:337–340, 1979.

241. Kivirikko KI, Myllylä R: The Hydoxylation of Prolyl and Lysyl Residues, in: Collagen In Health and Disease, Weiss JB and Jayson MIV, eds, pp 54–104, Churchill Livingstone, New York, 1982.

242. Berg RA and Prockop DJ: Purification of (14C) protocollagen and its hydroxylation by prolyl-hydroxylase. Biochem 12:3395–3401, 1973.

243. Kefalides NA: Basement membranes: Structural and biosynthetic considerations. J Invest Dermatol 65:85–92, 1975.

244. Kivirikko KI, Myllylä R: Collagen glycosyltransferases. Int Rev Connect Tissue Res 8:23–72, 1979.

245. Bailey AJ, Robins SP, Balian G: Biological significance of the intermolecular crosslinks of collagen. Nature (Lond.) 251:105–109, 1974.
246. Myllylä R, Tuderman L, Kivirikko KI: Mechanism of the prolyl hydroxylase reaction. 2. Kinetic analysis of the reaction sequence. Eur J Biochem 80:349–357, 1977.
247. Puistola U, Turpeennniemi-Hujanen TM, Myllylä R, et al.: Studies on the lysyl hydroxylase reaction. 1. Initial velocity kinetics and related aspects. Biochim Biophys Acta 611:40–50, 1980.
248. Hunt TK, Conolly WB, Aronson SB, et al.: Anaerobic metabolism and wound healing: A hypothesis for the initiation and cessation of collagen synthesis in wounds. Am J Surg 135:328–332, 1978.
249. Hunt TK, Knighton DR, Thakral KK, et al.: Studies on inflammation and wound healing: Angiogenesis and collagen synthesis stimulated in vivo by resident and activated macrophages. Surgery 96:48–54, 1984.
250. Green H and Goldberg B: Collagen and cell protein synthesis by an established mammalian fibroblast line. Nature 204:347–349, 1964.
251. Comstock JP and Udenfriend S: Effect of lactate on collagen proline hydroxylase activity in cultured L-929 fibroblasts. Proc Natl Acad Sci USA 66:552–557, 1970.
252. Levene CI and Bates CJ: The effect of hypoxia on collagen synthesis in cultures 3T6 fibroblasts and its relationship to the mode of action of ascorbate. Biochem Biophys Acta 444:446–452, 1976.
253. Sporn MB, Roberts AB, Shull JH, et al.: Polypeptide transforming growth factors isolated from bovine sources and used for wound healing in vivo. Science 219:1329–1330, 1983.
254. Zeitz M, Ruiz-Torres A, Merker HJ: Collagen metabolism in granulating wounds of rat skin. Arch Dermatol Res 263:207–214, 1978.
255. Werb Z, Mainardi CL, Vater CA, et al.: Endogenous activation of latent collagenase by rheumatoid synovial cells: Evidence for a role of plasminogen activator. N Engl J Med 296:1017–1023, 1977.
256. Werb Z, Burleigh MC, Barrett AJ, et al.: The interaction of α2-macroglobulin with proteinases: Binding and inhibition of mammalian collagenase and other neutral proteases. Biochem 139:359–368, 1974.
257. Montandon D, Gabbiani G, Ryan GB, et al.: The contractile fibroblast. Its relevance in plastic surgery. Plast Reconstr Surg 52:286–290, 1973.
258. Gabbiani G, Ryan GB, Majno G: Presence of modified fibroblasts in granulation tissue and their possible role in wound contraction. Experentia 27:549–550, 1971.
259. Hembry RM, Bernanke DH, Hayashi K, et al.: Morphologic examination of mesenchymal cells in healing wounds of normal and tight skin mice. Am J Pathol 125:81–89, 1986.
260. Doillon CJ, Hembry RM, Ehrlich HP, et al.: Actin filaments in normal dermis and during wound healing. Am J Pathol 126:164–170, 1987.
261. Ehrlich HP, Rajaratnam JB: Cell locomotion forces versus cell contractile forces for collagen lattice contraction: An in vitro model of wound contraction. Tissue Cell 22:407–417, 1990.
262. Willingham MC, Yamada SS, Davies PJA, et al.: Intracellular localization of actin in cultured fibroblasts by electron microscopic immunochemistry. J Histochem Cytochem 29:17–37, 1981.
263. Fujiwara K and Pollard TD: Fluorescent antibody localization of myosin in the cytoplasm, cleavage furrow, and mitotic spindle of human cells. J Cell Biol 71:848–875, 1976.
264. Lazarides E: Tropomyosin antibody: The specific localization of tropomyosin in nonmuscle cells. J Cell Biol 65:549–561, 1975.
265. Wang K: Filamin, a new high-molecular-weight protein found in smooth muscle and nonmuscle cells. Purification and properties of chicken gizzard filamin. Biochemistry 16:1857–1865, 1977.
266. Lazarides E, Burrdige K: α-actinin: Immunofluorescent localization of a muscle structural protein in nonmuscle cells. Cell 6:289–298, 1975.
267. Gabbiani G, Rungger-Brändle E: The fibroblast, in: Handbook of Inflammation: Tissue Repair and Regeneration, Glynn LE, ed., pp 1–50, Elsevier/North-Holland Biomedical Press, Amsterdam, 1981.
268. Rudolph R and Woodward M: Spatial orientation of microtubules in contractile fibroblasts in vivo. Anat Rec 191:169–182, 1978.
269. Gabbiani G, Rungger-Brändle E: The fibroblast, in: Handbook of Inflammation: Tissue Repair and Regeneration. Vol 3: pp 1–50, Glynn LE, ed., Elsevier/North-Holland Biomedical Press, Amsterdam, 1981.
270. Gabbiani G, Hirschel BJ, Ryan GB, et al.: Granulation tissue as a contractile organ. A study of structure and function. J Exp Med 135:719–734, 1972.

271. Singer II: The fibronexus: A transmembrane association of fibronectin-containing fibers and bundles of 5 nm microfilaments in hamster and human fibroblasts. Cell 16:675–685, 1979.
272. Heggeness MH, Ash JF, Singer SJ: Transmembrane linkage of fibronectin in intracellular actin-containing filaments in cultured human fibroblasts. Ann NY Acad Sci 312:414–417, 1978.
273. Ryan GB, Cliff WJ, Gabbiani GB, et al.: Myofibroblasts in human granulation tissue. Hum Pathol 5:55–67, 1974.

CHAPTER 3

Characteristics of Fetal Tissue Repair

N. Scott Adzick
Michael T. Longaker

Until recently, the womb protected the fetus from both observation and treatment. The development of ultrasonography allowed us to observe the fetus and fueled an explosion of knowledge about the fetus and its development (see Chapter 1). As a result of antenatal diagnosis, the fetus is now considered a patient.[1] The few life-threatening anatomic malformations that have been treated by hysterotomy and open fetal surgery include severe bilateral hydronephrosis,[2] congenital diaphragmatic hernia,[3] sacrococcygeal teratoma,[4] and cystic adenomatoid malformation of the lung. From the initial clinical series at The Fetal Treatment Program at The University of California, San Francisco, the observation was made that the human fetus appears to heal without scarring.[5] This experience confirms Rowlatt's observation that the mid-gestation human fetus heals by mesenchymal proliferation and without the scar formation normally seen in the adult.[6]

Recent experimental work supports these clinical observations. Studies in rats,[7] rabbits,[8–10] sheep,[11,12] and monkeys[13–15] all demonstrate distinct differences between fetal and adult skin wound healing. However, the nature of these differences remain unknown, and there are two general themes that could underlie them: differences in fetal cells, differences in the fetal wound environment, or a combination of the two. Ongoing research is just beginning to elucidate the mechanisms that endow the fetus with its unique healing qualities.

ADULT WOUND REPAIR

A brief summary of adult tissue repair provides the background for an overview of what is known about the biology of fetal wound healing (see Chapter 2). Adult wound healing is a response to injury ending in the restoration of tissue continuity.[16,17] While some amphibians heal by regeneration, adult mammalian tissue repair involves a complex series of biochemical events that ultimately ends in scar formation.

Adult wound repair includes the stages of hemostasis, inflammation, proliferation, and remodeling. Hemostasis includes vasoconstriction, platelet aggregation and degranulation, blood clotting, and fibrin formation. Inflammation represents a cellular cascade beginning with polymorphonuclear leukocytes (PMNs) followed by macrophages and lymphocytes. This stage is responsible for defending against bacteria and secretion of numerous growth factors, cytokines, and extracellular matrix (ECM) components. Of the inflammatory cells, the wound macrophage is the crucial effector cell that coordinates adult wound repair.[18–20] The proliferative stage involves multiplication of fibroblasts and endothelial and epithelial cells. The initial proteoglycan-rich fibrin matrix is replaced by collagen. In the final remodeling stage, collagen is cross-linked to form a mature scar. In abnormal wound healing conditions such as keloids, hypertrophic scars, strictures, and intra-abdominal adhesions, the final result of wound repair creates a cosmetic or functional problem.[21]

THE UNIQUE FETAL ENVIRONMENT

Amniotic Fluid

There are numerous intrinsic and extrinsic differences between the fetus and the adult that may dramatically influence wound healing. One major extrinsic difference is that fetal skin wounds are continually bathed in warm, sterile amniotic fluid known to be rich in growth factors that are crucial to fetal development (Figure 3.1).[22] Amniotic fluid is also a rich source for ECM components such as hyaluronic acid (HA) and fibronectin.[23,24] Amniotic fluid could modulate fetal skin wound repair simply by applying HA and fibronectin directly onto fetal skin

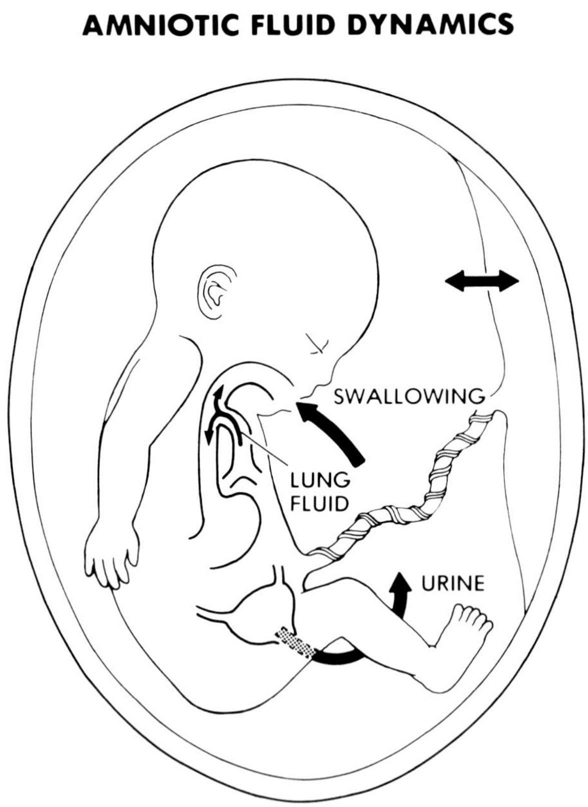

Figure 3.1 Amniotic fluid continually bathes fetal skin, and it is rich in growth factors. Amniotic fluid formation and resorption is a dynamic process. Fetal urine is the primary component of amniotic fluid, but actively secreted fetal lung fluid also constitutes a significant portion. Fetal swallowing is the principal means of amniotic fluid resorption.

wounds and by providing growth factors to stimulate fetal wound cells to make a unique wound matrix.[25]

To investigate the influence of the fetal environment on adult tissue repair, Longaker transplanted full-thickness sheep skin onto the backs of 60 day fetal lambs (term = 145 days).[121] Previous work has demonstrated that fetal lambs at less than 70 days gestation do not reject allogeneic skin grafts.[122] The adult skin graft is thus bathed in amniotic fluid and perfused by fetal blood (Figure 3.2); 40 days later (100 days gestation), incisional wounds were made on both the adult skin grafts and adjacent fetal skin, and immunohistochemical analysis was performed 7 and 14 days post-wounding (Figure 3.3). By 14 days the fetal wounds had healed without scarring, while the adult wound collagen pattern was in a typical scar pattern. Neither an amniotic fluid environment nor perfusion by fetal blood prevented scar formation in the wounded adult skin graft. This suggests that the ability of fetal skin to heal without scar formation may be a function of the fetal cells and matrix with or without a fetal environmental influence. Immunohistochemical studies of the fetal-adult tissue interface are currently underway.

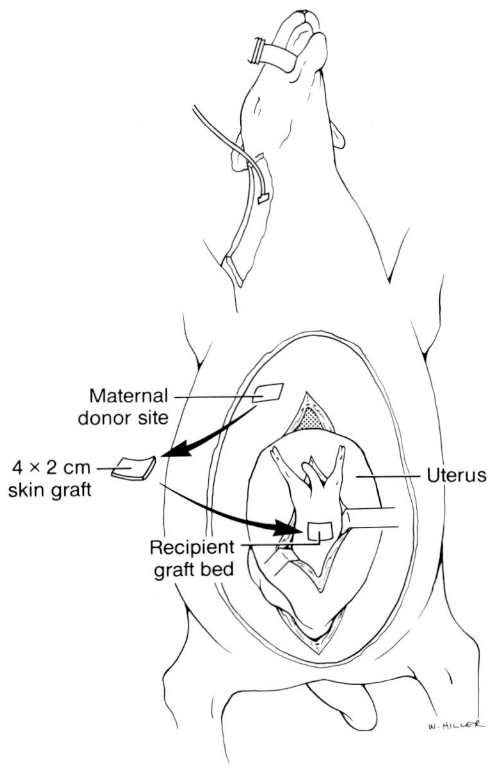

Figure 3.2 At 60 days gestation, a full-thickness maternal skin graft was harvested from the abdomen and was placed on a similar size defect on the back of a fetal lamb. After engraftment, the adult tissue was perfused by fetal blood and bathed in amniotic fluid.

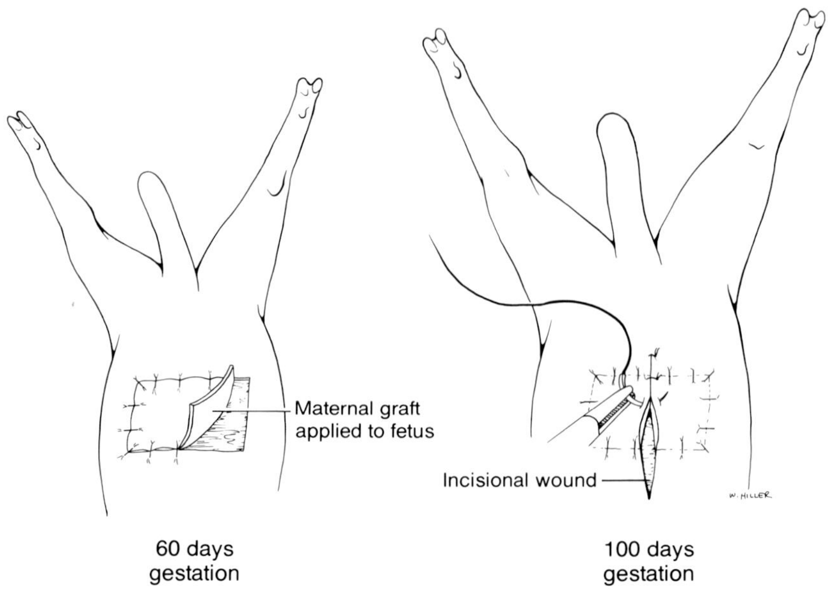

Figure 3.3 At 100 days gestation, an incisional wound was made through the maternal skin graft and into surrounding normal fetal skin. These wounds were examined histologically seven or 14 days later.

Oxygenation

Intrinsic environmental differences include fetal tissue oxygenation. The fetus depends on transplacental transport from the maternal circulation to meet its oxygen requirements (see Chapter 16). Because there is a large transplacental oxygen gradient between maternal arterial and umbilical venous blood, fetal arterial blood has a very low pO_2. In fact, the fetus appears to be markedly hypoxemic with an arterial pO_2 of 20 torr,[26] which is lower than a maskless mountaineer on top of Mt. Everest.[27] Partial compensation for the low pO_2 derives from the presence of fetal hemoglobin, which as a result of its high P_{50}, has a much greater affinity for O_2 than does adult hemoglobin. Although this is advantageous for O_2 uptake in the umbilical-placental circulation, this may interfere with O_2 delivery at the wound site.

It is well established that tissue perfusion and oxygenation are crucial during postnatal life for adequate healing and resistance to infection.[28] There is good evidence that adult healing can be accelerated by the addition of oxygen.[28] Consequently, the remarkable wound healing of the fetus seems paradoxical due to the low fetal arterial pO_2. Using a miniaturized oximeter probe, we have determined that the tissue pO_2 is 16 mm Hg in mid-gestation fetal lambs, whereas adult tissue pO_2 is approximately 45–60 mm Hg. It is intriguing that the fetus can heal so rapidly despite being relatively hypoxemic.

Fetal Skin Versus Other Fetal Tissues

Some of the properties of fetal skin wound healing may reflect the development of fetal skin (see Chapter 8). Lane determined that human fetal epidermis initially appears stratified (9 to 14 weeks gestation), followed by follicular keratinization (14 to 24 weeks), and finally by interfollicular keratinization after 24 weeks.[29]

Between four and 24 weeks gestation, human skin has an outermost layer called the periderm, which has the appearance of multiple microvilli projecting off the surface of the skin. It is possible that periderm has an absorption function as an amniotic fluid dialysate membrane. What effect the changing histology of fetal skin during development has on fetal wound healing remains unknown.

In Chapter 7, the sequence of events and timing of fetal fracture healing are reviewed. Fracture healing in the fetal lamb model occurs in a rapid and highly organized manner. Virtually no callus formation is present at any time during the healing process, and healed fracture sites are indistinguishable radiologically and histologically from uninjured bone. In addition, large bony defects in the fetus close but would be unhealable in infants and adults.

It is likely that not all fetal tissues share the remarkable regenerative qualities of fetal skin and bone wound healing. In experiments involving in utero repair of previously surgically created fetal diaphragmatic hernia, the fetal intestine was always densely adherent to the diaphragmatic defect, but no scar was evident on the previously made thoracic skin incision.[30] Clinical experience with human fetal surgery has shown extensive intra-abdominal adhesions following fetal diaphragmatic hernia repair.[31] Thus, fetal mesothelial wounds may heal differently from fetal skin wounds. In addition, amniotic fluid exposure may play an important role in the scarless healing of fetal skin wounds, but its effect on the healing of fetal mesothelial wounds has not been characterized.

To investigate these questions, our group created bilateral incisional diaphragmatic wounds on 100 day gestation fetal lambs (term = 145 days). The right thoracotomy wound was closed to exclude amniotic fluid. In contrast, an Eloesser flap was created at the left thoracotomy site, thus permitting the left diaphragmatic wound to be continually bathed in amniotic fluid (Figures 3.4, 3.5). Wounds were harvested at one, two, seven, or 14 days following wounding and analyzed by light microscopy and immunohistochemistry with antibodies to collagen types I, III, IV, and VI. Whether bathed in or excluded from amniotic fluid, the mesothelial-lined diaphragm healed with scar formation and without evidence of muscle

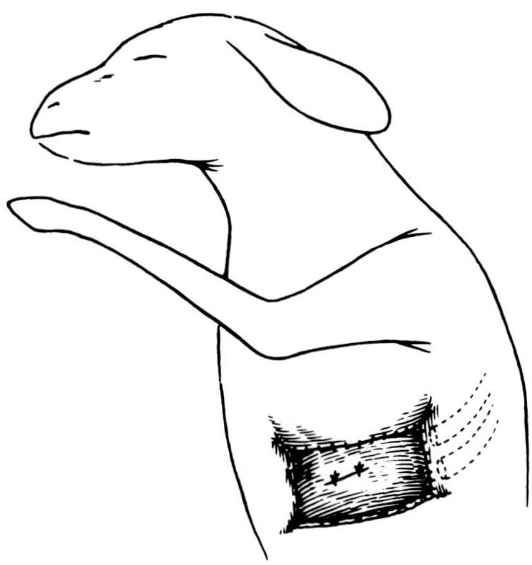

Figure 3.4 The left thoracotomy was fashioned into an Eloesser flap thoracoplasty to marsupialize the left diaphragmatic wound and permit continuous exposure of it to amniotic fluid.

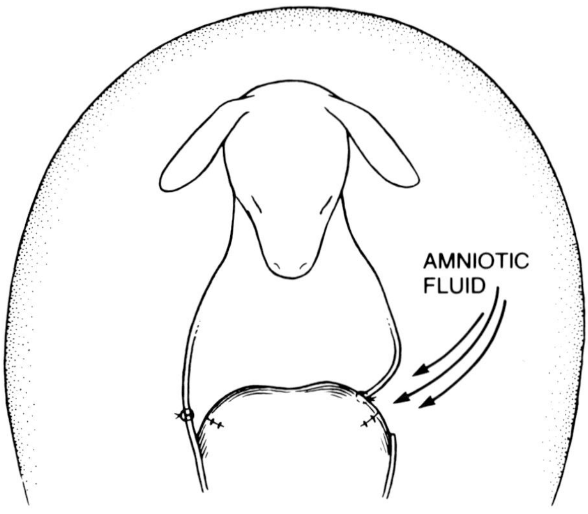

Figure 3.5 The right thoracotomy was closed to exclude the right diaphragmatic wound from amniotic fluid, and the left Eloesser thoracoplasty flap permitted the left diaphragmatic wound to be exposed to amniotic fluid.

regeneration.[120] Interestingly, wounds exposed to amniotic fluid were covered by a thick fibrous peel of collagen similar to that seen in gastroschisis bowel. These findings indicate that not all fetal tissues share the unique scarless healing properties of fetal skin.

Inflammation

Another intrinsic difference between the fetus and adult lies in the immune system. The fetal external environment is sterile. Until mid-gestation, the fetus is significantly neutropenic and has not developed self/nonself immunologic identity.[32] Histologically, there are very few, if any, PMNs in fetal wounds, and there may be a defect in immature PMN chemotactic ability.[33] Using antibodies to endogenous immunoglobulins as a marker for inflammation, Longaker found that fetal lamb wounds lacked the typical inflammatory response seen in adult sheep wounds.[12] Because of the prominent role that inflammation plays in adult tissue repair, the minimal fetal inflammatory response to injury may play a pivotal role in the unique fetal repair process (see Chapter 15).

Bracaglia evaluated the ontogeny of the inflammatory response in the rabbit fetus.[34] He injected the phlogistic agent carrageenan, a potent stimulant of inflammation, into the dermis on days 19, 23, and 27 of gestation (term = 31 days). In the youngest fetuses there was very little inflammation, but the cellular inflammatory response increased in the older fetuses and after birth. Schwartz showed similar results in fetal monkeys.[35] Fetal monkeys were subcutaneously injected with a variety of irritants at 60, 90, 120, or 150 days gestation (term = 165 days) and the response was compared to that of neonates and yearlings. The fetal response was different from the adult: a mononuclear cell infiltrate predominated in the young fetuses, whereas PMNs, fibrin, and edema were rare or absent.

Thomas determined that fetal rabbit neutrophils are capable of responding to the potent neutrophil chemoattractant formyl-methionyl-leucyl-phenylalanine

(FMLP).[36] Polyvinyl alcohol (PVA) sponges treated with FMLP were implanted into fetal rabbits on day 24 of gestation. Five days later the treated sponges showed histologic evidence of PMNs, fibroblasts, and collagen deposition. This study suggests that once present in a wound, fetal PMNs may initiate a sequence of events leading to scar formation. To further delineate whether the lack of fibrosis in fetal wounds is related to the lack of an acute inflammatory reaction, the same investigators first implanted PVA sponges subcutaneously into pregnant does for times varying from six to 36 hours, and then transferred the sponges into the fetuses of the does.[37] Implants were harvested from the fetuses from one to five days later. The fetal implants contained significantly more PMN cells than did control implants that were harvested from does but not implanted into fetuses, thus implying fetal PMN infiltration. Although the introduction of adult acute inflammatory cells into the fetus appeared to attract fetal PMNs to the wound site, an adult fibrotic type of healing response was not induced. These intriguing findings raise questions regarding what attracts fetal fibroblasts into wounds, how this differs between fetus and adult, and whether characteristic inflammatory mediators of adult wound healing are absent in fetal wounds.

The wound macrophage is the crucial inflammatory cell orchestrating adult wound healing.[18–20] Neutrophils can be eliminated from wound repair without a defect in granulation tissue but macrophages cannot.[18,38] Macrophages are essential regulatory cells that coordinate matrix debridement and turnover, and secrete mediators of inflammation, angiogenesis, and cell growth.[18,19] Adzick demonstrated a lack of PMNs and an abundance of macrophages by enzyme histochemistry in fetal rabbit wounds.[9] If fetal macrophages are recruited to the wound site, are they functioning in the same regulatory and debridement capacity that they have in adult wounds? Banda has preliminary evidence that fetal macrophages may act in a regulatory fashion by growth factor expression using highly sensitive mRNA phenotyping and polymerase chain reaction techniques.[39,40]

In addition to regulation through growth factor expression, wound macrophages are involved in matrix turnover through proteinase expression.[41] Their secretion of metalloproteinases (e.g. collagenase) and proteinase inhibitors coordinates the degradation and remodeling of the wound ECM. The observation that fetal lamb incisional wounds appear histologically indistinguishable from unwounded skin within two weeks suggests that fetal wound matrix turnover and repair are rapid and efficient.[12]

Fetal Growth

The fetus grows and develops at an astounding rate. In order to support this growth rate, fetal physiology may be primed by a rich milieu of growth factors and developmental gene expression.[42,43] The fetus can be physically wounded, but physiologically does not respond to the injury in an adult-like fashion. All of these factors in the unique fetal milieu may affect the cellular and connective tissue response to injury. Fetal tissue repair may be a process more closely resembling regeneration and growth rather than healing by scar formation.

MODELS AND METHODS

Many different animal models for studying fetal wound healing have been used (see Chapter 4) including the chick embryo,[44] mice,[45,46] rat,[7,47–50] guinea pig,[51] opossum,[52] rabbit,[8–10] sheep,[11–12,59] monkey,[13–15] and man.[5,6] In addition, numerous wound implant techniques have been used to study fetal tissue repair.[53–57] In all species studied, fetal wound healing is fundamentally different from wound healing in the adult. Hallock demonstrated in both fetal mice and monkeys that lip wounds heal by complete re-epithelialization and without scarring.[15,45] Burrington and Longaker using fetal sheep,[11,12] Viljanto, Adzick, and Krummel[8–10] in rabbits, and Rowsell and Robinson in rats,[49,50] all demonstrated scarless skin healing without a PMN infiltrate. Dixon[47] and Longaker[12] showed a spectrum to fetal wound healing as a function of gestational age: skin wound healing in the rat or the lamb fetus becomes adult-like with scar formation late in gestation.

THE ROLE OF THE EXTRACELLULAR MATRIX

Hyaluronic Acid (see Chapters 12–14)

Krummel[10] and DePalma[60,61] demonstrated that the fetal wound matrix is rich in the glycosaminoglycan (GAG), hyaluronic acid (HA). They implanted PVA sponges into fetal rabbits on day 24 of gestation as well as in adult rabbits and harvested them one to six days later. The GAG content of fetal sponges was significantly greater on day 2-6 when compared to adult sponges, and was 10 times the content of GAG found in unwounded fetal skin. The major GAG component represented HA as determined by cellulose acetate electrophoresis followed by alcian blue staining. From this pioneering work, an understanding of the role that fetal wound matrix plays in the repair process is beginning to unfold.

Hyaluronic acid is a key structural and functional component of the ECM whenever there is rapid tissue proliferation, regeneration, and repair. HA fosters a permissive environment that promotes cell proliferation.[62,63] It is now clear that HA is laid down early in the matrix of both fetal and adult wounds but that sustained deposition of HA is unique to fetal wound healing. A prolonged presence of HA in fetal wounds may provide the matrix signal orchestrating healing by regeneration rather than by scarring.

To delineate the mechanisms for HA deposition in fetal wounds, Longaker[25,64,65] studied the ability of fetal sera, wound fluid, and amniotic fluid to stimulate HA synthesis using a newly developed in vitro assay.[66] Fetal lamb and bovine serum contain an elevated HA-stimulating activity (HASA) that, in both species, peaks in mid-gestation, whereas there is little HASA in postnatal sera. The HASA from fetal sera has been recently characterized as a 55 kD glycoprotein.[66]

Analysis of wound fluid obtained from Hunt-Schilling wire mesh cylinders (Figure 3.6) implanted in mid-gestation fetal lambs for one to 14 days demonstrated that HASA levels were markedly elevated in fetal wound, whereas there was no HASA in adult wound fluid. This phenomena may underlie the rich deposition of HA in the ECM of fetal wounds. The activity of fetal wound fluid also had a bimodal distribution. One explanation for this may be that the first peak (days one to four) reflects HASA from fetal serum. The second peak (days eight to 14) may represent local production of HASA by wound fibroblasts.

One of the differences between the external environment of fetal and adult wounds is the amniotic fluid that bathes fetal skin wounds. Amniotic fluid has been shown to contain high concentrations of HA,[23] and sheep amniotic fluid also

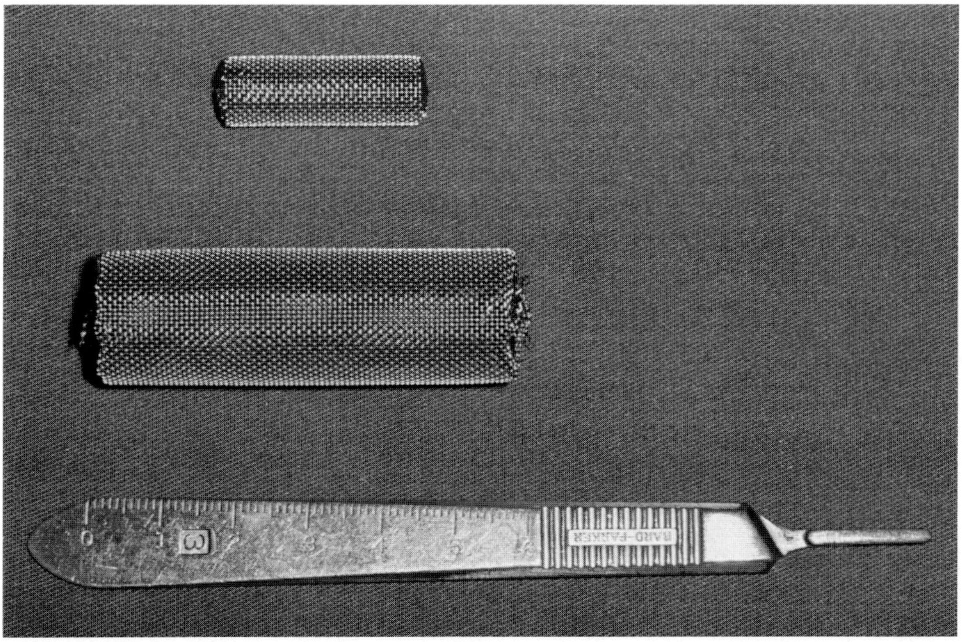

Figure 3.6 Photograph of wire mesh wound cylinders. These cylinders have relatively large mesh pores and separate the tissue, creating a dead space that fills with wound fluid. Top: fetal cylinder. Bottom: adult cylinder. *Reprinted with permission.*[65]

has markedly elevated HASA.[25] Unlike fetal sera, the peak activity of HASA in amniotic fluid is at term. This probably reflects the increased contribution of fetal urine to amniotic fluid, since fetal urine is a particularly rich source of HASA.[67] Since fetal skin wounds are bathed in amniotic fluid that contains both an HASA and HA, these factors provide additional mechanisms by which HA is deposited in the matrix of fetal skin wounds.

This series of studies demonstrated that HASA is present in the fetal wound for a prolonged period of time from a variety of sources, which results in a prolonged HA-rich response in fetal wounds, a mechanism entirely absent in the adult wound. HA is deposited only briefly at the earliest stages of adult wound healing.[68,69] Following the initial deposition of HA in adult wounds, hyaluronidase is produced, HA is removed, and the wound matrix is replaced by collagen.[70] In the adult wound, local deposition of HA by the platelet plug and fibrin clot obviates the need for an exogenous mechanism for stimulating local HA production.[71] These findings suggest that the mechanism for eliciting the early HA-rich response in adult wounds is different from the prolonged HA-rich response in fetal wounds. A fetal wound matrix rich in HA fosters an ECM environment permissive for cell motility and proliferation that may contribute to the unique properties observed in fetal wound healing.

Collagen

The mechanisms that underlie the lack of scarring in fetal wounds are unknown but probably relate to the control of collagen synthesis and fibrillogenesis (see Chapter 11). The role of collagen in the fetal wound matrix is controversial, and histologic techniques in fetal rabbits and sheep have conflicting results.[10,12] Krummel implanted a PVA sponge within a perforated silastic cylinder into fetal rabbits and could not detect collagen using Masson's trichrome staining. In contrast, an immunohistochemistry study using antibodies to collagen types I, III, IV, and VI showed collagen was rapidly deposited in the wounds of 75, 100, and 120 day gestation fetal lambs. The collagen staining pattern of incisional wounds in the 75 and 100 day fetal lambs was exactly the same as unwounded fetal skin by two weeks following wounding. Interestingly, there was a switch to an adult-like healing late in gestation with a dense dermal collagen scar present in the wounded 120-day fetuses.

To provide quantitative analysis of fetal wound collagen, a variety of techniques and animal models have been used. Merkel and Hallock pooled tissue extracts from excisional fetal rat wounds and showed similar ratios of type I and III collagen to that found in normal unwounded fetal skin.[72,73] In the fetal rabbit model, Adzick[9] and Siebert[74] used a Gore-Tex implant and Viljanto[8] used a viscose cellulose sponge implant; all showed evidence of collagen in fetal rabbit wounds by a variety of techniques. In contrast, Krummel and DePalma[10,61] implanted a PVA sponge within a perforated silastic cylinder into fetal rabbits and could not detect collagen using a highly sensitive HPLC assay. These conflicting results most likely reflect different wound sampling techniques. Using the versatile fetal lamb model, Burd examined collagen deposition in PVA sponge implants using histologic, biochemical, and wound breaking strength methods.[75] Sponges were implanted into 75 and 100 day fetuses as well as in non-pregnant adults. The sponges were harvested in all three groups at five, 10, 15, and 20 days following implantation. Masson's trichrome staining documented abundant collagen deposition in the fetal implants, and the hydroxyproline content of implants in both fetal groups was greater than in the adult group at all time points. Additionally, using a modification of the PVA sponge where it is bisected and then stapled together, an estimate of wound bursting strength was calculated by the force required to pull the sponges apart following harvesting and staple removal. All three groups showed a rise in wound breaking strength, although the adult wounds were strongest at 20 days post-implantation. Thus, the deposition of collagen without scarring in the fetal lamb model has been firmly established using a variety of techniques.

In vitro studies suggest that fetal fibroblasts are more proficient than their adult counterparts at collagen synthesis (see Chapter 19). Thomas compared the relative collagen synthesis of first and second passage fetal and adult rabbit fibroblasts.[76] The relative collagen synthesis of fetal fibroblasts was much higher than adult fibroblasts during both first and second passage. However, all values were significantly lower in second passage cells. In addition to total collagen synthesis, fetal fibroblasts produced more type III and V collagen than their adult counterparts. The facility of fetal fibroblasts to synthesize collagen in vitro is supported by Duncan's recent work examining the ontogeny of fetal prolyl hydroxylase, an important rate-limiting step in collagen biosynthesis.[77] Using an in vitro assay system and early passage human fetal and adult dermal fibroblasts, he demonstrated that prolyl hydroxylase activity in fetal fibroblasts is much higher compared to adult fibroblasts up until 20 weeks gestation; later in gestation the fetal fibroblast prolyl hydroxylase activity begins to fall toward adult levels. Prolyl hydroxylase in fetal cells, unlike adult cells, appears to be controlled by poly-ADP-ribose synthetase, an enzyme that has been implicated in the regulation of tumorigenesis and cell repair.[78] These recent studies suggest that the fetal intrinsic mechanism for collagen synthesis is not only functional but appears to be up-regulated compared to the adult.

Since collagen is the major component of scar tissue in postnatal animals, how does the fetus lay down a collagen-rich repair matrix and yet heal without scarring? Scarless healing is likely related to the organization of the fetal wound matrix. An HA-rich matrix may provide a permissive environment for orderly deposition of collagen fibrils in fetal wounds,[79] whereas the collagen fibrils in an adult wound matrix are aligned in a distorted unorganized scar pattern (see Chapter 10). Scott and colleagues noted that early in development, bovine and chick collagen fibrils were of a smaller diameter at a time when HA was abundant.[80] A rapid increase in collagen fibril diameter in mid-gestation coincided with a decrease in HA and chondroitin sulfate content. Of particular interest is the apparent enhancement of postnatal wound matrix reorganization by topically applied tissue-extracted HA.[81]

Adhesion Molecules

The critical differences between fetal and adult wound healing appear beginning at the very earliest stages of the two processes. Some of these differences could potentially be accounted for by other ECM components besides HA and collagen, particularly the adhesion glycoproteins as well as their receptors, known as "integrins."[82]

During the process of embryogenesis as well as in wound healing, specific interactions between migratory cells and the ECM occur. The ECM provides the scaffolding for cell attachment, adhesion, and migration. Various adhesion glycoprotein components found in the ECM such as fibronectin, thrombospondin, and tenascin may mediate such functions. For instance, Tonnesson found that fibronectin was more abundant in fetal skin than neonatal or adult skin.[83] This suggests that fibronectin deposition is enhanced during embryogenesis and morphogenesis, providing a favorable microenvironment for cell migration and proliferation.

During adult wound healing, fibroblasts and epidermal cells deposit large amounts of fibronectin.[84,85] Fibronectin is associated with the fibrin clot early during adult wound healing, and the fibronectin deposited is of the embryonic type (see Chapter 19). Fibronectin is contained in platelet alpha granules and is also brought to the wound site by serum.[86–88] When applied topically, fibronectin accelerates wound healing in rats.[84,89]

To detect the presence of these adhesion molecules histologically in fetal and adult rabbit wounds, Longaker used antibodies to the adhesion glycoproteins, fibronectin and laminin.[90] He showed that fibronectin is deposited earlier in fetal than in adult rabbit skin wounds; laminin deposition showed no difference. Amniotic fluid, which contains fibronectin, coats fetal skin wounds continuously and may be an important mechanism for fibronectin deposition.[24] Using similar immunohistochemical techniques, Whitby has determined in both fetal mice and sheep that tenascin is deposited earlier in fetal than in adult wounds (see Chapter 10).[91] Tenascin, an ECM glycoprotein, has been implicated in epithelial-mesenchymal interactions during fetal development where its deposition precedes cell migration. Tenascin antagonizes the adhesion properties of fibronectin and permits cells to detach from the wound matrix and migrate.[91,92] Thus, the deposition of fibronectin and tenascin occurs quickly in the fetal wound matrix and these phenomena may underlie rapid re-epithelialization in fetal wounds.

DO FETAL WOUNDS CONTRACT?

Adult excisional wounds heal by secondary intention, which includes wound contraction (see Chapter 9). Krummel[10,58,93] confirmed Somasundarum's original observation[94] that fetal rabbit skin excisional wounds gape open and actually increase in size. Neither contraction nor healing by secondary intention was seen in open fetal rabbit wounds. Hayes[95] investigated whether open fetal rabbit wounds contain myofibroblasts, which some consider an important cellular element for wound contraction. There was no evidence for the presence of myofibroblasts by either myofibroblast-specific anti-muscle actin antibody or electron microscopy. We should note, however, that myofibroblasts may not be a necessary component of contraction.[96]

Explanations for the lack of fetal rabbit wound contraction include an absence of myofibroblasts, a defect in fetal fibroblast contractility, or the presence of an amniotic fluid inhibitor of wound contraction. Studies using the fibroblast-populated collagen lattice (FPCL) demonstrated that fetal rabbit dermal fibroblasts contracted either the fetal or adult collagen lattices to a greater degree than did adult fibroblasts.[58] Since contractile forces are demonstrated by FPCL, the failure of fetal rabbit wounds to close by secondary intention is not due to either a defect in the contractility of fetal fibroblasts or in the contractability of the fetal collagen matrix. The effect of amniotic fluid on lattice contraction was then determined. Interestingly, amniotic fluid inhibited lattice contraction using either fetal or adult fibroblasts in a dose-dependent fashion, suggesting that amniotic fluid may contain a wound contraction inhibitor. These in vitro findings may explain Somasundaram's[97] observation that fetal rabbit skin excisional wounds excluded from amniotic fluid by a silastic patch healed within eight days. Whether the silastic patch promoted re-epithelialization by excluding amniotic fluid or functioned as a wound template for regenerating epidermis remains unknown.[98]

In contrast to the rabbit findings, Burrington[11] studied excisional wounds in fetal lambs and showed rapid wound healing with evidence of wound contraction. More recently, myofibroblasts have been identified by both anti-muscle actin antibody and transmission electron microscopy in fetal lamb excisional wounds that have a wound matrix rich in HA.[99]

There is limited data on primate excisional wound healing. Sopher investigated excisional fetal wound healing in third trimester cynomologus monkeys,[13,14] and demonstrated that the wounds failed to epithelialize and contract. Because of the obvious limitations in determining whether human fetal wounds contract, the FPCL model has recently been used to evaluate the effect of amniotic fluid on human fetal and adult fibroblast contraction.[100] Both fetal and adult fibroblast contraction was inhibited by human amniotic fluid. Fractionation of human amniotic fluid may uncover an inhibitor of wound contraction. This work has potential clinical applicability in treating pathologic wound contraction.

GROWTH FACTORS AND FETAL WOUND HEALING

Explosive fetal growth combined with the prominent role of growth factors in both development[42,101] and adult wound repair[102,103] suggest that peptide growth factors may play an important regulatory role in fetal wound healing (see Chapters 6, 10, 12, 13, 15). In contrast to peptide hormones, peptide regulatory factors act either locally on adjacent cells (paracrine effect) or in the same cell that secreted them (autocrine effect). For example, transforming growth factor-beta (TGF-β) is produced by multiple wound cell types and its biologic activities are protean and variable depending on the target cell and the local environment. It can stimulate proliferation in some cells, especially in connective tissue, while being a potent inhibitor of proliferation in others, such as epithelial cells. A common theme is that TGF-B can stimulate the synthesis of ECM components such as fibronectin, proteoglycans, and collagen.[104] Local application of TGF-β accelerates wound healing and increases wound breaking strength in rats.[105]

Krummel[106] reported that the addition of TGF-B to PVA sponge implants placed into fetal rabbits on day 24 of gestation resulted in histologic evidence of acute inflammatory cells and fibrosis. Using an elegant flow cytometry technique, Durham[107] demonstrated that as rabbit fibroblasts differentiate during development from embryo to fetus and on to adult, there is a progressive reduction in the number of TGF-β cell surface receptors as well as an apparent decrease in TGF-β binding affinity. Fetal fibroblasts are thus capable of responding to exogenous TGF-β by fibroblast proliferation and collagen synthesis,[104] but the role of TGF-β in the local fetal wound environment remains unclear.

Delozier[108] studied the effect of a single local dose of epidermal growth factor (EGF) on excisional fetal rabbit wounds. EGF is a mitogen that stimulates epithelialization in adults.[109–111] Treated wounds re-epithelialized to a significantly greater extent when compared to control wounds, suggesting that re-epithelialization can be accelerated in fetal rabbit wounds by EGF. Similarly, Ditesheim[112] treated fetal rabbit excisional wounds with transforming growth factor-alpha (TGF-α), a growth factor that closely resembles EGF. The TGF-α was locally applied via either a single application or a slow release pellet. Wounds were either exposed to amniotic fluid or excluded from it by a silastic patch and harvested six days later. Both treated groups (single application and slow release pellet) showed mesenchymal cell infiltrates without re-epithelialization whether they were exposed to or excluded from amniotic fluid. Future studies may give clues to the role of growth factors in cellular proliferation, interaction, and differentiation during fetal wound healing.

IN VITRO ORGAN CULTURE STUDIES

One approach to simplify the complexity of in vivo healing is to examine the healing process in vitro (see Chapters 14, 17, 18, 20). Kistler[113] developed a model of fetal limb organ culture in fetal rats. Incisional wounds were made on the outer side of the lower fore-limb of rat fetuses at day 19 of gestation. The whole limb was then placed in culture. The principal observation of this study was that fetal skin, cultured as whole-limb organ culture, differentiated and showed healing without scarring similar to in vivo fetal rat skin healing.

Burd[114] developed an in vitro explant model using fetal lamb skin. In this model mid-gestation full-thickness fetal lamb skin was excised, placed into culture and wounded by a standard incision. He found that after four days in culture the epidermis had completely re-epithelialized, and by seven days, the dermal defect was smaller, but still present. This model preserves normal dermal-epidermal architecture in vitro, allows for the examination of epithelial-mesenchymal interactions, and can be used to analyze fetal sheep skin wound healing in a controlled fashion. Excisional and incisional wounds can be compared, and the effects of fetal serum, wound fluid, amniotic fluid, ECM components, and numerous growth factors can be studied systematically.

FUTURE RESEARCH

Adult wound healing entails a complex series of events involving many cell types and products that ultimately end in scar formation. In comparison, we are only beginning to understand fetal wound healing. Fetal wound healing studies may help surgeons understand what accounts for scarring and, perhaps more importantly, how scar formation can be modulated. During the prenatal stage of life, rules are established for cellular growth and differentiation of the postnatal organism. So, to understand why things go wrong in children and adults, we need to know how they are constructed in the first place.

The possibility of fetal surgery to correct craniofacial anomalies such as cleft lip is intriguing (see Chapter 5). The fetal surgeon could take advantage of the unique qualities of scarless fetal healing. Results of prenatal correction of cleft lip may offer insight into the questions regarding an intrinsic or extrinsic mechanism underlying the nasal and maxillary deformity in cleft lip.[46,115,116] However, open fetal surgery has only been performed for life-threatening defects, and at the current time fetal surgery for craniofacial anomalies hardly justifies the inherent risks of open fetal surgery to both mother and fetus.[15,45,46,117–119]

Much work remains before we can understand how the fetus heals in such a remarkable manner. A variety of methods and animal models exist that permit wound analysis at the histologic, biochemical, and molecular biological levels. In vitro techniques including cell and organ culture and collagen lattices may give valuable information on fetal cell-cell and cell-matrix interactions. Of particular interest will be insights on how the fetal wound matrix synthesizes and organizes wound collagen without scar formation. Modern techniques for analyzing the roles of amniotic fluid, angiogenesis, proto-oncogene expression, growth factors, macrophage regulation, ECM remodeling, and HA-collagen interactions may provide insight into the mechanisms of fetal tissue repair.

Unraveling the secrets of fetal wound healing may provide a blueprint for ideal tissue repair (see Chapter 21). Since scarring and fibrosis dominate some diseases in almost every medical specialty, the greatest potential of this work lies with modulation of postnatal scar formation.

REFERENCES

1. Harrison MR, Golbus MS, Filly RA (Eds): The Unborn Patient. WB Saunders, 1990.
2. Crombleholme TM, Harrison MR, Langer JC, et al.: Early experience with open fetal surgery for congenital hydronephrosis. J Pediatr Surg 23:1114, 1988.
3. Harrison MR, Adzick NS, Longaker MT et al.: Successful repair in utero of a fetal diaphragmatic hernia after removal of herniated viscera from the left thorax. NEJM 322:1582, 1990.
4. Langer JC, Harrison MR, Schmidt KG, et al.: Fetal hydrops and demise from sacrococcygeal teratoma: Rationale for fetal surgery. Amer J Obstet Gynecol 160:1145, 1989.
5. Harrison MR: Personal communication, January, 1990.
6. Rowlatt V: Intrauterine wound healing in a 20-week human fetus. Virchow's Arch 381:353, 1979.
7. Goss AN: Intrauterine healing of fetal rat oral mucosal, skin and cartilage wounds. J Oral Pathol 6:35, 1977.
8. Viljanto J, Thomasson B, Pikkarainen T, et al.: Foetal connective tissue regeneration. Acta Chir Scan 141:85, 1975.
9. Adzick NS, Harrison MR, Glick PL, et al.: Comparison of fetal, newborn and adult wound healing

by histologic, enzyme-histochemical, and hydroxyproline determination. J Pediatr Surg 20:315, 1985.
10. Krummel TM, Nelson JM, Diegelmann RF, et al.: Fetal response to injury in the rabbit. J Pediatr Surg 22:640, 1987.
11. Burrington JD: Wound healing in the fetal lamb. J Pediatr Surg 6:523, 1971.
12. Longaker MT, Whitby DJ, Adzick NS, et al.: Studies in fetal wound healing: VI. Second and early third trimester fetal wounds demonstrate rapid collagen deposition without scar formation. J Pediatr Surg 25:63, 1990.
13. Sopher D: A study of wound healing in the foetal tissues of the cynomologus monkey. Lab Animals Handbook 6:327, 1975.
14. Sopher D: Future prospects for fetal surgery, in Poswillo D (ed). Teratology: Trends and applications. Springer-Verlag, pp 165.
15. Hallock GG, Rice DC, McClure HM: In utero lip repair in the rhesus monkey: An update. Plas Reconstr Surg 80:855, 1987.
16. Hunt TK, Goodson WH: Wound healing. In: Way LW (ed). Current Surgical Diagnosis and Treatment (8th ed.). San Mateo, CA, Appleton and Lange, 1988, pp 86.
17. Cohen IK, Diegelmann RF: Wound healing in cosmetic surgery: An overview. In: Ross R (ed): Problems in Aesthetic surgery: Biological Causes and Clinical Solutions. St. Louis, MO, CV Mosby Co., 1986.
18. Leibovich SJ, Ross R: The role of the macrophage in wound repair. A study with hydrocortisone and antimacrophage serum. Am J Path 78: 71, 1975.
19. Knighton DR, Fiegel UD: The macrophage: Effector cell in wound repair. Prog Clin Biol Res 299:217, 1989.
20. Diegelmann RF, Cohen IK, Kaplan AM: The role of macrophages in wound repair: A review. Plast Reconstr Surg 68:107, 1981.
21. Rockwell WB, Cohen IK, Ehrlich HP: Keloids and hypertrophic scars: A comprehensive review. Plas Reconstr Surg 84:827, 1989.
22. Mulvihill SJ, Stone MM, Fonkalsrud EW: Trophic effects of amniotic fluid on fetal gastrointestinal development. J Surg Res 40:291, 1986.
23. Dahl L, Hopwood JJ, Laurent BG, et al.: The concentration of hyaluronate in amniotic fluid. Biochemical Medicine 30:280, 1983.
24. Harris MC, Mennuti MT, Kline JA, et al.: Amniotic fluid fibronectin concentrations with advancing gestational age. Ob Gyn 72:593, 1988.
25. Longaker MT, Adzick NS, et al.: Studies in fetal wound healing. VII: Fetal wound healing may be modulated by elevated hyaluronic acid stimulating activity in amniotic fluid. J Pediatr Surg 25:430, 1990.
26. Nelson NM.: Respiration and circulation before birth, in Smith CA, Nelson NM (eds): The Physiology of the Newborn Infant, 4th Ed. Thomas, Springfield, Illinois, 1976.
27. Hock RJ: The physiology of high altitude. Sci Amer 22:52, 1970.
28. Hunt TK, Zederfeldt B, Goldstick TK: Oxygen and healing. Amer J Surg 118:521, 1969.
29. Lane AT: Human fetal skin development. Pediatric Dermatology 3:487, 1986.
30. Adzick NS, Outwater KM, Harrison MR, et al.: Correction of congenital diaphragmatic hernia in utero IV. An early gestational fetal lamb model for pulmonary vascular morphometric analysis. J Pediatr Surg 20:673, 1985.
31. Harrison MR, Langer JC, Adzick NS, et al.: Correction of congenital diaphragmatic hernia in utero. V. Initial clinical experience. J Pediatr Surg 25:47, 1990.
32. Flake AW, Harrison MR, Adzick NS, Zanjani ED: Transplantation of fetal hematopoietic stem cells in utero: The creation of hematopoietic chimeras. Science 233:776, 1986.
33. Miller ME: Chemoattractant function in the human neonate: Humoral and cellular aspects. Pediatr Res 5:487, 1971.
34. Bracaglia R, Montemari G, Rotoli M, et al.: Variation in acute phlogistic reaction in the skin of rabbit fetuses. Ann Plast Surg 9:175, 1988.
35. Schwartz LW, Osburn BI: An ontogenic study of the acute inflammatory reaction in the fetal rhesus monkey. Lab Invest 31:441, 1974.
36. Thomas BL, Krummel TM, Nelson JM, et al.: Fetal wound healing can be switched to an adult type of response by the attraction of neutrophils to the site of injury. Presented at the 33rd Annual Meeting of the Plastic Surgery Research Council, San Francisco, California, 1988.
37. Borchelt BD, Krummel TM, Cawthorn JW, et al: Transposition of an early adult wound site does not result in recruitment of fibroblasts. Surgical Forum 40:555, 1989.

38. Simpson DM, Ross R: The neutrophilic leukocyte in wound repair. A study with antineutrophil serum. J Clin Invest 51:2009, 1972.
39. Banda MJ: Personal communication. December, 1990.
40. Rappolee DA, Mark D, Banda MJ, Werb Z: Wound macrophages express TGF-Alpha and other growth factors in vivo: Analysis by mRNA phenotyping. Science 241:708, 1988.
41. Banda MJ, Rice AG, Griffin GL, et al.: Alpha1-proteinase inhibitor is a neutrophil chemoattractant after proteolytic inactivation by macrophage elastase. J Biol Chem 263:4481, 1988.
42. Heine UI, Munoz EF, Flanders KC, et al.: Role of transforming growth factor-b in the development of the mouse embryo. J Cell Biol 105:2861, 1987.
43. Downs KM, Martin GR, Bishop JM: Contrasting patterns of myc and N-myc expression during gastrulation of the mouse embryo. Genes Develop 3:860, 1989.
44. Weiss P, Matoltsy AG: Wound healing in chick embryos in vivo and in vitro. Dev Biol 1:302, 1959.
45. Hallock GG: In utero cleft lip repair in A/J mice. Plast Reconstr Surg 75:785, 1985.
46. Sullivan WG: In utero cleft lip repair in the mouse without an incision. Plast Reconstr Surg 84:723, 1989.
47. Dixon JB: Inflammation in the foetal and neonatal rat: The local reactions to skin burns. J Path Bact 80:73, 1960.
48. Sopher D: The response of rat fetal membranes to injury. Ann Royal Coll Surg (England) 51:240, 1972.
49. Rowsell AR: The intra-uterine healing of foetal muscle wounds: experimental study in the rat. Br J Plast Surg 37:635, 1984.
50. Robinson BW, Goss AN: Intrauterine healing of fetal rat cheek wounds. Cleft Palate J 18:251, 1981.
51. Hess A: Reactions of mammalian fetal tissues to injury. II. Skin. Anatomic Res 119:435, 1958.
52. Block M: Wound healing in the newborn opossum. Nature 187:340, 1960.
53. Schilling JA, Joel W, Shurley HM: Wound healing: A comparative study of the histochemical changes in granulation tissue contained in stainless steel wire mesh and polyvinyl sponge cylinders. Surgery 48:702, 1959.
54. Diegelmann RF, Lindblad WJ, Cohen IK: A subcutaneous implant for wound healing studies in humans. J Surg Res 40:229, 1986.
55. Viljanto J: Cellstic: A device for wound healing studies in man: Description of the method. J Surg Res 20:115, 1976.
56. Goodson WH III, Hunt TK: Development of a new miniature method for the study of wound healing in human subjects. J Surg Res 33:394, 1982.
57. Hunt TK, Twomey P, Zederfelt B, et al.: Respiratory gas tensions and pH in healing wounds. Am J Surg 114:302, 1967.
58. Krummel TM, Ehrlich HP, Nelson JM, et al.: Fetal wounds do not contract in utero. Surgical Forum 40:613, 615, 1989.
59. Harrison MR, Jester JA, Ross NA: Correction of congenital diaphragmatic hernia in utero. I. The model: Intrathoracic balloon produces fatal pulmonary hypoplasia. Surgery 88:174, 1980.
60. DePalma RL, Krummel TM, Nelson JM, et al.: Fetal wound matrix is composed of proteoglycan rather than collagen. Surg Forum 38:626, 1987.
61. DePalma RL, Krummel TM, Durham LA III, et al.: Characterization and quantitation of wound matrix in the fetal rabbit. Matrix 9:224, 1989.
62. Kujawa MJ, Tepperman K: Culturing chick muscle cells on glycosaminoglycan substrates: attachment and differentiation. Dev Biology 99:277, 1983.
63. Kujawa MJ, Pechak DG, Fiszman MY, et al.: Hyaluronic acid bonded to cell culture surfaces inhibits the program of myogenesis. Dev Biology 113:10, 1986.
64. Longaker MT, Crombleholme TM, Langer JC, Verrier ED, Harrison MR, Stern R: Studies in fetal wound healing: I. A fetal factor modulates extracellular matrix synthesis. J Pediatr Surg 24:789, 1989.
65. Longaker MT, Chiu ES, Harrison MR, et al.: Studies in fetal wound healing: IV. Hyaluronic acid stimulating activity of fetal versus adult wound fluid. Annals of Surgery 210:667, 1989.
66. Decker M, Chui ES, Dollbaum C, et al.: Hyaluronic acid stimulating factor in serum from the bovine fetus and from breast cancer patients. Cancer Research 49:3499, 1989.
67. Williams SI, Longaker MT, Harrison MR, Stern R: Hyaluronic acid stimulating factor: Fetal urine is the source for this trophic factor in amniotic fluid. J Cell Biol 107:593a, 1988.
68. Dunphy JE, Upuda KN: Chemical and histochemical sequences in the normal healing of wounds. N Engl J Med 253:847, 1953.

69. Alexander SA, Donoff RB: The glycosaminoglycans of open fetal wounds. J Surg Res 29:422, 1980.
70. Bertolami CN, Donoff RB: Hyaluronidase activity during open wound healing in rabbits: A preliminary report. J Surg Res 25:256, 1978.
71. Weigel PH, Fuller GM, LeBoeuf RD: A model for the role of hyaluronic acid and fibrin in the early events during the inflammatory response and wound healing. J Theor Biol 119:219, 1986.
72. Hallock GG, Merkel JR, DiPaolo BR: Analysis of collagen content in the fetal wound. Ann Plast Surg 21:310, 1988.
73. Merkel JR, Dipaolo BR, Hallock GG, Rice DC: Type I and type III collagen content of healing wounds in fetal and adult rats. Proc Soc Exp Biol Med 187:493, 1988.
74. Siebert JW, Burd DAR, McCarthy JG, et al.: Fetal wound healing: A biochemical study of scarless healing. Plast Reconstr Surg 85:495, 1990.
75. Burd DAR, Longaker MT, Adzick NS, Harrison MR, Ehrlich HP: Fetal wound healing in a large animal model: The deposition of collagen is confirmed. Br J Plast Surg 43:571, 1990.
76. Thomas BL, Krummel TM, Melang M, et al.: Collagen synthesis and type expression by fetal fibroblasts in vitro. Surgical Forum 39:642, 1988.
77. Duncan BW, Adzick NS, Longaker MT, Bhatnagar R: The ontogeny of fetal prolyl hydroxylase activity. Presented at The Tenth Annual Pediatric Surgery Resident's National Meeting. Buffalo, NY, October 1989.
78. Hussain Z, Hunt TK: Inhibition of prolyl hydroxylase by poly (ADP-ribose) and phosphoribose-AMP. J Biol Chem 264:7850, 1989.
79. Vogel KG, Trotter JA: The effect of proteoglycans on the morphology of collagen fibrils formed in vitro. Collagen Rel Res 7:105, 1987.
80. Scott JE, Hughes EW: Proteoglycan-rich relationships in developing chick and bovine tendons: Influence of the physiologic environment. Conn Tis Res 14:267, 1986.
81. Hellstrom S, Laurent C: Hyaluronan and healing of tympanic membrane perforations. An experimental study. Acta Otolaryngology Suppl 442:54, 1987.
82. Hynes RO: Integrins: A family of cell surface receptors. Cell 48:549, 1987.
83. Tonnesen MG, Jenkins D, Siegel SL, et al.: Expression of fibronectin, laminin, and factor VII-related antigen during development of the human cutaneous microvasculature. J Invest Dermatol 85:564, 1985.
84. Grinnell F, Billingham RE, Burgess L: Distribution of fibronectin during wound healing in vivo. J Invest Derm 76:181, 1981.
85. Clark RA: Potential roles of fibronectin in cutaneous wound repair. Arch Dermatol 124:201, 1988.
86. Ginsberg M, Plow EF: Fibronectin expression on the platelet surface occurs in concert with secretion. J Supramol Struct 17:91, 1981.
87. Ginsberg MH, Painter RG, Birdwell C, et al.: The detection, immunofluorescent localization, and thrombin induced release of human platelet-associated fibronectin antigen. J Supramol Struct 11:167, 1979.
88. Zucker MB, Moesson MW, Broekman MJ, et al.: Release of platelet fibro-nectin (cold-insoluble globulin) from alpha granules induced by thrombin or collagen: Lack of requirement for fibronectin in ADP-induced platelet aggregation. Blood 54:8, 1979.
89. Cheng CY, Martin DE, Legget CG, et al.: Fibronectin enhances healing of excised wounds in rats. Arch Dermatol 124:221, 1988.
90. Longaker MT, Whitby DJ, Crombleholme TM, et al.: Studies in fetal wound healing: III. Early deposition of adhesion molecules distinguishes fetal from adult wounds. J Pediatr Surg 24:799, 1989.
91. Whitby DJ, Longaker MT, Adzick NS, et al.: Early deposition of tenascin characterizes fetal wound healing. Presented at 34th Annual Meeting of The Plastic Surgery Research Council. Atlanta GA, 1988.
92. Mackie B, Tucker RP, Halfter W, Chiquet-Ehrensmann, Epperlein: The distribution of tenascin coincides with pathways of neural crest migration. Development 102:237, 1988.
93. Krummel TM, Ehrlich HP, Nelsen JM, et al.: Fetal wounds do not contract in utero (Manuscript submitted).
94. Somasundaram M, Prathap K: Intrauterine healing of the skin wounds in rabbit foetuses. J Pathol 100:81, 1970.
95. Hayes JH, Krummel TM, Schatzki PF, et al.: Open wound histology in the fetal rabbit. Surg Forum 40:558, 1989.
96. Ehrlich HP: The role of the connective tissue matrix in wound healing. In: Growth factors and other aspects of wound healing: Biological and clinical implications. New York, AR Liss, Inc., 1988, pp 243–258.

97. Somasundaram M, Prathap K: The effects of exclusion of amniotic fluid on intra-uterine healing of skin wounds in rabbit foetuses. J Pathol 107:127, 1972.
98. Ditesheim JA, Delozier JB, Rees RS, et al.: Covered fetal excisional wounds heal by tissue regeneration. Surgical Forum 40:615, 1989.
99. Longaker MT, Burd DAR, Yen TSB, et al.: Mid-gestation fetal wounds contract in utero. Presented at The 35th Annual Meeting of The Plastic Surgery Research Council. Washington, DC, April 1990.
100. Chang B, Longaker MT, Tuchler RE, et al.: Do human fetal wounds contract? Presented at The 35th Annual Meeting of The Plastic Surgery Research Council. Washington, DC, April 1990.
101. Rappolee DA, Brfenner CA, Schultz R, et al.: Developmental expression of PDGF, TGF-a, and TGF-B genes in preimplantation mouse embryos. Science 241:1823, 1988.
102. Pessa ME, Bland KI, Copeland EM: Growth factors and the determinants of wound repair. J Surg Res 42:207, 1987.
103. Barbul A, Pines E, Caldwell M, Hunt TK (Eds): Progress in Clinical and Biologic Research. Growth factors and other aspects of wound healing. AR Liss, New York, 266:243–258, 1988.
104. Roberts AB, Sporn MB, Assoian RK, et al.: Rapid induction of fibrosis and angiogenesis in vivo and stimulation of collagen formation. PNAS 83:4167, 1986.
105. Mustoe TA, Pierce GF, Thomason A, et al.: Accelerated healing of incisional wounds in rats induced by transforming growth factor-B. Science 237:1333, 1987.
106. Krummel TM, Nelson JM, Diegelmann RF, et al.: Fetal response to injury and its modulation with transforming growth factor-beta. Surg Forum 38:622, 1987.
107. Durham LA, Krummel TM, Cawthorn JW, Thomas BL, Diegelmann RF: Analysis of TGF-beta receptor binding in embryonic, fetal, and adult rabbit fibroblasts. J Pediatric Surg 24:784, 1989.
108. Delozier J, Nanney LB, Hago K, Rees RS: Epidermal growth factor enhances fetal reepithelialization. Surgical Forum 623, 1987.
109. Niall M, Ryan GB, O'Brian BJ: The effects of epidermal growth factor on wound healing in mice. J Surg Res 33:164–169, 1988.
110. Brown GL, Curtsinger JR, Brightwell DM, et al.: Enhancement of epidermal regeneration by biosynthetic epidermal growth factor. J Exp Med 163:1319, 1986.
111. Schultz GS, White M, Mitchell G, et al.: Epidermal wound healing enhanced by transforming growth factor alpha and vacciniagrowth factor. Science 235:350, 1987.
112. Ditesheim JA, Delozier JB, Rees RS, et al.: Fetal excisional wounds can respond to intrauterine injury. Presented at The American Society of Plastic and Reconstructive Surgery, San Francisco, CA, October 1989.
113. Kistler A, Utsugi R, Ihara S: Wound healing in fetal limb organ culture. Ann Plast Surg 21:303, 1988.
114. Burd DAR, Longaker MT, Adzick NS, Harrison MR, Ehrlich HP: Fetal wound healing: An in vitro explant model. J Pediatr Surg 25:898, 1990.
115. Stark RB, Kaplan JM: Development of the cleft lip nose. Plast Reconstr Surg 51:413, 1973.
116. Sadove R, Ladaga L, Magee WP: Cartilaginous histology of the cleft lip nose: proving the extrinsic etiology. Plast Reconstr Surg 18:655, 1988.
117. Duncan BW, Adzick NS, Bradley SM, et al.: An in utero model of craniosynotosis. Surg Forum 40:608, 1989.
118. Christ JE: Fetal surgery: A frontier for plastic surgery. Plast Reconstr Surg 77:645, 1986.
119. Dado DV, Kernahan DA, Gianopoulos JG: Intrauterine repair of cleft lip: What's involved. Plast Reconstr Surg 85:461, 1990.
120. Longaker MT, Whitby DJ, Jennings RW, et al.: Fetal diaphragmatic wounds heal with scar formation. J Surg Res 50:375, 1991.
121. Longaker MT, Whitby DJ, Jennings RW, et al.: Adult skin in the fetal environment heals with scar formation. Surg Forum 41:639, 1990.
122. Silverstein AM, Prendergast RA, Kraner KL: Fetal response to antigenic stimulus: IV. Rejection of skin homografts by the fetal lamb. J Exp Med 119:955, 1964.

CHAPTER **4**

Fetal Animal and Wound Implant Models

N. Scott Adzick

Our clinical experience with open fetal surgery has demonstrated that fetal skin wound healing occurs rapidly and without the scar formation seen in adult tissue repair.[1–5] Experimental work, although limited, supports these clinical observations. Studies in the chick embryo,[6] guinea pig,[7] mouse,[8,9] rat,[10–12] opossum,[13] rabbit,[14–16] sheep,[17,18] and monkey,[19–21] all demonstrate distinct differences between the fetal and adult tissue response to injury.

Numerous techniques have been used to study fetal tissue repair. The least artificial method is wound histology using light and electron microscopy or immunohistochemistry. While supplying much descriptive information, these methods do not provide quantitative biochemical data representative of the various stages of wound repair. Several wound implants have been used to analyze the various parameters of fetal wound healing. These include the polyvinyl alcohol (PVA) sponge,[22] PVA sponge within a perforated silicone tube implant,[16,23] Cellstic,[14,24] polytetrafluoroethylene tube,[15,25] and the Hunt-Schilling wire mesh wound cylinder.[26,27]

There have been differences in the nature, size, location, assessment, and findings in various fetal wound models. For example, excisional skin wounds contract and heal in fetal lambs, whereas this does not happen in fetal rabbits.[17,28] There are also advantages and disadvantages to each animal model. Whereas small animal models are relatively inexpensive, their short gestation limits analysis to late in the third trimester, and their small size precludes significant surgical manipulation. Large, long gestation animals such as sheep permit fetal wound healing analysis throughout gestation, easy fetal surgical manipulation, and resistance to abortion after fetal surgery. This chapter summarizes experimental fetal wound healing observations by species.

CHICK EMBRYO

Chick embryo wound healing studies can be performed both in vivo or in organ culture, but this model has the drawback of not being mammalian. Weiss and Matoltsy[6] studied dermal and corneal wounds in White Leghorn chick embryos both in vivo and in vitro between the fourth and seventeenth day of incubation (hatching occurs at day 21). In vivo studies demonstrated that wound closure in both skin and cornea is absent during the first half of the embryonic period, the critical date being the tenth day of incubation. The inability of early skin to heal appeared to be secondary to a failure of cell migration, since cells proliferated and piled up at the wound edge but did not spread to cover the denuded wound defect. Wounds made after the tenth day of incubation healed completely within four days. In contrast, in vitro skin and cornea explants at all days of incubation exhibited prompt epithelial migration and wound closure within three days. The authors speculated that by the tenth day of incubation in the whole chick embryo, wound epithelium acquired the ability to migrate, and that this migratory capability was supported by the adult chicken plasma on which the in vitro explants were grown.

More recently, Martin and Lewis have studied the mechanics of wound closure in a chick embryo limb-bud wound model.[29] For excisional lesions on the dorsum of a chick limb bud, the wound closure process began without any noticeable lag and the wound edges closed in at 10–20 um/hr, eventually overrunning slightly to produce a small transient pile-up of epidermal cells at the site of closure. By contrast with conventional descriptions of adult wound healing, there was no sign of any lamellipodial migratory activity by epidermal cells at the wound margin. Instead, scanning electron microscopy studies identified a thick and taut cable of actin around the perimeter of the wound. This actin cable apparently elicits a purse-string effect to facilitate epithelial movement and wound contraction (see Chapter 18).

GUINEA PIG

The first animal model for fetal surgery was developed in the guinea pig over 70 years ago.[30] In 1958, Hess studied fetal guinea pig wound healing between 37 and 47 days gestation (term = 67 days), and noted that healing occurred more rapidly than in postnatal animals.[7] He also demonstrated a lack of hair follicle regeneration in open fetal wounds. The fetal guinea pig has not been a very popular model because of the difficulty in obtaining reliably time-dated pregnancies.

MOUSE

Reports that fetal wounds heal without scarring have stimulated interest in the possibility of fetal surgery for congenital defects such as cleft lip and palate. Hallock[8] and Sullivan[9] performed in utero repair of cleft lip defects in A/J mice on day 17 (term = 19 days). The defects were induced by maternal diphenylhydantoin administration. Interestingly, Sullivan simply closed the drug-induced cleft without "freshening up" the edges. Both studies demonstrated that fetal cleft lip repair is technically feasible, that the pregnancy is not disrupted by this intervention, and that histologically there is absence of scar formation in the healed wound.

More recently, Whitby and Ferguson conducted a detailed immunohistochemical study of the extracellular matrix produced in fetal mouse wounds (see Chapter 10).[31] Upper lip wounds were made in fetal mice at days 14, 16, and 18 of gestation, and in neonates and adults. The wound tissue was harvested at multiple time points from one hour to 12 days postoperatively. Cryosections were analyzed using indirect immunostaining for specific collagen types, cell adhesion molecules, glycosaminoglycans and endogenous immunoglobulins. Immunostaining was also carried out for the following growth factors: transforming growth factor-alpha (TGF-α), transforming growth factor-beta type 1 (TGF-β_1), epidermal growth factor (EGF), platelet-derived growth factor (PDGF), and fibroblast growth factor (FGF).

The authors documented rapid scarless deposition of collagen in a regenerative fashion in fetal wounds, whereas adult wounds showed typical scar formation. Epithelialization was markedly faster in the fetus than in the adult, which may be related to the early appearance of tenascin in the fetal wound; other studies have shown that tenascin can initiate cell migration in wounds.[32] Chondroitin sulfate deposition was seen only in fetal wounds, and there was no immunoglobulin deposition in fetal wounds.

Finally, PDGF was present in fetal and adult wounds but TGF-β_1, and FGF were only detectable in adult wounds. Multiple studies have demonstrated that TGF-β stimulates collagen production during wound healing,[33,34] and addition of platelet-derived TGF-β to fetal rabbit wounds induces fibrosis[35]—thus regeneration of a normal collagen pattern may relate to the absence of TGF-β_1 in the fetal wound. FGF has potent angiogenic properties and neovascularization is a prominent feature of the healing adult wound but was not seen in the fetal wound.

RAT

Wound healing in the fetal rat has been studied by several investigators. In 1960, Dixon described the healing of burn wounds inflicted by a heated needle.[11] She found a lack of an acute inflammatory response (no polymorphonuclear leukocytes) and an absence of new capillary buds in fetal wounds. Epithelial regeneration was inversely proportional to the gestational age at time of wounding, and the cellular component of the wound matrix was characterized by local mononuclear mesenchymal cells. Finally, a spectrum of fetal rat wound healing occurred as a function of gestational age; healing switched to an adult-type healing pattern late in gestation.

Goss made orofacial wounds in fetal Sprague-Dawley rats at day 19 of gestation.[10] He demonstrated rapid and complete epithelialization of oral and skin wounds, and a complete lack of an acute inflammatory response or scab formation. Nasal cartilage wounds showed rapid reformation of perichondrium without callus formation. Further studies of the intra-uterine healing of fetal rat cheek wounds by Robinson and Goss confirmed the absence of scarring and polymorphonuclear leukocytes in fetal wounds.[36] Rowsell made upper lip wounds in Wistar rats on day 18 and examined them one to three days later.[37] The wounded muscle healed by regeneration, no inflammatory response was seen, and no collagen was detected using the van Gieson staining technique. To provide quantitative analysis of fetal wound collagen, Merkel and Hallock[38,39] pooled tissue extracts from excisional fetal rat wounds and showed similar ratios of collagen types III and I to that found in normal unwounded fetal skin. Both fetal and adult granulation tissues have elevated type III collagen content, but normal fetal tissue had a much higher content of type III than does normal adult tissue.

OPOSSUM

At birth, the opossum is physiologically and anatomically a fetus, and remains attached to the mother's nipple for four to five weeks before weaning. Thus the "fetal" development of the marsupial continues in the nonsterile environment of the pouch/nipple and in the absence of an amniotic fluid milieu. A comparison of wound healing in adult and pouch marsupials may therefore reveal interesting insights into the differences between adult and fetal-type wound healing.

In 1960, Block studied sterile needle burn wounds and nonsterile linear wounds in the newborn opossum.[13] Before six days of life, there was almost a complete absence of inflammatory reaction, whereas after six days an intense mononuclear inflammatory response was elicited. Recently, Howarth and Ferguson examined newborn opossum wound healing using histological and immunohistochemical techniques.[40] Their thorough and original description of dermal wound healing in pouch young and adult marsupials is presented in Chapter 6. In brief, wound repair in the neonate occurred more rapidly than in the adult, the inflammatory response was less extensive, no angiogenesis was documented, wound contraction was seen, and there was no scar formation. Neonatal collagen studies documented very rapid deposition of collagen fibrils that were uniformly oriented parallel to the wound surface. The pattern of wound healing in neonatal marsupials suggests that the absence of inflammation and scar formation in fetal wounds is not due solely to the lack of infection or the fluid uterine environment. The contraction of neonatal opossum wounds suggests that contact with amniotic fluid may play a role in the absence of wound contraction in some other fetal wound healing models.

RABBITS

The rabbit has been the most widely used animal model for fetal wound healing studies.[41] As with all small animal models, the major limitation of the fetal rabbit model is the relatively short gestation (31 days). This confines studies to the third trimester since surgery prior to 23 days gestation is fraught with difficulties including size limitations and high fetal wastage.

Thomasson used a viscose cellulose sponge implant and enzyme histochemical techniques to study granulation tissue ingrowth into fetal and adult rabbit wounds.[42] He found much more rapid granulation tissue ingrowth in the fetal wounds and noted a mesenchymal cellular reaction in the fetus in contrast to the adult leukocytic response. The most striking histochemical difference was the constantly more intense alkaline phosphatase activity in the fetus. Adzick used a miniaturized wound cylinder of expanded polytetrafluoroethylene to compare fetal, newborn, and adult rabbit wound healing (Figure 4.1).[15] Histology and enzyme histochemical techniques documented the most rapid tissue ingrowth into the fetal implants with abundant macrophages but no polymorphonuclear leukocytes (Figure 4.2). The absence of an acute inflammatory response in fetal wounds was attributed to documented fetal neutropenia. Perhaps the characteristic inflammatory mediators of adult wound healing are absent in fetal wounds.

The role of collagen in the fetal wound matrix is controversial. Adzick[15] and Siebert[43] used a Gore-Tex implant and Viljanto[14] used a viscose cellulose sponge implant; all showed evidence of collagen in fetal wounds by a variety of techniques. In contrast, Krummel[16] implanted a PVA sponge within a perforated silastic cylinder into fetal rabbits and could not detect collagen using a sensitive high-pressure liquid chromatography assay. These conflicting results most likely reflect different wound sampling techniques.

Krummel[16] and DePalma[44] demonstrated that the fetal rabbit wound matrix is rich in the glycosaminoglycan, hyaluronic acid (HA). HA is a key structural and functional component of the extracellular matrix whenever there is rapid tissue

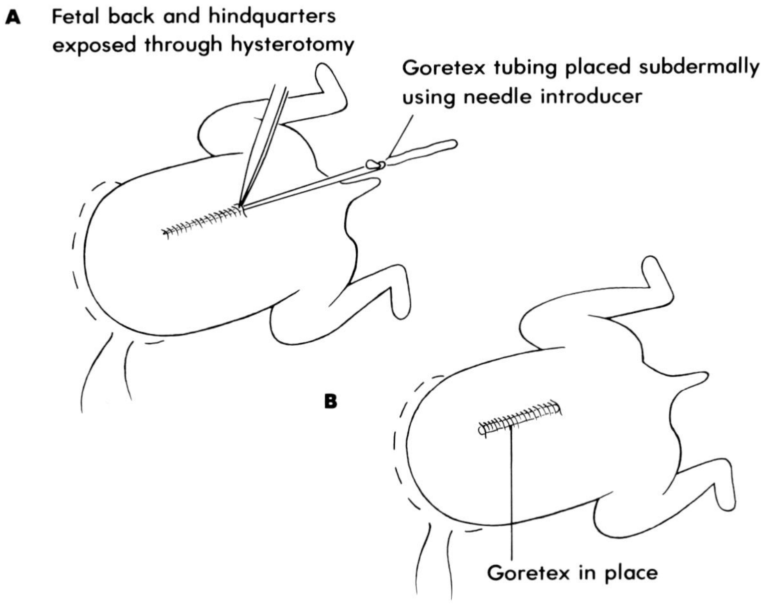

Figure 4.1 Technique of Gore-Tex insertion in the fetal rabbit. *Reprinted with permission.*[15]

proliferation, regeneration, and repair. HA fosters a permissive environment that promotes cell proliferation and dedifferentiation.[45,46] It is now clear that HA is laid down early in the matrix of both fetal and adult wounds but that sustained deposition of HA is unique to fetal wound healing.[61] The prolonged presence of HA in fetal wounds may provide a unique environment that promotes a highly organized wound matrix.

In addition to hyaluronic acid and collagen, other extracellular matrix com-

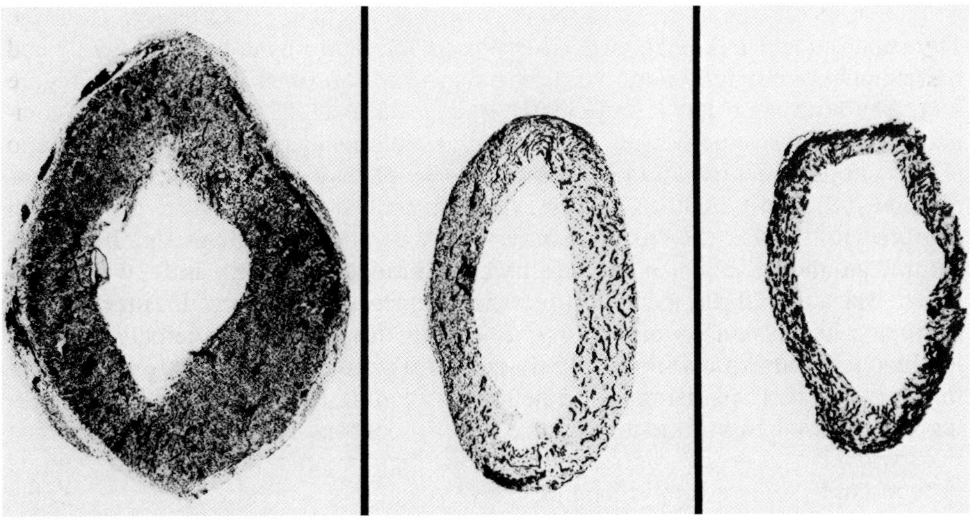

Figure 4.2 Comparison of cellular infiltration into the Gore-Tex tubing at 7 days in each group. The fetal group (far left) had far greater amounts of granulation tissue ingrowth than the newborn (middle) and adult (far right) groups. *Reprinted with permission.*[15]

ponents may be important in fetal wound healing, particularly the adhesion glycoproteins such as fibronectin and laminin. Fibronectin deposition is enhanced during embryogenesis and morphogenesis, providing a favorable microenvironment for cell migration and proliferation.[47] Longaker[48] used immunohistochemical techniques to detect the presence of fibronectin and laminin in fetal and adult rabbit wounds. Whereas there was no difference in the tempo of laminin deposition between fetal and adult wounds, fibronectin deposition occurred very quickly in the fetal wound matrix and this phenomenon may underlie rapid re-epithelialization in fetal wounds. Further support for this concept comes from the work of Cheng that demonstrated that when fibronectin is applied topically, it accelerated wound healing in rats.[49]

Adult excisional wounds heal by secondary intention, which includes wound contraction. Somasundarum and Prathrap reported that neither contraction nor healing by secondary intention occurred in open fetal rabbit wounds.[50] In contrast, open wounds that were excluded from amniotic fluid with a silastic patch healed within eight days.[51] These findings have been confirmed by Krummel and colleagues, who have also demonstrated that fetal rabbit amniotic fluid inhibits contraction of fibroblast-populated collagen lattices in vitro.[28] These studies raise the intriguing possibility that amniotic fluid may contain factors that inhibit wound contraction.

Rapid fetal growth combined with the prominent role of growth factors in both development[52] and adult wound repair[53,54] suggest that peptide growth factors may play an important regulatory role in fetal wound healing. Krummel[35] reported that the addition of TGF-β to PVA sponge implants placed into fetal rabbits on day 24 of gestation resulted in histologic evidence of acute inflammation and fibrosis. Delozier[55] studied the effect of a single dose of epidermal growth factor (EGF) on excisional fetal rabbit wounds. Treated wounds re-epithelialized to a significantly greater extent when compared to control wounds, suggesting that re-epithelialization can be accelerated in fetal rabbit wounds by EGF.

SHEEP

The sheep model has been extensively used for fetal physiology studies,[56] and the techniques for fetal lamb surgery have been described previously[57] (Figure 4.3). The fetal lamb has a sufficiently long gestation (145 days) to permit comparison of fetal wound healing at different gestational ages, is of adequate size to permit surgical manipulation with minimal risk of fetal loss or abortion, and can provide sufficient wound tissue for extensive analysis.

Burrington[17] was the first to study fetal wound healing in sheep. Incisional sutured wounds, excisional wounds, and full-thickness skin autografts were made on 60, 90, and 120 day gestation fetal lambs. He described an absence of scar formation in incisional wounds. Polymorphonuclear leukocytes appeared in the fetal wound matrix only in the 120 day gestation animals, and he speculated that this merely reflected rising blood neutrophil counts late in gestation. Fetal autografts showed engraftment within 3 days. In contrast to fetal rabbit excisional open wounds that do not contract or heal, Burrington noted that excisional wounds in fetal lambs showed rapid healing with evidence of wound contraction. Some investigators have suggested that myofibroblasts are an important cellular element of wound contraction.[58] This hypothesis is supported by the finding that myofibroblasts have been identified by both anti-muscle actin antibody and transmission

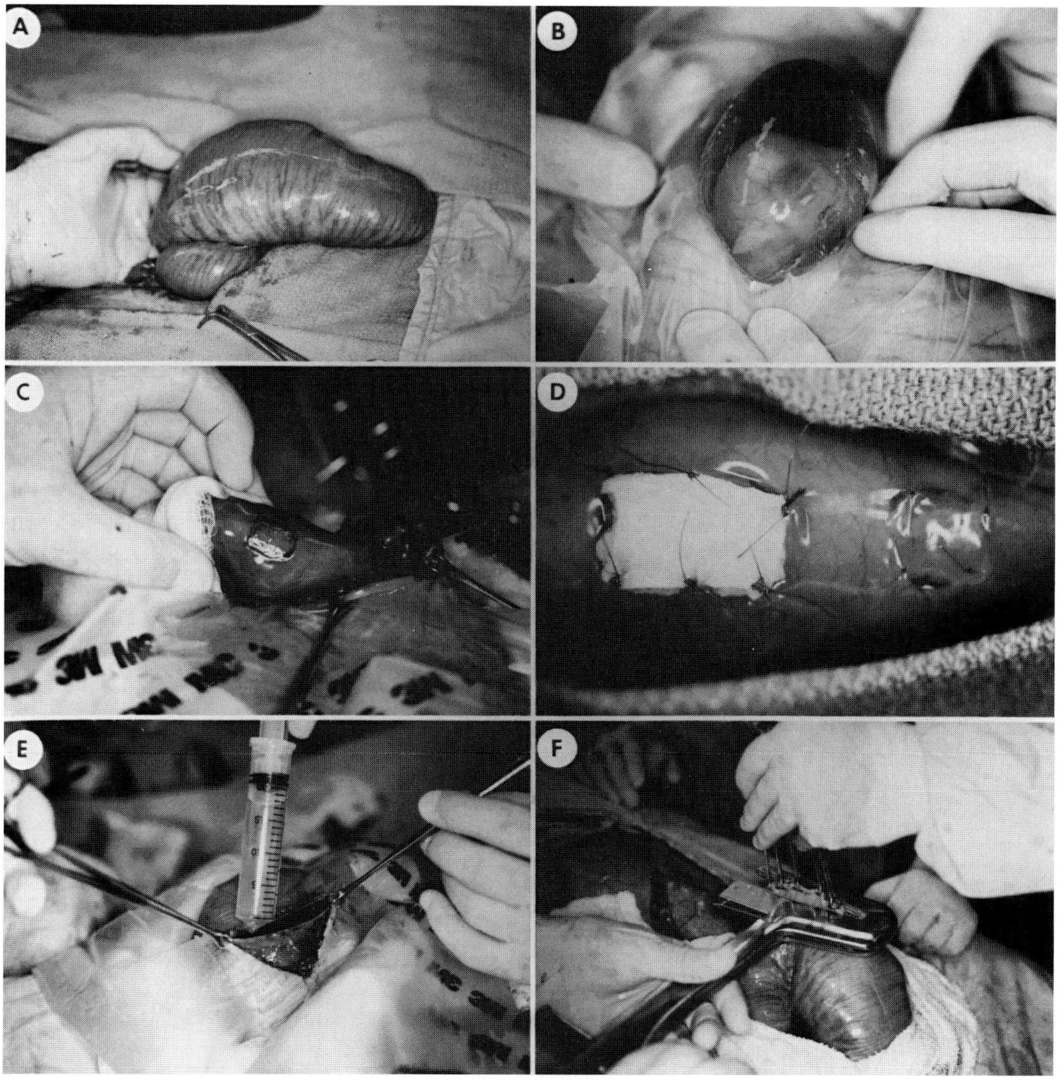

Figure 4.3 Photographic description of surgery. A. Bicornuate sheep uterus delivered into the surgical field via a maternal laparotomy. B. Following incision of uterine muscular layers, the tiny fetal lamb head is seen within the amniotic bubble. C. Hindquarters of 60-day gestation fetal lamb exposed and skin excised creating a recipient graft bed. D. Maternal (left) and auto-transplanted fetal (right) skin grafts sutured onto the fetal back. Note the differences in the adult and fetal skin phenotypes. E. Amniotic fluid was kept warm and returned to the uterus upon completion of the fetal procedure. F. The uterus is shown being closed using a TA-90 stapler which seals the amniotic membranes to the myometrium.

electron microscopy in fetal lamb excisional wounds,[59] whereas these cells are absent in fetal rabbit open wounds.[60]

A prolonged presence of hyaluronic acid (HA) in fetal wounds may provide the matrix signal orchestrating healing by regeneration rather than by scarring. Analysis of wound fluid from Hunt-Schilling wire mesh wound chambers implanted in mid-gestation fetal lambs for one to 21 days revealed that adult wound fluid had a rapid rise in HA, which peaked at three days, and fell to zero by seven

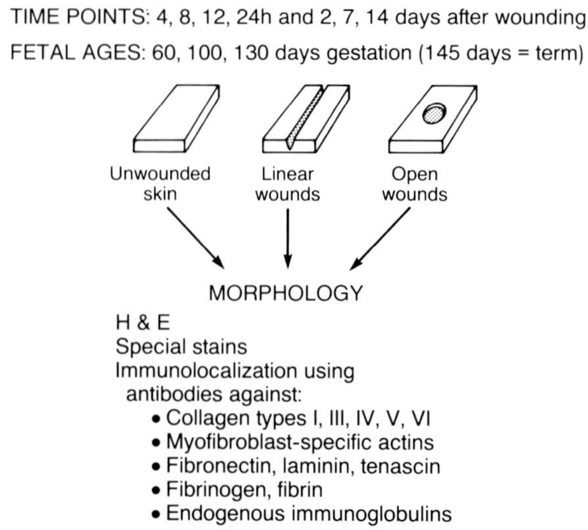

Figure 4.4 Histologic and immunohistochemical studies in the fetal lamb model.

days. In contrast, levels of HA in fetal wound fluid rose rapidly and remained significantly elevated for three weeks.[61] Longaker helped delineate the mechanisms for HA deposition in fetal wounds by studying the ability of fetal sera, wound fluid, and amniotic fluid to stimulate HA synthesis using a newly developed in vitro assay.[62] Fetal lamb serum contains an elevated HA-stimulating activity (HASA) that peaks in mid-gestation, whereas there is little HASA in postnatal sera.[63] Analysis of fetal and adult wound fluid demonstrated that HASA levels were markedly elevated in fetal wound fluid, whereas there was no HASA in adult wound fluid.[27] Finally, one of the crucial differences between the external environment of fetal and adult wounds is the amniotic fluid that continually bathes fetal skin wounds. It is now clear that fetal skin wounds are bathed in amniotic fluid that contains both HASA and HA.[64,65] All of these phenomena may contribute to the rich deposition of HA in the extracellular matrix of fetal wounds.

Wound healing studies using the versatile fetal lamb model have helped elucidate the role of fetal wound collagen and other extracellular matrix components (Figure 4.4). An immunohistochemistry study using antibodies to collagen types I, III, IV, and VI showed collagen was rapidly deposited in the wounds of 75, 100, and 120 day gestation fetal lambs.[18] The collagen staining pattern of incisional wounds in the 75 and 100 day fetal lambs was exactly the same as unwounded fetal skin by two weeks following wounding, whereas there was a switch to an adult-like healing late in gestation with a dense dermal collagen scar present in the wounded 120 day fetuses. Burd documented collagen deposition in PVA sponge implants placed in 75 and 100 day gestation lambs using histologic, biochemical, and wound breaking strength methods.[22] Since the deposition of collagen without scarring in the fetal lamb model has been firmly established using a variety of techniques, the absence of scarring must be due to the *organization* of collagen within the fetal wound matrix.

MONKEY

The nonhuman primate is an extremely rigorous model for fetal intervention. Like the human, the gravid monkey uterus is very susceptible to preterm labor with late gestation fetal loss. Prior to attempting open fetal surgery in human fetuses, we first developed a successful technique for anesthetic, surgical, and tocolytic management of monkeys undergoing fetal surgery.[66] Uterine electromyographic activity was then analyzed to determine the effect of hysterotomy, fetal surgery, and tocolytic agents on the induction of preterm labor in monkeys.[67] We subsequently devised models for congenital hydronephrosis and congenital hydrocephalus and studied the efficacy of in utero decompression.[68,69] Finally, from our series of 102 fetal surgical procedures on time-dated pregnant, we examined the maternal complications, the potential for future pregnancy, and the effects of uterine staples used for hysterotomy and uterine closure.[70] For wound healing studies, the fetal monkey model has the drawbacks of high expense and the need for postoperative monitoring and tocolysis to prevent preterm labor.

Wound healing in the fetal cynomolous monkey has been studied by Sopher.[19,20] Both incisional and excisional wounds were created five to seven weeks prior to term and were studied one day to four weeks later. Open wounds failed to heal or to contract. While sutured fetal wounds did not show evidence of acute inflammation, it is intriguing that open wounds did show leukocytic infiltration within 24 hours of birth. This suggests that the lack of bacterial contamination in the sterile uterine environment may partially account for the lack of PMN infiltration in utero. Hallock studied in utero cleft lip repair in the rhesus monkey.[21] The only evidence of lip repair at subsequent examination was a slight depression at the surgical site. Histologic study revealed that complete re-epithelialization had occurred across the oral mucosal and skin wounds, but there was no evidence of regeneration of ectodermal elements at the site of repair. Preliminary studies from our laboratory indicate that midgestational fetal rhesus monkey excisional wounds contract and heal, and that a transition to healing with scar formation occurs at about 100 days gestation.

SUMMARY

Recent experimental and clinical evidence suggests that the fetus responds to injury in a fashion fundamentally different from that of the adult. Using a variety of animal models and techniques, numerous investigators have begun to analyze the constituents of the fetal wound healing process in an attempt to understand the control mechanisms that endow the fetus with unique healing abilities.

REFERENCES

1. Harrison MR, Golbus MS, Filly RA (Eds.): The Unborn Patient. WB Saunders, Philadelphia, 1990.
2. Crombleholme TM, Harrison MR, Langer JC, et al.: Early experience with open fetal surgery for congenital hydronephrosis. J Pediatr Surg 23:1114, 1988.
3. Harrison MR, Adzick NS, Longaker MT et al.: Successful repair in utero of a fetal diaphragmatic hernia after removal of herniated viscera from the left thorax. N Engl J Med 322:1582, 1990.
4. Langer JC, Harrison MR, Schmidt KG, et al.: Fetal hydrops and demise from sacrococcygeal teratoma: Rationale for fetal surgery. Amer J Obstet Gynecol 160:1145, 1989.
5. Harrison MR, Adzick NS, Jennings RW, et al.: Antenatal intervention for congenital cystic adenomatoid malformation. Lancet 336:965, 1990.
6. Weiss P, Matoltsy AG: Wound healing in chick embryos in vivo and in vitro. Dev Biol 1:302, 1959.
7. Hess A: Reactions of mammalian fetal tissues to injury: II. Skin. Anatomic Res 119:435, 1958.
8. Hallock GG: In utero cleft lip repair in A/J mice. Plast Reconstr Surg 75:785, 1985.
9. Sullivan WG: In utero cleft lip repair in the mouse without an incision. Plast Reconstr Surg 84:723, 1989.
10. Goss AN: Intrauterine healing of fetal rat oral mucosal, skin and cartilage wounds. J Oral Pathol 6:35, 1977.

11. Dixon JB: Inflammation in the foetal and neonatal rat. The local reactions to skin burns. J Path Bact 80:73, 1960.
12. Sopher D: The response of rat fetal membranes to injury. Ann Royal Coll Surg (England) 51:240, 1972.
13. Block M: Wound healing in the newborn opossum. Nature 187:340, 1960.
14. Viljanto J, Thomasson B, Pikkarainen T, et al.: Foetal connective tissue regeneration. Acta Chir Scan 141:85, 1975.
15. Adzick NS, Harrison MR, Glick PL, et al.: Comparison of fetal, newborn and adult wound healing by histologic, enzyme histochemical, and hydroxyproline determination. J Pediatr Surg 20:315, 1985.
16. Krummel TM, Nelson JM, Diegelmann RF, et al.: Fetal response to injury in the rabbit. J Pediatr Surg 22:640, 1987.
17. Burrington JD: Wound healing in the fetal lamb. J Pediatr Surg 6:523, 1971.
18. Longaker MT, Whitby DJ, Adzick NS, et al.: Studies in fetal wound healing: VI. Second and early third trimester fetal wounds demonstrate rapid collagen deposition without scar formation. J Pediatr Surg 25:63, 1990.
19. Sopher D: A study of wound healing in the foetal tissues of the cynomologus monkey. Lab Animals Handbook 6:327, 1975.
20. Sopher D: Future prospects for fetal surgery in teratology: Trends and applications. Springer-Verlag, pp 165.
21. Hallock GG, Rice DC, McClure HM: In utero lip repair in the rhesus monkey: An update. Plast Reconstr Surg 80:855, 1987.
22. Burd DAR, Longaker MT, Adzick NS, Harrison MR, Ehrlich HP: Fetal wound healing in a large animal model: The deposition of collagen is confirmed. Br J Plast Surg 43:571, 1990.
23. Diegelmann RF, Lindblad WJ, Cohen IK: A subcutaneous implant for wound healing studies in humans. J Surg Res 40:229, 1986.
24. Viljanto J: Cellstic: A device for wound healing studies in man: Description of the method. J Surg Res 20:115, 1976.
25. Goodson WH III, Hunt TK: Development of a new miniature method for the study of wound healing in human subjects. J Surg Res 33:394, 1982.
26. Schilling JA, Joel W, Shurley HM: Wound healing: A comparative study of the histochemical changes in granulation tissue contained in stainless steel wire mesh and polyvinyl sponge cylinders. Surgery 48:702, 1959.
27. Longaker MT, Chiu ES, Harrison MR, et al.: Studies in fetal wound healing: IV. Hyaluronic acid stimulating activity of fetal versus adult wound fluid. Annals of Surgery 210:667, 1989.
28. Krummel TM, Ehrlich HP, Nelson JM, et al.: Fetal wounds do not contract in utero. Surgical Forum 40:613, 1989.
29. Martin P, Lewis J: The mechanics of embryonic skin wound healing: Limb-bud lesions in mouse and chick embryos. Presented at the British Society of Cell Biology meeting. Manchester, England, April 1990.
30. Mayer A: Ueber die Moglichkeit opertiver Eingriffe Bevin lebender Sangeiterp-fetus. Zentrabl Gynakol 42:773, 1918.
31. Whitby DJ, Ferguson MWJ: The extracellular matrix and soluble growth factors in fetal and adult mouse wound healing. Presented at the British Society of Cell Biology meeting. Manchester, England, April 1990.
32. Mackie EJ, Halfer W, Liverani D: Induction of tenascin in healing wounds. J Cell Biology 107:2757, 1988.
33. Roberts AB, Sporn MB, Assoian RK, et al.: Rapid induction of fibrosis and angiogenesis in vivo and stimulation of collagen formation. PNAS 83:4167, 1986.
34. Mustoe TA, Pierce GF, Thomason A, et al.: Accelerated healing of incisional wounds in rats induced by transforming growth factor-B. Science 237:1333, 1987.
35. Krummel TM, Nelson JM, Diegelmann RF, et al.: Fetal response to injury and its modulation with transforming growth factor-beta. Surg Forum 38:622, 1987.
36. Robinson BW, Goss AN: Intrauterine healing of fetal rat cheek wounds. Cleft Palate J 18:251, 1981.
37. Rowsell AR: The intra-uterine healing of foetal muscle wounds: experimental study in the rat. Br J Plast Surg 37:635, 1984.
38. Hallock GG, Merkel JR, DiPaolo BR: Analysis of collagen content in the fetal wound. Ann Plast Surg 21:310, 1988.

39. Merkel JR, DiPaolo BR, Hallock GG, et al.: Type I and type III collagen content of healing wounds in fetal and adult rats. Proc Soc Exp Biol Med 187:493, 1988.
40. Howarth G, Ferguson MWJ: A comparison of wound healing in adult and pouch young of Monodelphis Domestica. Presented at the British Society of Cell Biology meeting. Manchester, England, April 1990.
41. Adzick NS, Harrison MR: Surgical techniques in the fetal rabbit. In: Nathanielsz PW (ed): Animal Models in Fetal Medicine. Perinatology Press, Ithaca NY, 1986.
42. Thomasson B, Viljanto J, Jaaskelainen T, et al.: Enzyme histochemical observations on the formation of granulation tissue in rabbit fetuses and does. Acta Chir Scan 139:327, 1973.
43. Siebert JW, Burd DAR, McCarthy JG, et al.: Fetal wound healing: A biochemical study of scarless healing. Plast Reconstr Surg 85:495, 1990.
44. DePalma RL, Krummel TM, Durham LA III, et al.: Characterization and quantitation of wound matrix in the fetal rabbit. Matrix 9:224, 1989.
45. Kujawa MJ, Tepperman K: Culturing chick muscle cells on glycosaminoglycan substrates: attachment and differentiation. Dev Biology 99:277, 1983.
46. Kujawa MJ, Pechak DG, Fiszman MY, et al.: Hyaluronic acid bonded to cell culture surfaces inhibits the program of myogenesis. Dev Biology 113:10, 1986.
47. Tonnesen MG, Jenkins D, Siegel SL, et al.: Expression of fibronectin, laminin, and factor VII-related antigen during development of the human cutaneous microvasculature. J Invest Dermatol 85:564, 1985.
48. Longaker MT, Whitby DJ, Crombleholme TM, et al.: Studies in fetal wound healing: III. Early deposition of adhesion molecules distinguishes fetal from adult wounds. J Pediatr Surg 24:799, 1989.
49. Cheng CY, Martin DE, Legget CG, et al.: Fibronectin enhances healing of excised wounds in rats. Arch Dermatol 124:221, 1988.
50. Somasundaram M, Prathap K: Intrauterine healing of the skin wounds in rabbit foetuses. J Pathol 100:81, 1970.
51. Somasundaram M, Prathap K: The effects of exclusion of amniotic fluid on intra-uterine healing of skin wounds in rabbit foetuses. J Pathol 107:127, 1972.
52. Rappolee DA, Brenner CA, Schultz R, et al.: Developmental expression of PDGF, TGF-a, and TGF-B genes in preimplantation mouse embryos. Science 241:1823, 1988.
53. Pessa ME, Bland KI, Copeland EM: Growth factors and the determinants of wound repair. J Surg Res 42:207, 1987.
54. Barbul A, Pines E, Caldwell M, Hunt TK (Eds): Progress in Clinical and Biologic Research. Growth factors and other aspects of wound healing. AR Liss, New York, Vol 266:243–258, 1988.
55. Delozier J, Nanney LB, Hago K, et al.: Epidermal growth factor enhances fetal re-epithelialization. Surgical Forum 38:623, 1987.
56. Rudolph AM, Heymann MA: Methods for studying the circulation of the fetus in utero. In: Nathanielsz PW (ed.): Animal Models in Fetal Medicine. Elsevier/North-Holland Biomedical Press, 1980.
57. Adzick NS, Outwater KM, Harrison MR, et al.: Correction of congenital diaphragmatic hernia in utero. IV. An early gestational fetal lamb model for pulmonary vascular morphometric analysis. J Pediatr Surg 20:673, 1985.
58. Vande Berg JS, Rudolph R: Cultured myofibroblasts: A useful model to study wound contraction and pathological contracture. Ann Plast Surg 14:111, 1985.
59. Longaker MT, Burd DAR, Yen TSB, et al.: Midgestation fetal wounds contract in utero. Presented at The 35th Annual Meeting of The Plastic Surgery Research Council. Washington, DC, April 1990.
60. Hayes JH, Krummel TM, Schatzki PF, et al.: Open wound histology in the fetal rabbit. Surg Forum 40:558, 1989.
61. Chiu E, Longaker MT, Adzick NS, et al.: Hyaluronic acid patterns in fetal and adult wound fluid. Surg Forum 41:336, 1990.
62. Decker M, Chui ES, Dollbaum C, et al.: Hyaluronic acid stimulating factor in serum from the bovine fetus and from breast cancer patients. Cancer Research 49:3499, 1989.
63. Longaker MT, Crombleholme TM, Langer JC, Verrier ED, Harrison MR, Stern R: Studies in fetal wound healing: I. A fetal factor modulates extracellular matrix synthesis. J Pediatr Surg 24:789, 1989.
64. Dahl L, Hopwood JJ, Laurent BG, et al.: The concentration of hyaluronate in amniotic fluid. Biochemical Medicine 30:280, 1983.

65. Longaker MT, Adzick NS, et al.: Studies in fetal wound healing. VII: Fetal wound healing may be modulated by elevated hyaluronic acid stimulating activity in amniotic fluid. J Pediatr Surg 25:430, 1990.
66. Harrison MR, Anderson J, Rosen MA, et al.: Fetal surgery in the primate. I. Anesthetic, surgical, and tocolytic management to maximize fetal-neonatal survival. J Pediatr Surg 17:115, 1982.
67. Nakayama DK, Harrison MR, Berger MS, et al.: Correction of congenital hydrocephalus in utero. I. The model: Intracisternal kaolin produces hydrocephalus in fetal lambs and fetal monkeys. J Pediatr Surg 18:331, 1983.
68. Glick PL, Harrison MR, Halks-Miller M, et al.: Correction of congenital hydrocephalus in utero. II. Efficacy of in utero shunting. J Pediatr Surg 19:851, 1984.
69. Nakayama DK, Harrison MR, Serone-Ferre M, et al.: Fetal surgery in the primate. II. Uterine electromyographic response to operative procedures and pharmacologic agents. J Pediatr Surg 19:333, 1984.
70. Adzick NS, Harrison MR, Glick PL, et al.: Fetal surgery in the primate. III. Maternal outcome after fetal surgery. J Pediatr Surg 21:477, 1986.

CHAPTER **5**

Fetal Models for Craniofacial Surgery: Cleft Lip/Palate and Craniosynostosis

Michael T. Longaker
Leonard B. Kaban

The field of craniofacial surgery has rapidly evolved during the past 30 years. In the 1960s and early 1970s, craniofacial surgeons were occupied with understanding the pathologic anatomy of congenital craniofacial anomalies such as Crouzon and Apert syndromes, hypertelorbitism, hemifacial microsomia, and Treacher-Collins syndrome.[1–7] Professor Paul Tessier pioneered the operative techniques for correction of these morphologic defects and brought them to university centers all over the world. Multidisciplinary craniofacial teams were established and surgeons gained experience correcting end-stage deformities with reduced operative time, uniformly good results, and fewer complications.[1–12]

Craniofacial surgeons, in the 1980s, began to correct certain anomalies during infancy and early childhood in an effort to improve growth potential, minimize secondary distortion, and aid in body image development.[13–15] Computed tomography of the craniofacial skeleton has led to improved diagnosis and treatment planning.[16]

Future challenges for investigators and clinicians in this complex field will be to improve understanding of the developmental biology of normal and abnormal facial morphology, to further elucidate the genetics of craniofacial anomalies, and to develop new therapeutic methods that will enhance growth of the abnormal skeleton and soft tissue.

The observation that fetuses heal without inflammation and fibrosis has led investigators to consider the possibility of fetal surgery to correct craniofacial anomalies. For example, if prenatal repair of cleft lip would result in healing without scar formation, then secondary midface hypoplasia, common in cleft patients, might be diminished or entirely prevented.

Since craniofacial anomalies are non-fatal morphologic defects and postnatal corrective procedures are currently available, there is no urgency to develop prenatal treatments. However, fetal models may improve our understanding of the pathogenesis of craniofacial deformities. For example, in the case of cleft lip/palate, comparison of prenatal and postnatal repair may provide valuable insight for the prevention of secondary mid-face growth deformities. Before fetal surgery can be applied to humans with craniofacial anomalies, considerable experimental work must be done to demonstrate the biologic basis and benefits of the procedures and to demonstrate safety for the fetus and the mother. In the future it might be more practical to use the information we derive from fetal wound healing studies to manipulate postnatal wounds and make them more fetal-like. This might produce a result similar to fetal surgery with fewer patient and no maternal risks.

We have developed fetal models for cleft lip/palate and craniosynostosis. These models will potentially:

1. Improve our understanding of the pathogenesis of secondary mid-face growth defects in cleft lip/palate patients;
2. Help characterize the differences in fetal and postnatal wound healing;
3. Improve our understanding of the pathogenesis of craniosynostosis;
4. Allow us to compare facial growth after prenatal versus postnatal repair of craniosynostosis and cleft lip/palate.

CLEFT LIP AND PALATE

Cleft lip and cleft lip/palate are the most common congenital facial anomalies with an incidence of one in 800 live births in Caucasians. The inheritance is multifactorial with genetic predisposition and environmental factors both playing a role. Cleft lip and palate are associated with multiple progressive abnormalities as the child grows: a) 25%–35% have abnormal speech requiring a secondary operation on the palate and speech therapy, b) nasal deformity consisting of depression of the alar base and tip and deviation of the septum (unilateral cleft lip/palate) and bilateral widening of the alar base and short columella (bilateral), c) mid-face growth deficiency resulting in maxillary retrusion and relative mandibular prognathism, d) recurrent otitis media (cleft palate) secondary to abnormal eustachian tube function and e) dental anomalies consisting of missing teeth, extra teeth, and malpositioned teeth.

Experimental models for the study of cleft lip/palate have existed for many years.[17–23] These have been used primarily to document the embryologic events leading to development of the deformity. In addition, cleft lip/palate models have

A 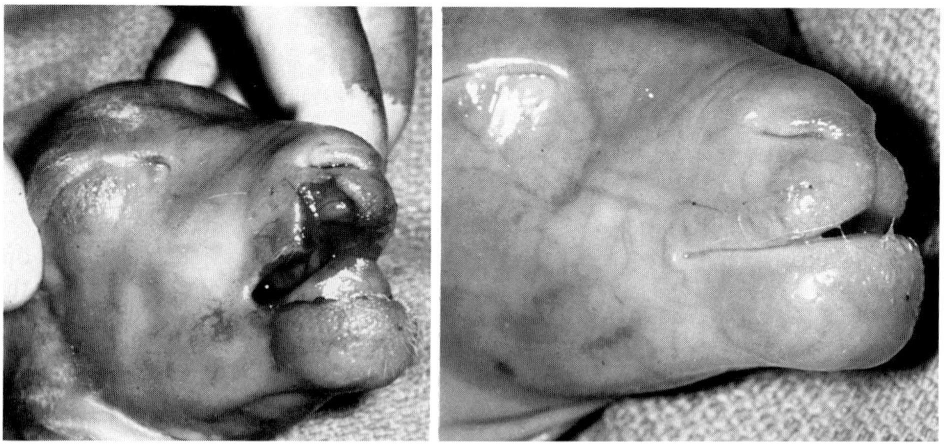 B

Figure 5.1 **(a)** Photograph of a large surgically created cleft in the upper lip of a 75 day gestation fetal lamb. The wound was closed by interrupted sutures. **(b)** Photograph of wound in Figure 1A two weeks following repair. Note the tiny suture present and a lack of scar formation. This fetus has the typical relative prognathism seen in unoperated control lambs at this gestational age.

been used to document the secondary growth effects of postnatal cleft lip/palate repair. More recently investigators have examined the feasibility of fetal cleft lip repair.[21–24]

It is well known that mid-face retrusion and deficiency in maxillary width are often the result of surgically induced scar formation. Bardach has demonstrated that increased lip pressure following postnatal repair of cleft lip in animals is associated with progressive mid-face hypoplasia.[17–20] Several studies in animal models have shown that fetal wound healing is fundamentally different from that in adults. As detailed in Chapter 3, the fetal process does not involve inflammation and/or scarring.[25–29] Hallock has demonstrated in utero repair of cleft lip is possible in mice and monkeys.[21,22] Sullivan has recently reported that a drug-induced cleft lip can be repaired in utero simply by reapposing the cleft edges without a surgical incision.[23] Our fetal surgery laboratory has developed techniques for in utero cleft lip repair in larger animals with a longer gestation.

A simple linear repair of cleft lip in utero might result in healing without scar formation. The resultant oral sphincter, with intact muscle, would provide a normal "functional matrix" for the growing fetus. The esthetic result would be greatly improved (Figure 5.1a and b). The major advantage, however, would be unimpaired facial growth without the adverse effect of the lip and/or palate scar.

Animal Models

Fetal Rabbit

We have recently developed a fetal model for cleft lip repair using rabbits.[30] Time-dated pregnant New Zealand white rabbits at 24 days gestation (term = 31 days) are sedated by a ketamine HCl/acepromazine maleate mixture (0.5 cc intramuscular injection followed by 0.5 cc intravenously into an ear vein). General anesthesia (0.5% halothane/O_2) is achieved by mask. Penicillin G (3×10^5 u) is given as an intramuscular injection. The maternal abdomen is shaved and scrubbed with Betadine[R]. A sterile mid-line laparotomy is used to expose the bicornuate uterus. Each pregnant doe carries at least four fetuses (Figure 5.2). On one side of the bicornuate uterus, a pursestring is placed in the uterine wall and a hysterotomy is made using electrocautery. Clamps are used to secure the amniotic membranes and the fetal head is exposed. Under surgical loupe magnification (6×) a 1mm section of fetal lip and anterior maxillary alveolus is excised halfway between the mid-line and labial commissure. The excision creates a full thickness oronasal fistula. In one group, the lip is repaired with two 9-0 nylon interrupted sutures through skin, muscle, and mucosa. Meticulous technique is used to align the vermillion border and nasal sill during the closure. In another fetus, on the opposite side of the uterus, the lip is left unrepaired. The fetus is returned to the uterus, sterile saline is used to replace the amniotic fluid, and the pursestring is tied to close the hysterotomy. For controls, fetuses are exposed and returned to the uterus without having an operation.

For harvesting, the does are sedated and anesthetized in a similar fashion as for the initial operation. The mid-line laparotomy is reopened and the uterus and operated fetuses are exposed. The fetuses are removed, observed, weighed, and photographed to compare size and facial morphology to control (unoperated) fetuses. After documenting the viability of the control and experimental fetuses, they are killed by pentobarbital overdose.

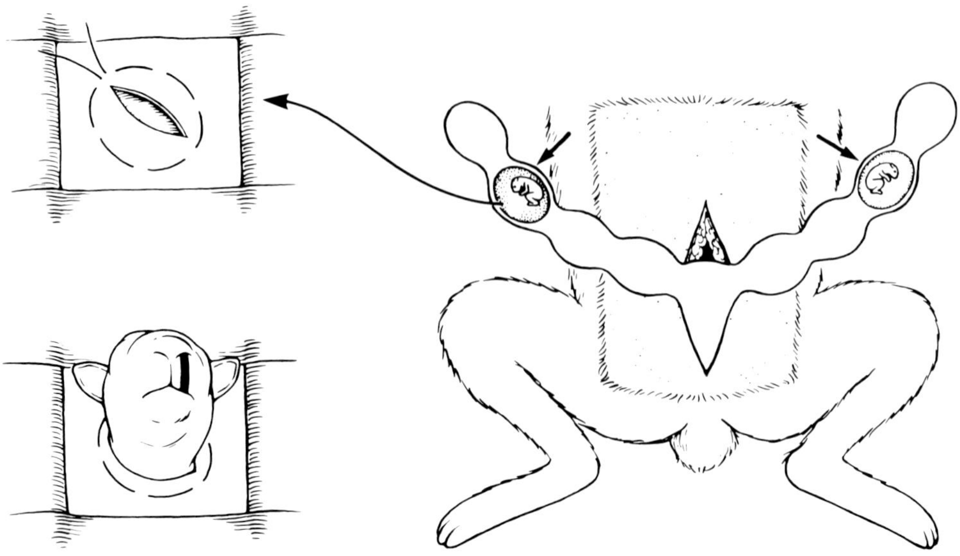

Figure 5.2 Operative anatomy. **Right:** Representative line drawing demonstrating bicornuate uterus. There are usually multiple fetuses. Arrows indicate relative position of the two fetuses selected for in utero cleft lip model. **Top left:** Pursestring suture shown surrounding the hysterotomy. **Bottom left:** Head exposed showing full-thickness left-sided oronasal fistula created by excision of a 1mm paramedian section of fetal lip halfway between the mid-line and labial commissure. *Reprinted with permission.*[30]

Fetal Rabbit Cleft Lip Model—Results

Forty-seven fetuses, in 25 pregnant does, underwent the cleft lip procedure; 36 fetuses survived the operation and were alive at the time of harvest, for a survival rate of 76.6%. This included 15 out of 20 fetuses in the repaired group (75% survival), 11 out of 17 fetuses in the unrepaired group (64.7% survival), and 10 out of 10 controls (100% survival). There was no statistically significant difference in survival rates between the repaired and unrepaired fetuses.

The first group of fetuses was harvested at four days postoperatively (28 days gestation). There was a marked facial asymmetry in the unrepaired group. This consisted of retraction of the lip segments into the underlying full thickness defect and elevation and flattening of the nose on the cleft side. The cleft lip edges were epithelialized, but the lip remained open. There was no epithelialization or scar formation across the gap. In the repaired fetuses, at 28 days gestation, there was epithelial continuity across the cleft lip and the facial asymmetry was less severe than the unrepaired group.

The second group of fetuses was sacrificed at birth (seven days postoperatively) after spontaneous vaginal delivery. In the unrepaired fetuses, the cleft remained open, without scar or epithelial bridging. The cleft side of the nose remained flat and depressed. In repaired fetuses, there was epithelialization across the cleft, which was closed and the facial asymmetry was less than that at four days postoperatively.

The third group of fetuses also delivered spontaneously per vagina. These fetuses were cared for by the mother as long as all normal newborns were removed from the litter except for one control. With multiple normal fetuses in the litter, the cleft animals were cannibalized or neglected. By 12 days after birth (19 days postoperatively), gross observation revealed that the unrepaired cleft animals had slight flattening and asymmetry of the nose. The cleft remained open. It was epithelialized at the edges but there was no continuity across the cleft. In repaired animals, the nose was symmetrical and the lip was full. There was a linear depression in the area of the previous cleft, but this was covered with epithelium and there was no scar. There was normal hair distribution in the area of the repaired cleft. The distance from the mid-line to the commissure was decreased on the cleft side as a result of the magnitude of resection and not by the formation of scar tissue.

Histologic analysis of serial horizontal sections of cleft wounds was carried out following formalin fixation and plastic embedding. Hematoxylin and eosin stained sections confirmed that, in both sutured and unrepaired wounds, the fetal rabbit cleft healed without inflammatory cell infiltration or scar formation. In the unsutured cleft, epithelialization occurred at the edges but a defect remained within the connective tissue. In the sutured cleft, there was no scar formation and there was regeneration of skin (with normal appendages), muscle and mucosa across the cleft (Figure 5.3).

Fetal Repair and Maxillary Growth

To determine the effect of fetal cleft lip repair on postnatal facial growth, we used the fetal rabbit model.[31] At birth, the litter was examined to identify the operated and control newborn rabbits. The remainder of the newborns were sacrificed to reduce competition for food and water. The newborn rabbits were weighed, pho-

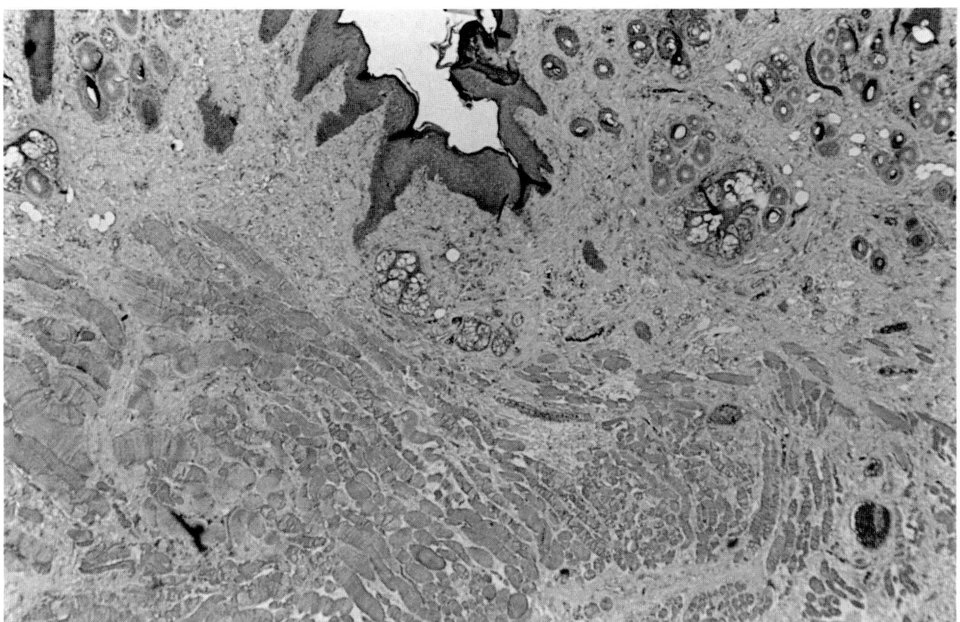

Figure 5.3 Histology of fetal rabbit cleft lip/palate repair at 26 weeks stained for hematoxylin and eosin. Epithelial continuity is present of both the oral mucosa and skin. There is no scar and there is evidence for muscle regeneration across the wound.

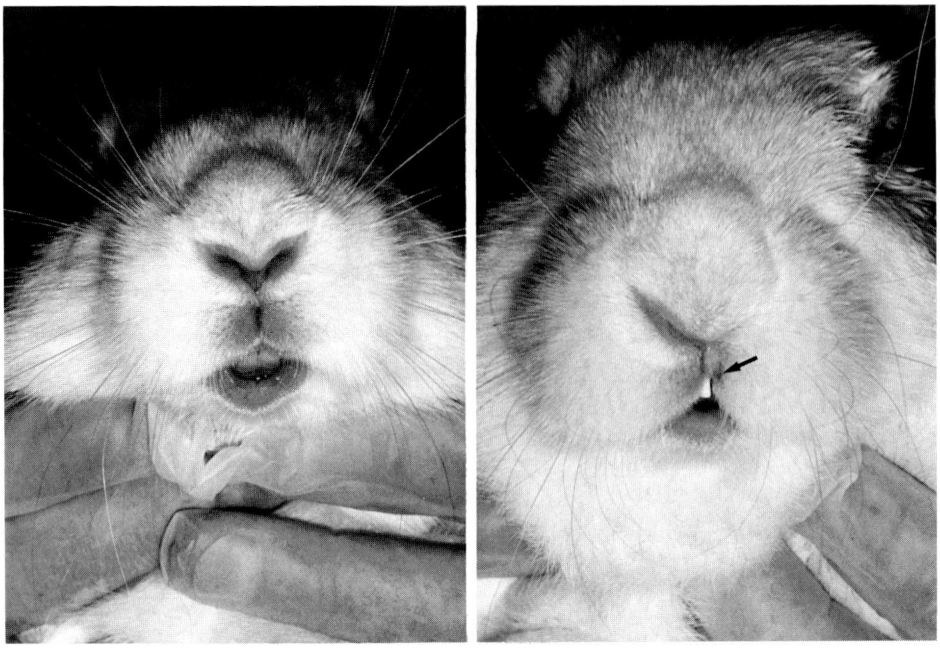

A B

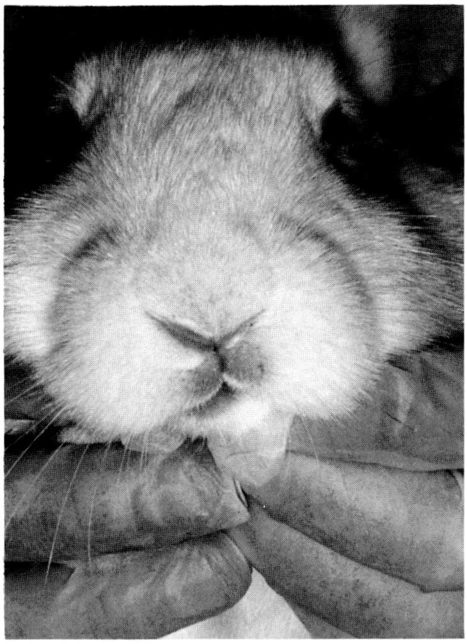

C

Figure 5.4 Facial morphology following fetal cleft lip procedure: six months of age. **(a)** Unoperated control. Note the symmetry of nares, midline natural cleft and symmetry of lateral labial commissures. **(b)** Unrepaired animal. There is flattening and asymmetry of nose. The cleft (arrow) remains open, epithelialized at the edge, but without continuity across the cleft and there is decreased distance from the midline to the labial commissure on the affected side. **(c)** Repaired animal. The nose is symmetrical. The lip is full on the cleft side. There is no scar. The distance from midline to commissure is also decreased on the cleft side, a reflection of the resected tissue. *Reprinted with permission.*[31]

tographed, and divided into three sets. Each set of rabbits included two unrepaired specimens (U-CL), two repaired specimens (R-CL), and four unoperated controls.

One set of animals was sacrificed at four, 12, and 26 weeks after birth. Four weeks after delivery, all three sets of rabbits were sedated, weighed, and photographed. One set of rabbits was sacrificed; 12 weeks after delivery, the two remaining sets of rabbits were sedated, weighed, and photographed. A second set of rabbits was sacrificed; 26 weeks after delivery, the last set of rabbits was sedated, weighed, and photographed (Figure 5.4a–c). Rabbits complete facial growth by 26 weeks.[32,33]

Following sacrifice, rabbit heads were cleaned and bleached dry. The nasal septum was examined and direct skull cephalometry was performed on the dried skulls. Multiple measurements were performed to assess maxillary length and width (Figure 5.5a–c).

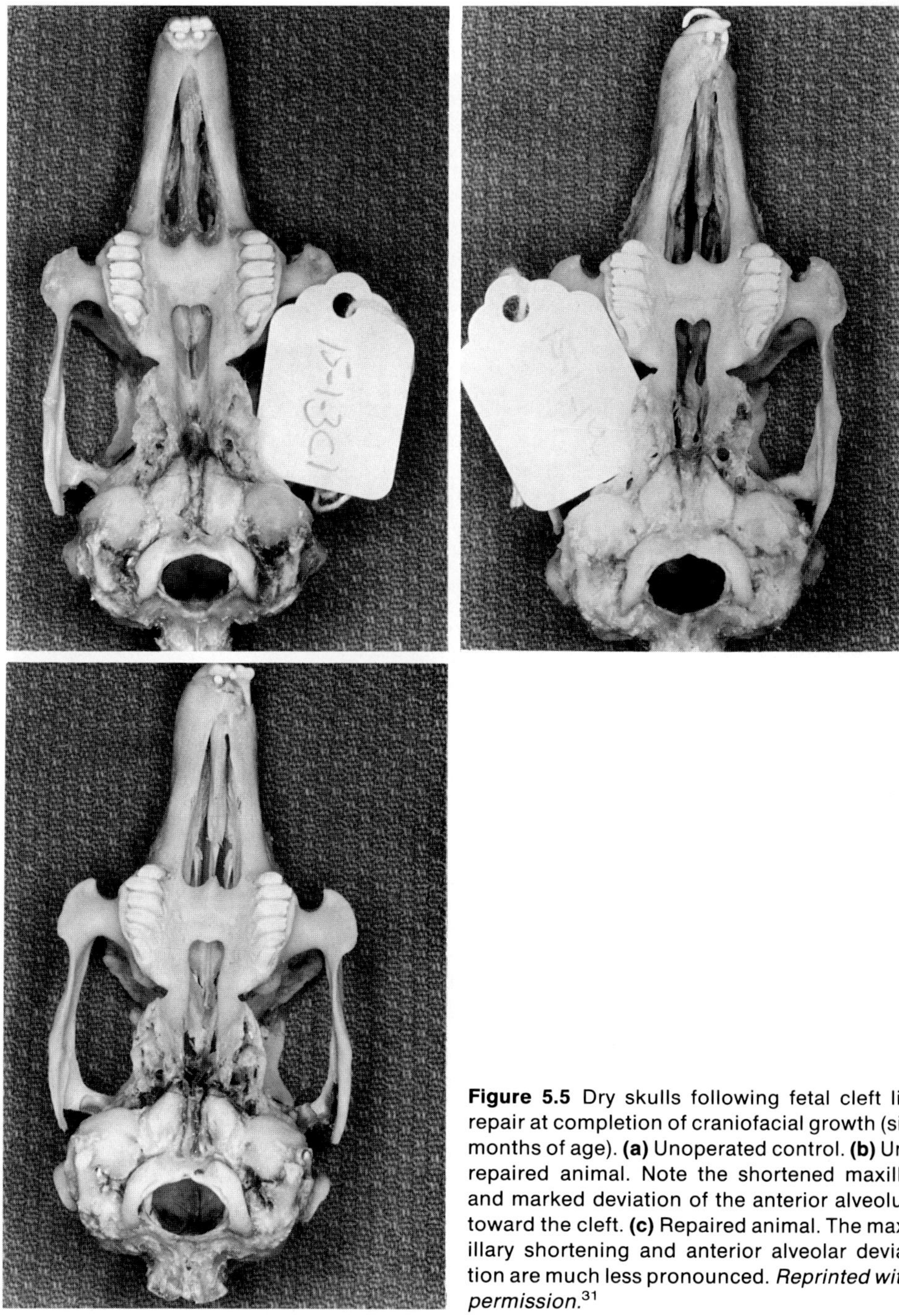

A B C

Figure 5.5 Dry skulls following fetal cleft lip repair at completion of craniofacial growth (six months of age). **(a)** Unoperated control. **(b)** Unrepaired animal. Note the shortened maxilla and marked deviation of the anterior alveolus toward the cleft. **(c)** Repaired animal. The maxillary shortening and anterior alveolar deviation are much less pronounced. *Reprinted with permission.*[31]

There was minimal deviation of the nasal septum toward the cleft side in both the repaired and unrepaired specimens at all time points: four, 12 and 26 weeks. Clinical examination and direct cephalometric measurements of anterior maxillary width, premaxillary width, and maxillary width, revealed no significant evidence of anterior maxillary growth inhibition in rabbits who underwent the fetal cleft lip procedure. However, subjectively there appeared to be more asymmetry in the unrepaired than repaired animals. We are in the process of accumulating more specimens for growth measurements to obtain statistically valid results.

This preliminary study was the first to report results of long-term facial growth in rabbits after fetal repair of cleft lip. The findings of minimal maxillary growth retardation in fetal rabbits who had in utero repair of cleft lip are in direct contrast to published findings in postnatal animals. Following cleft lip repair these animals demonstrate significant mid-face growth retardation, presumably on the basis of scarring secondary to the operative procedure.[17,34]

Our results using the fetal rabbit model support the hypothesis that in utero repair of cleft lip/palate would result in healing without scarring and would avoid the adverse effects on mid-face growth produced by postnatal repair.

Fetal Lamb

The fetal rabbit model is limited by the rabbit's small size and short gestation. Therefore, the effects of fetal cleft lip repair can only be studied in mid–third trimester. In light of the observation that there may be a spectrum of fetal wound healing with a transition to adult type healing late in gestation, we have recently developed a model for cleft lip repair in fetal lambs. The advantages of this animal model include a long gestation (term = 145 days) and a larger fetus that allows us to compare cleft lip repair in both the second and third trimesters. Using this model we can define the latest gestational age at which a fetal cleft lip can be repaired and heal without scar formation.

We have surgically created cleft lip and palate defects in four 75-day gestation fetal lambs using surgical techniques previously described for fetal lambs.[35] Two of these lesions were repaired and two were left unrepaired. All fetuses survived the operation and two fetuses (one repaired and one unrepaired) were harvested 14 days later, and the remaining two were harvested 21 days postoperatively.

At 14 days postoperatively, the unrepaired fetuses demonstrated a persistent cleft lip and an oronasal fistula. There was slight flattening of the nasomaxillary area producing a mild facial asymmetry. The repaired fetuses demonstrated a healed cleft lip with sutures remaining in place. They had a symmetrical facial appearance with no nasal asymmetry. At 21 days, the unrepaired animals remained with an unhealed, persistent cleft lip and an oronasal fistula. The nasomaxillary region remained slightly flatter on the cleft side, maintaining the facial asymmetry. The repaired animals had a healed cleft lip that was not visible except for sutures. There was no scar and the nose and facial appearance were symmetrical.

We plan to use the fetal lamb model to study fetal cleft lip and cleft palate repair. The large size and long gestation of fetal lambs will allow for both histologic and biochemical analysis of wound healing at various gestational ages. We will also determine the effect of fetal cleft lip and/or cleft palate repair on subsequent facial growth.

CRANIOSYNOSTOSIS

The estimated incidence of craniosynostosis is one in 1000 live births. The facial skeleton is affected in approximately 9% to 10% of cases.[36,37] In this anomaly, premature fusion of cranial sutures prevents expansion of the skull in response to growth of the brain, resulting in deformities that depend on the suture involved. These include scaphocephaly (mid-sagittal suture, long, narrow skull), oxycephaly, acrocephaly, turricephaly (coronal suture, tall or "tower" skull), trigonocephaly (metopic suture, triangular skull) and, most commonly, plagiocephaly or asymmetric skull. Obstructive hydrocephalus is commonly seen in plagiocephaly and trigonocephaly but rarely in Crouzon and Apert syndromes.

For many years, it was believed that cranial sutures were primary growth sites of the skull. Moss, however, demonstrated that skull growth is determined by expansion of the underlying brain—his "functional matrix" concept.[38–40] The pathophysiology is not entirely clear, however, because anatomical dissections of infants with craniosynostosis suggest that the focus of abnormal skeletal morphogenesis is in the cranial base and the calvarial deformities are probably secondary.[41]

In 1912, Crouzon first described a group of patients with craniosynostosis and severe mid-face hypoplasia.[42] Oxycephaly and brachycephaly are the most common skull types seen in Crouzon syndrome. The bony orbits are shallow, resulting in exorbitism. Divergent strabismus may lead to progressive visual loss during the first three years of life.[43] With time, exposure keratitis and corneal damage become a threat. The maxilla is deficient in three dimensions producing relative prognathism (the mandible is normal) and the characteristic drooping lower lip. The nose has a typical "parrot's beak" appearance.

In 1906, Apert described patients with craniosynostosis, mid-face hypoplasia, and peculiar extremity deformities—a syndrome known today as acrocephalosyndactyly.[44] The facial deformities of Apert syndrome are in many ways similar to Crouzon syndrome. However, Apert patients more frequently exhibit: (a) cleft palate; (b) asymmetric exorbitism; (c) severe lateral canthal dystopia; and (d) isolated involvement of the coronal suture producing oxycephaly and a transverse forehead skin furrow.[5] The major distinguishing feature of Apert's syndrome is the complex mirror-image syndactyly of the hand and/or feet.

Fetal Rabbit Model

Nappen, et al. have reported an animal model for craniosynostosis in five-week-old rabbits.[45] They found that mechanical immobilization of the suture did not produce osseous union, but application of methyl-2-cyanoacrylate to the overlying periosteum caused a bony ridge to develop across the suture. This suggests that the periosteum plays a role in craniosynostosis.

Our laboratory has attempted to immobilize cranial sutures by a variety of techniques: staples, silk suture, and glue. These methods have not resulted in bone formation across the gap because the immobilization effect was only transient and did not remain during the entire period of rapid brain and skull growth. We have recently excised the soft tissue between cranial sutures and placed demineralized bone matrix into the resultant defect. Demineralized bone matrix (DBM) is known for its osteoinductive effect in a variety of clinical and experimental models.[46] We hypothesized that it would be possible to excise a cranial suture, fill the defect with demineralized bone powder (DBP), and thereby produce craniosynostosis across the gap.

We recently developed a fetal model for craniosynostosis using DBP and fetal rabbits.[47] The DBP was prepared from the long bones of adult rabbits. The bones were dissected free of soft tissue, washed, defatted, and pulverized to a particle size of 75 to 250 um. This bone powder was demineralized by extraction with 0.5N HCl.[48]

Time-dated fetal rabbits on day 25 of pregnancy (term = 31 days) were used in this study. The technique for exposure of the fetus (one on each side of the uterus) was similar to that described previously for cleft lip/palate. Through a coronal incision, anterior and posterior scalp flaps were elevated and a bilateral strip craniectomy was performed to completely excise the coronal suture under 6× loupe magnification. DBP was placed in the craniectomy defect. The scalp incision was closed with 7-0 prolene suture, and the maternal hysterotomy and laparotomy incisions were closed. Pregnancies continued to term, and the newborn rabbits were delivered per vagina.

Experimental offspring were examined for overall growth and development. The newborns were sacrificed on days six, 10, 21, and 28 days following in utero surgery for histologic analysis. Computerized tomography (CT) was performed on the offspring at 28 days following surgery. The coronal sections were used to create three-dimensional CT reconstructions of the skulls. Computerized measurements of cranial vault height, lateral dimension, and area were made.

There were 36 fetuses in 18 pregnant does; 17 of these fetuses (47%) survived the procedure and were delivered vaginally; 10 of the 17 fetuses survived long-term for full evaluation. The experimental animals had a grossly normal appearance and feeding behavior when compared to their littermates. At the time of sacrifice, the sagittal and lambdoidal sutures were normal but the coronal sutures were fused with DBP induced bone.

Histologically, DBP-induced bone formation across the gap was produced by coronal suture excision. The results of this preliminary study establish the feasibility of creating bony fusion across cranial sutures by osteoinduction in an in utero model. This model produces surviving experimental newborn rabbits in an acceptable percentage of cases. Histologic studies show that three weeks after birth there was substantial bony fusion across the excised coronal sutures. Preliminary CT results indicate that there is a difference in calvarial shape in experimental versus control animals. Additional confirmatory studies and long-term follow-up are needed to assess the validity of the model.

This model may be used to improve our understanding of the mechanism, the pathologic anatomy, and the abnormal craniofacial growth in craniosynostosis. By increasing our understanding of the pathophysiology of craniosynostosis, it is possible that fetal repair may become feasible in the future.

SUMMARY

In this chapter we have discussed two fetal models for craniofacial anomalies: cleft lip/palate and craniosynostosis. Wound healing and facial growth studies indicate that prenatal cleft lip repair results in less mid-face hypoplasia when compared to postnatal repair. In the craniosynostosis model we have demonstrated bone formation across an excised coronal suture. We are currently pursuing this model by excising multiple cranial sutures in an effort to produce changes in skull shape that mimic the clinical deformities.

REFERENCES

1. Tessier P: Osteotomes totales de la foce; syndrome de Crouzon; syndrome d'Apert; oxycephalies, scaphocephalies, tarricephalies. Ann Chir Plast 12:273, 1967.
2. Tessier P: Relationship of craniostenosis to craniofacial dysostosis and to faciostenosis. Plast Reconstr Surg 48:224, 1971.
3. Tessier P: The definitive plastic surgical treatment of the severe facial deformities of craniofacial dysostosis. Plast Reconstr Surg 48:419, 1971.
4. Tessier P: Orbital hypertelorism: I. Successive surgical attempts, materials, and methods, causes and mechanisms. Scan J Plast Reconstr Surg 6:135, 1972.
5. Tessier P: Experiences in the treatment of orbital hypertelorism. Plast Reconstr Surg 53:1, 1974.
6. Tessier P, Guiot B, Derome P: Orbital hypertelorism: II. Definitive treatment of orbital hypertelorism by craniofacial or extracranial osteotomies. Scand J Plast Reconstr Surg 7:39, 1973.
7. Tessier P, Guiot B, Rougerie J, et al.: Osteotomies cranio-naso-orbito-faciales hypertelorisme. Ann Chir Plast 12:113, 1967.
8. Converse JM, Wood-Smith D, McCarthy JG, et al.: Craniofacial surgery. Clin Plast Surg 1(3):499, 1974.
9. Murray JE, Swanson LT, Strand RD, et al.: Evaluation of craniofacial surgery in the treatment of facial deformities. Ann Surg 182:240, 1975.
10. Murray JE, Mulliken JB, Kaban LB, et al.: Twenty year experience with maxillo-cranio-facial surgery. Ann Surg 190:320, 1979.
11. Kaban LB, Mulliken JB, Murray JE: Craniofacial abnormalities, in Welch KJ, Randolph JG, Ravitch M, et al. (eds): Pediatric Surgery, 4th Edition, Chicago, Yearbook Medical Publishers, Inc.; pp 423–439, 1986.
12. Whitaker LA, Munro IR, Salyer KE, et al.: Combined report of problems and complications in 793 craniofacial operations. Plast Reconstr Surg 64:198, 1979.
13. Kaban LB, Mulliken JB, Murray JE: Three-dimensional approach to analysis and treatment of hemifacial microsomia. Cleft Palate J 18:90, 1981.
14. Marchac D, Renier D: Craniofacial Surgery for Craniosynostosis. Boston, Little, Brown & Company, p 93, 1982.
15. Murray JE, Kaban LB, Mulliken JB: Analysis and treatment of hemifacial microsomia. Plast Reconst Surg 74:186, 1984.
16. Marsh J, Vannier MW: The "third" dimension in craniofacial surgery. Plast Reconstr Surg 71:756, 1983.
17. Bardach J, Roberts DM, Yale R, et al.: The influence of simultaneous cleft lip and palate repair on facial growth in rabbits. Cleft Palate J 17:309, 1980.
18. Bardach J, Klousner EC, Eisbach KJ: The relationship between lip pressure and facial growth after cleft lip repair: an experimental study. Cleft Palate J 16:137, 1979.
19. Bardach J, Mooney MP: The relationship between lip pressure following lip repair and craniofacial growth. An experimental study in beagles. Plast Reconstr Surg 73:544, 1984.
20. Bardach J, Bakowska J, McDermott-Murray J, et al.: Lip pressure changes following lip repair in infants with unilateral clefts of the lip and palate. Plast Reconstr Surg 74:476, 1984.
21. Hallock GG: In utero cleft lip repair in A/J mice. Plast Reconstr Surg 75:785, 1985.
22. Hallock GG, Rice DC, McClure HM: In utero lip repair in the rhesus monkey: An update. Plast Reconstr Surg 80:855, 1987.
23. Sullivan WG: In utero cleft lip repair in the mouse without an incision. Plast Reconstr Surg 84:723, 1989.
24. Dado DV, Kernahan DA, Gianopoulos JG: Intrauterine repair of cleft lip: What's involved. Plast Reconstr Surg 85:461, 1990.
25. Burrington JD: Wound healing in the fetal lamb. J Pediatr Surg 6:523, 1971.
26. Robinson BW, Goss AN: Intrauterine healing of fetal rat cheek wounds. Cleft Palate Journal 18:251, 1987.
27. Roswell A: The intrauterine healing of foetal muscle wounds: experimental study in the rat. Br J Plastic Surg 37:635, 1984.
28. Krummel TM, Nelson JM, Diegelmann RF, et al.: Fetal response to injury in the rabbit. J Pediatr Surg 22:640, 1987.

29. Longaker MT, Whitby DJ, Adzick NS, et al.: Studies in fetal wound healing: VI. Second and early third trimester fetal wounds demonstrate rapid collagen deposition without scar formation. J Pediatr Surg 25:63, 1990.
30. Longaker MT, Dodson TB, Kaban LB: A rabbit model for cleft lip repair. J Oral Maxillofac Surg 48:714, 1990.
31. Dodson TB, Kaban LB, Schmidt B, Longaker MT: Fetal cleft lip repair in rabbits: II. Post-natal facial growth after repair. J Oral Maxillofac Surg 49:603–611, 1991.
32. Urbanus NAM: The significance of skull growth studies for the treatment of cleft lip patients. Acta Morphol Neerl-Scand 23:369, 1985.
33. Engdahl E: Bone regeneration in maxillary defects. Scand J Plast Reconstr Surg 8(suppl):1, 1972.
34. Bardach J, Mooney M, Giedrojc-Juraha ZI: A comparative study of facial growth following cleft lip repair with or without soft tissue undermining: An experimental study in rabbits. Plast Reconstr Surg 69:745, 1982.
35. Harrison MR, Jester JA, Ross NA: Correction of congenital diaphragmatic hernia in utero. I. The model: Intrathoracic balloon produces fatal pulmonary hypoplasia. Surgery 88:174, 1980.
36. Bertelson TL: The premature synostosis of the cranial sutures. Acta Ophthalmol (Suppl) 51:47, 1958.
37. Shillito J, Matson DD: Craniosynostosis: a review of 519 surgical patients. Pediatrics 41:829, 1968.
38. Moss ML: The pathogenesis of premature cranial synostosis in man. Acta Anat 37:351, 1959.
39. Moss ML: Twenty years of functional cranial analysis. Am J Orthod 61:479, 1972.
40. Moss ML: New studies of cranial growth. Birth Defects 11(7):283, 1975.
41. Ousterhout DK, Melsoe B: Cranial base deformity in Apert's syndrome. Plast Reconstr Surg 69:254, 1982.
42. Crouzon D: Dyostose cranio-faciale hereditaire. Bull Soc Med Hop 33:545, 1912.
43. Wood-Smith D, Epstein F, Morello D: Transcranial decompression of the optic nerve in the osseous canal in Crouzon's disease. Clin Plast Surg 3(4):621, 1976.
44. Apert E: De l'acrocephalosyndoctylie. Bull Soc Med Hop 23:1310, 1906.
45. Nappen DL, Kokich VG: Experimental craniosynostosis in growing rabbits. J Neurosurg 58:101, 1983.
46. Urist MR: Bone formation by autoinduction. Science 150:893, 1965.
47. Duncan BD, Adzick NS, Bradley SM, et al.: An in utero model for craniosynostosis. Surg Forum 40:608, 1989.
48. Huang DST, Kao RT, Shteyer A, et al.: Mitogenic response of cells in culture to demineralized bone matrix. J Oral Maxillofac Surg 46:460, 1988.

CHAPTER 6

Marsupial Models of Scarless Fetal Wound Healing

Mark W. J. Ferguson
Georgina F. Howarth

INTRODUCTION

Fetal dermal incisional wound healing differs from adult healing in a number of important parameters, summarized in Table 6.1. These differences may reflect, and indeed be caused by, the differing environments present in the fetal versus adult dermis (Table 6.2). Broadly, such differences may be a reflection of factors extrinsic to the animal such as the presence of amniotic fluid and a uniform higher temperature in fetal wound healing. Equally, differences between fetal and adult dermal incisional wound healing may reflect processes intrinsic to the animal such as the less differentiated state of the wounded tissues, a more rapid turnover and growth of tissue components, and a relatively immature immune system in the fetus. Investigation of the factors responsible for the differences between fetal and adult wound healing is an important objective and an essential prelude to devising strategies of manipulating adult wound healing to minimize scarring. There are already data to suggest that both extrinsic and intrinsic factors may be important. Thus, the rapid healing of fetal wounds may reflect the higher levels of cell division and migration and the lower levels of cell differentiation analogous to the age-related decline in the speed of wound healing in old versus young postnatal animals.[1] Equally, the absence of a scab in fetal wounds is probably a result of healing in a fluid environment.[2] Evidence for intrinsic effects, even in the adult, stems from observations that regionally discrete tissues or cells that display embryonic characteristics, e.g., oral mucosa or hair follicles[3] exhibit fetal-like, scar-free healing when wounded in the adult.[4]

Marsupials possess numerous advantages as experimental models to dissect apart not only fundamental mechanisms of fetal versus adult wound healing, but also the relative importance of extrinsic versus intrinsic differences in these two modes of wound healing. These advantages largely accrue from the fact that marsupial embryos are born at a very early developmental stage and that the equivalent fetal period of eutherian mammalian embryonic development occurs while attached to the nipple in the absence of amniotic fluid. However, the newborn marsupial skin is highly keratinized while the cranial end of the embryo is at an advanced developmental stage compared to both eutherian mammalian embryos and the caudal end of newborn marsupial embryos. Thus, in marsupial embryos, some tissues are highly differentiated (e.g., skin keratinization) and similar to the

TABLE 6.1 Comparison of Fetal Versus Adult Dermal Incisional Wound Healing (for references see Chapter 10)

Fast
No scab
Poor inflammatory response
Lower growth factor profile
Rapid epithelialization
Reduced angiogenesis
Higher rates of cell division and migration
Different wound metabolism, pH, and pO_2
Quantitative and qualitative differences in extracellular matrix molecules
Reduced wound tension and contraction
Enhanced regeneration of epithelial and mesenchymal tissues
No scar tissue formation

adult, while others such as the immune system are poorly differentiated like a eutherian mammalian embryo. Moreover, marsupial embryos show very early tissue function such as suckling on the nipple and crawling from the vagina up the mother's fur, to attach to the nipple (see Fig. 6.1 in color section) by use of the precociously developed forelimb (Fig. 6.2a–d), while the pouch young embryos are generally 1–2°C lower in temperature compared to the mother.

Marsupial pouch young may therefore be advantageous for wound healing studies, not only because of easy accessibility (compared to the in utero development of eutherian mammalian embryos), but also because they possess a unique combination of fetal-like and adult-like extrinsic and intrinsic characteristics. This facilitates analysis of the relative importance of these factors in the differences between fetal and adult wound healing.

Why Marsupials?

The feature that most clearly distinguishes marsupials from most other mammals is the immaturity of their young at birth.[5] Only newly hatched monotremes such as the duck-billed platypus or echidna are as immature at birth, whereas even the most altricial young of eutherian mammals (bears and insectivores) are more advanced than any marsupial. In essence, marsupials have substituted lactation for placentation.

In eutherian mammals, the complex structure and function of the placenta interposed between the embryo and the mother throughout development makes it difficult to investigate the early development of physiological, neurological, and biochemical systems. Such problems do not apply to marsupials where the young

TABLE 6.2 Comparison of the Fetal Dermal Environment With That of the Adult

Moist healing in amniotic fluid, rich in growth (and other) factors
Uniform higher temperature
Less differentiated mesenchymal and epithelial cells
Skin less keratinized ± periderm
Extracellular matrix of dermis less spatially ordered
Rapid tissue turnover and growth
Immature fetal immune system
Lower tissue oxygenation
Decreased tissue function

are born at a much earlier stage of development (usually weighing at birth less than 0.01% of the mother's weight) and where numerous aspects of development occur in the easily accessible pouch environment.[5] Moreover, the simple yolk sac placenta of marsupial embryos means that they can be more successfully cultured in vitro.[6–9] In recent years, methods have been developed for growing rat and mouse embryos in whole embryo culture during early stages of organogenesis.[10] Unfortunately, such techniques do not allow embryos to be supported in vitro for long periods of time, nor to develop to late fetal stages or beyond.[10] The limiting factor is the failure of the complex allantoic placenta to develop in culture, thereby restricting nutrition to the embryo resulting in death. Marsupials do not have a complex allantoic placenta and rely almost entirely on a simple yolk sac placenta that grows well in culture.[6–9] In marsupials, such as the opossum, the allantois is present only as a simple sac that enlarges with urine during the last three days of gestation and probably has no placental function.[6,7] This means that marsupial embryos, unlike those of eutherian mammals, can be grown in vitro during all the later stages of organogenesis and, in theory, until the time the animal would normally be born. Paradoxically, there have been relatively few investigations of marsupial embryonic development in vitro.[6–9] Interestingly, techniques have been developed for the in vitro fertilization and culture of early marsupial embryos.[11] However, there appears to be a block in development around the four to eight cell stage in vitro corresponding to a time when development may normally be arrested in vivo.[5,8,9,11] If marsupial embryos are recovered just after this stage in vivo, then they can be cultured in vitro to developmental stages approximating those present at birth. Therefore, if this developmental arrest could be overcome in vitro, it ought to be possible to develop marsupial embryos in culture all the way from in vitro fertilization to birth. It may even be possible to place such embryos on the nipples of surrogate mothers to allow for their subsequent weaning and growth! Such strategies would make marsupials an extremely powerful system for experimentally investigating many aspects of mammalian development.

Moreover, the fact that much marsupial development occurs when the animal is attached to the mother's teat means that the importance of particular molecules in development can be determined by introducing them directly to the pouch young by placing a narrow oral-gastric cannula parallel to the nipple.[12,13] Analysis of the milk composition itself gives interesting insights into the biochemical and nutritional requirements of the developing marsupial.[12] The milks of eutherian mammalian species differ widely from each other but hardly change during the course of lactation, whereas the milk composition of all marsupials changes dramatically throughout the course of lactation.[12] The content of solids increases progressively, the carbohydrate content decreases, there is a reciprocal increase in lipid content, and a large number of subtle changes occur in individual molecules and fractions.[12] This changing composition of the milk reinforces a consensus that much of what is considered to be embryonic and fetal development in eutherian mammals occurs during the first phase of postnatal development in marsupials. The second phase of postnatal development in marsupials corresponds to weaning during the neonatal period of eutherian mammals.

The accessibility of the postnatal marsupial and its relatively poor state of development make it an unrivalled model for the experimental study of early development, including wound healing. Moreover, there is an asynchrony in the development of particular tissues and functions in marsupials compared to eutherian mammals, despite the extreme immaturity of most marsupial systems at birth. Paradoxically, the neonatal marsupial is better developed than its corresponding eutherian counterpart in specific tissues and systems. Thus, the locomotor system of the upper limb is sufficiently well developed to enable it to move, the general sensory system is well enough developed to enable it to locate a teat and attach, and the muscles of the tongue and oral cavity are sufficiently developed and coordinated to enable it to suckle (Figs. 6.1 and 6.2). Moreover, the lung is sufficiently mature to permit gaseous exchange, while the skull bones are sufficiently ossified both to provide attachments for functioning muscles and to protect the developing brain. All of these systems develop much earlier than the comparable stages of development in eutherian mammals.

By contrast, the newborn marsupial has very poor development of its brain and special sense organ systems.[14] Nearly the entire developmental programs for the neo-cortex and the primary visual pathways occur after birth,[15,16] the hind

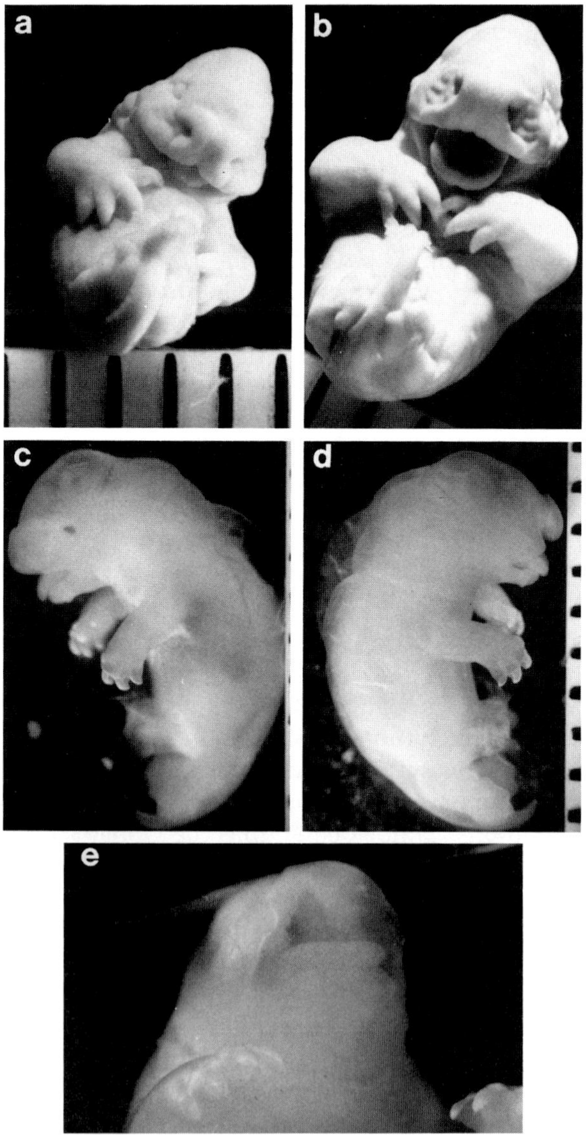

Figure 6.2 (a) Day 11 embryo of the marsupial *Didelphis virginiana.* Note the precocious development of the upper limb and hands, poorly developed eye, the well developed nostrils and protuberant tongue. mm scale. (b) Day 12 opossum *Didelphis virginiana* embryo (the day of birth). Note the well developed upper limb, poorly developed lower limb, large protuberant tongue and broad nasal region: the latter two facilitating attachment to the mother's nipple. mm scale. (c) Lateral view of a day 14 *Monodelphis domestica* embryo (the day of birth). Note the well developed upper limbs with ossified claws, the protuberant tongue and the under developed eye. (d) Lateral view of a day 14 embryonic *Monodelphis domestica* indicating a unilateral cleft in the upper lip. mm scale. (e) Higher power view of the unilateral cleft lip and palate of the day 14 *Monodelphis domestica* embryo, illustrated in (Fig. 6.2d).

limb is at a much earlier bud stage of development (Figs. 6.1 and 6.2), the skeleton in the caudal end of the embryo is poorly developed, the thyroid and other endocrine glands are poorly developed and a newborn marsupial is not homeothermic. Endothermy develops during pouch life unlike eutherian mammals where it is present at birth. Sexual differentiation has not occurred at birth while the secondary sexual characteristics of marsupials are genetically, rather than hormonally determined,[17,18] the immune system of the newborn marsupial is poorly developed and the animals are immunologically incompetent.[19] In general, the development of the marsupial thymus takes place almost entirely after birth, active immunological responses are not made until several days after birth, and there is a prolonged period during pouch life when antibodies from the mother's milk are absorbed through the gut, into the circulation of the pouch young to protect it by passive immunity.[19] This is in marked contrast to most eutherian mammals that have mature active immune responses at birth. From the above, it will be obvious that marsupials exhibit a cranio-caudal gradient at birth in terms of the state of tissue differentiation: the head in general being more advanced than the tail. This poses interesting problems in relation to differential growth: for example, the upper limb is well developed and at an advanced stage of differentiation, while the hind limb is extremely retarded (Fig. 6.2a–d); yet in the adult, both limbs are either the same size or the asymmetry is reversed with larger hind limbs (Fig. 6.1). Clearly, there is coordinated differential growth of the upper and lower limbs within the same hormonal milieu of the pouch young. Equally, although the skin of the newborn marsupial is heavily keratinized (to prevent dehydration in the extra uterine environment) the skin is highly transparent and very vascular, capillaries often lying within 100 microns of the surface.[20] Newborn marsupials appear bright red as a result (Fig. 6.1b). Moreover, this anatomical arrangement greatly facilitates the topical application of a number of compounds, e.g., hormones to the developing pouch young.[18]

Although marsupials offer major advantages for a variety of experimental investigations, owing to their easy accessibility during critical periods of development (so facilitating serial sampling of body fluids or tissues, surgery on the young without affecting the mother, and easy administration of test molecules, either topically or via the milk), nonetheless, they have been poorly exploited and investigated.[5] There are two possible reasons for this paradox. First, many investigators perceive marsupials as primitive mammals of no particular relevance to biomedical studies, and important only because they are rare, unusual, and therefore of phylogenic and conservation interest. Such a perception is based largely on ignorance. Second, many marsupials have proved difficult to maintain and breed in routine laboratory conditions. This latter obstacle has recently been overcome, largely by investigations of *Monodelphis domestica,* the gray short-tailed opossum from South America. This species has proved easy to keep under routine laboratory conditions[21] and major breeding colonies exist in the United States (Dr. J. L. Vandeberg, South West Foundation of Biomedical Research, San Antonio, Texas—1,500 animals) and in Europe (Professor M. W. J. Ferguson, University of Manchester—200 breeding pairs, Dr. H. Moore, Zoological Society of London—250 animals).

Monodelphis domestica as a Laboratory Animal

Monodelphis domestica is one of the American opossums in the superfamily Didelphoidea, which comprises a sizable array of living and fossil mammals.[22]

They are of particular interest to students of evolution and biology because some of the living taxa are thought to approximate many of the features seen in early therians (mammal-like reptiles) and they include the ancestral stem of the metatheria, representing the early stalk from which the diversification of American, European, and Australasian marsupials took place.

The Monodelphis short-tailed opossums are a polytypic genus of small, pouchless, terrestrial animals, ranging from Panama to the southern pampas of Argentina.[22] They inhabit open grasslands, savanna, and dense forests: *Monodelphis domestica* derives its specific name from its habit of frequenting human habitations where it is normally welcomed because it feeds on rodent and insect pests. All species feed on small rodents, insects, fruits, seeds and carion.[21,22] Seventeen living species of Monodelphis are recognized, including *Monodelphis domestica*.[22] Monodelphis is nocturnal and outside human dwellings is terrestrial or semi-arboreal, reportedly living near water and building nests among rocks and in hollow logs.[21] The short tail, which characterizes all members of the genus, is slightly prehensile and used for carrying nesting material and for support during climbing.

Adult *Monodelphis domestica* have a head and body length of 170–200 mm with an additional tail length of 60–80 mm (Fig. 6.1). Adult males weigh 90–155 g and females 80–100 g. Their fur is grayish-brown in color, with lighter ventral coverings (Fig. 6.1). In both the wild and captivity, *Monodelphis domestica* breed throughout the year and produce litters of approximately four to 12 offspring. Monodelphis is a pouchless genus and the neonates and juveniles (collectively referred to as pouch young in keeping with general marsupial terminology) at first adhere directly to the underside of the mother's belly attached to the teats but later often ride on the dam's back, clinging to her fur (Fig. 6.1). The animals can be successfully maintained and bred for a number of generations in captivity under housing and feeding regimes not terribly different from normal laboratory rodents.[21]

Breeding occurs throughout the year in captivity and the specific activities observed at various points during the mating routine have been extensively described.[24] The oestrus cycle in *Monodelphis domestica* is approximately 28 days and oestrus can be induced in mature females by a system of pairing with an unfamiliar male.[21,23] Ovulation occurs about 18 hours after first mating and video recording of the behavioral events at this time allows for the recovery of known-age embryos.[23] The in utero gestation period is 14–15 days after which the mother gives birth to a litter of 5–12 offspring. The newborn opossums are 8–10 mm long and weigh less than one hundreth of a gram (Figs. 6.1 and 6.2). They are bright red and quickly climb up the mother's abdomen to attach to her teats, often in a circular cluster (Fig. 6.1). The advanced development of the cranial end of the newborn (coinciding with the need for teat attachment, suckling, coordinated crawling movements, and olfaction) is evidenced by ossification in the mandible and several skull bones, advanced middle-ear development, precociously developed forearms with ossified claws that grab the mother's fur and often puncture her skin (Figs. 6.1 and 6.2). Conversely, the caudal end of the embryo is poorly developed with characteristic paddle-shaped limbs and pendulum-like rump. The oral and nasal cavities are separated by a well-developed palate and the nostrils are flattened, facilitating simultaneous breathing and suckling while attached on the nipple (Fig. 6.2). The young remain continuously attached to the nipples for about two weeks (by which time they weigh 2–3 g). After this initial period, the young continue to nurse, but will detach from the nipples and either re-attach spontaneously or with the assistance of the mother. Detached pouch young monodelphis emit a high-pitched squeaking noise, attracting the mother's attention. The young begin to wean and eat solid food at approximately four to five weeks after birth and can be separated from the mother around seven weeks after birth. The precise sequence of events at the time of birth in macropodid marsupials has been described,[25] but not in the same detail for monodelphis. Cleft lip and palate occur spontaneously and can be teratogenically induced in *Monodelphis domestica* (Fig. 6.2d and e).

For the reasons outlined earlier, we investigated incisional dermal wound healing in pouch young monodelphis, aged two, 14, and 28 days and compared it with healing in adult male animals, at least 16 months old. The purpose of these investigations was to determine the nature of the wound healing response in the early pouch young monodelphis and specifically to investigate if this was of the fetal scar-free variety.

Materials and Methods

Wounding Technique

Female *Monodelphis domestica* with litters aged two and 14 days were anaesthetized using halothane/nitrous oxide/oxygen ventilation before surgery was performed on their young. Females with litters aged 28 days were sedated by injecting 0.04 ml ketamine intramuscularly; the pouch young were then separated from the mother and anaesthetized using halothane/nitrous oxide/oxygen ventilation before surgery. Adult male *Monodelphis domestica* were locally shaved after inhalational anesthesia. Full thickness linear incisions were created longitudinally down the lateral sides of both flanks in the pouch young and adults. The incisions went to the depth of the Panniculus carnosus muscle and were approximately 0.5 cm long in the two and 14 day pouch young and 1 cm long in the 28 day pouch young and the adult. Wounds were neither sutured nor covered.

Specimen Preparation

Pouch young and adults were killed by chloroform overdose at the time of surgery and one to seven and 28 days postoperatively. The two wounds and the surrounding skin were excised. Normal unwounded skin was also excised from several control animals. One specimen was fixed in 10% formal saline, dehydrated, and embedded in paraffin wax, followed by serial sectioning at 6 microns and staining with hematoxylin and eosin, Weigert's iron hematoxylin and Van Gieson or Mallory's trichrome. The other specimen of intact skin and wound tissue was frozen in OCT compound using liquid nitrogen, stored at −80°C and serially sectioned at 7 microns using a cryostat. These sections were then immunocytochemically stained, using antibodies to laminin, fibronectin, tenascin, chondroitin sulphate, and collagen types I, III, VI. The antibodies and procedures used are identical to those described in Chapter 10. In addition, specimens were stained for leukocytes and macrophages, using antibodies against the common leukocyte antigen and macrophage specific markers (Serotec). Frozen sections were also used to demonstrate alkaline phosphatase activity histochemically and the orientation of collagen fibers using polarizing microscopy.

Quantifications

Leukocytes and macrophages were identified using a ×25 objective lens on the microscope and the total number of positive cells in at least 10 spaced histological sections counted. The results were expressed as total average number per slide, plus or minus a standard deviation. Quantitative evaluation of wound re-epithelialization was performed as shown in Fig. 6.3.[26] A measure of the degree of scarring was obtained using microspectrophotometry. Histological sections of re-epithelialized wounds stained with Mallory's trichrome were selected. The intensity of methyl blue staining in these sections was determined using a Leitz microspectrophotometer.[27] The microspectrophotometer measurements of the absorbancy of methyl blue dye were taken using a 617 nanometre filter (maximum absorbancy of methyl blue dye occurs at 620 nanometres). 100% transmission was determined in clear regions adjacent to each section. The area of the mi-

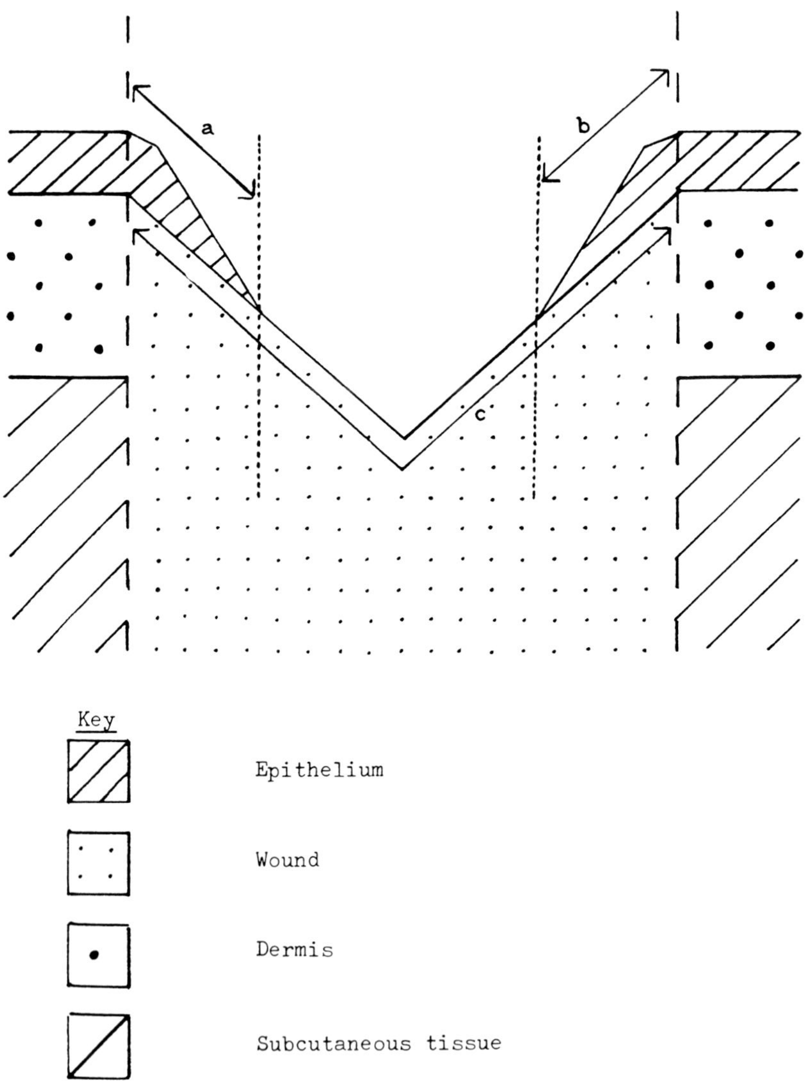

Figure 6.3 Diagram illustrating the quantitative evaluation of wound re-epithelialization. In every fifth section, the total length of the wound (C) and the length of the epithelialized surfaces (A,B) are measured using an image analyzer. The percentage re-epithelialization equals $[a + b)/c] \times 100$.

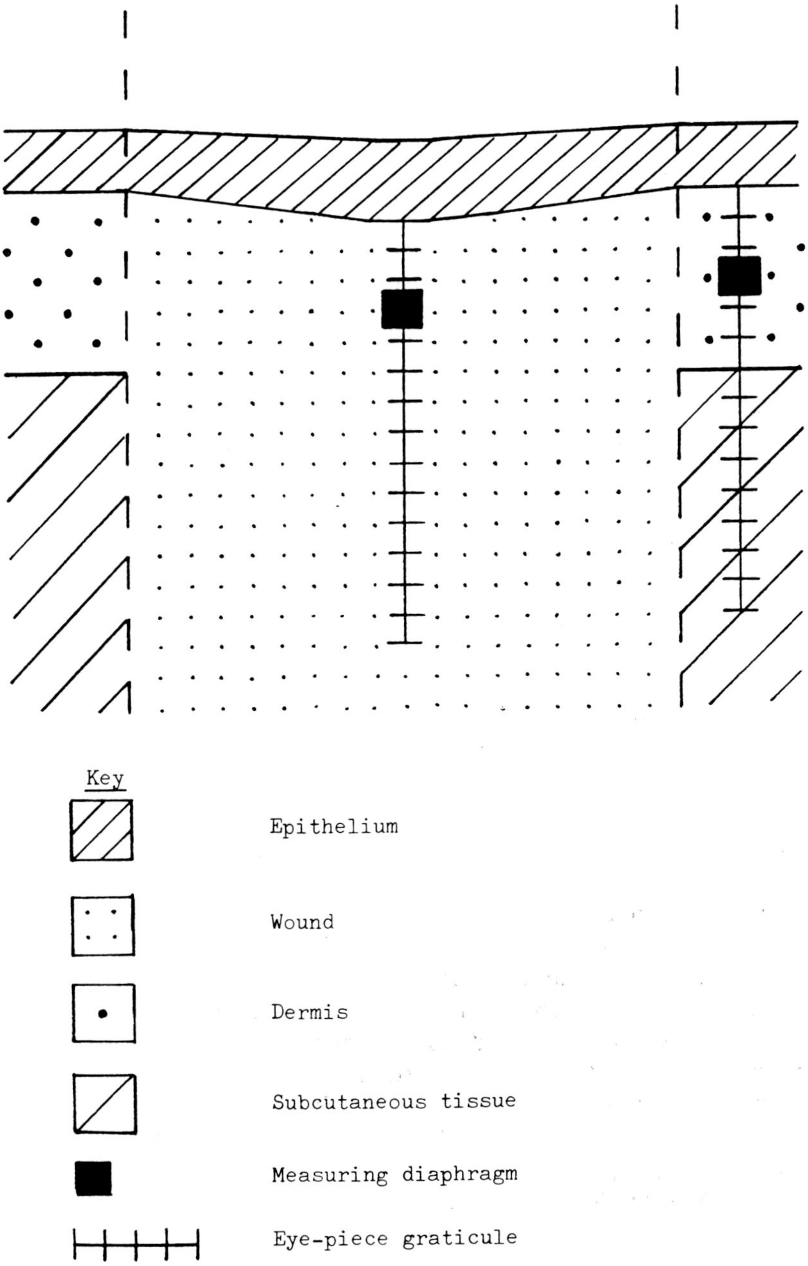

Figure 6.4 Diagram illustrating the quantitative evaluation of methyl blue staining by the scar tissue and adjacent normal tissue using microspectrophotometry.

crospectrophotometer measuring diaphragm was 80 square microns. Within any given section, the measuring diaphragm was placed at increasing distances from the epithelium in both the wound area and the adjacent intact skin (Fig. 6.4). Characteristic absorption values for each re-epithelialized wound were obtained from at least 10 sections. The absorbancy measurements within the intact skin were divided by those of the wounded area at the same distance from the epithelium (Fig. 6.4). A ratio of one indicated an absence of scar tissue. The average value of this ratio at different levels within the sections was plotted against the percentage distance of the measurement from the epithelium. This analysis depends critically on the binding of methyl blue dye being linearly related to the concentration of collagen and proteoglycans and on the absorbancy measurements being an accurate reflection of dye concentrations. These prerequisites were established in preliminary experiments where drops of serially diluted known concentrations of rattail collagen and proteoglycans were air dried onto slides, fixed, stained using the same protocol, and then measured using the microspectrophotometer. A linear relationship was established.

RESULTS

Although there is no pouch in *Monodelphis domestica,* we will follow the marsupial convention of referring to the animals attached to the mother's teat as pouch young.

Normal Development of the Skin

The morphology of the skin of *Monodelphis domestica* changes markedly during the four to five weeks on the nipple. In both pouch young and adult the skin is very lax and not firmly attached to the underlying tissue.

At birth, the skin is heavily keratinized and there is little subsequent increase in the number of keratin layers. However, the skin thickens considerably: the skin of day two pouch young is 0.18 mm thick, increasing in thickness threefold to 0.51 mm by pouch day 35. As the epidermis of day two pouch young is composed of approximately six to seven cell layers and the thickness of the epidermis hardly alters; the increase in thickness of the skin reflects the development of the dermis and subcutaneous tissues.

In one to nine day old pouch young, the dermis constitutes approximately 40% of the total skin thickness. The dermis is predominantly cellular, the mesenchymal cells being separated by a fine reticular matrix of predominantly type III collagen. The dermis is very homogeneous and neither dermal appendages nor hair follicles have developed. The dermis is well delineated from the subcutaneous tissue, blood vessels predominating at the junction between these two regions. By pouch day 14, the dermis, though still cellular, has a greatly increased content of collagen, the reticular and papillary regions are distinguishable, and dermal appendages and hair follicles are beginning to form.

In later pouch young (day 21–35) the dermis represents only 35% of the total cutaneous thickness. The density of cells within the dermis decreases gradually, the collagen content increases, and the collagen is arranged into larger fibers, reflecting the higher content of type I collagen. The hair follicles continue to develop and increase in density, as do the sebaceous glands which form around the bases of the hair follicles. White adipose tissue begins to accumulate in the subcutaneous tissues.

Wound Healing

Survival

Only 40% of the day two and day 14 pouch young survived the surgical procedures: death was due entirely to maternal cannibalism of the wounded young; 75% of the day 28 pouch young and 100% of the adults survived the surgical procedures.

Wound healing is very different in the early day two pouch young *Monodelphis domestica,* compared with the older day 28 pouch young and the adult. Day two pouch young wounds were nearly completely healed within two days after surgery and there was no apparent scar formation. By contrast, the day 28 pouch young and the adult wounds were nearly completely healed by seven days postsurgery and the residual scar persisted after injury.

Scab Formation

The skin wound was evident in both the pouch young and adult animals. Microscopic observations revealed that the scissors had created full thickness skin wounds, involving the epidermis, dermis, and subcutaneous tissues down to the level of the panniculus carnosus muscle. The wound breach was filled with hemorrhagic debris in both the adult and pouch young. One day after surgery, a macroscopic scab was evident on the surface of all pouch young and adult wounds. Immunocytochemistry revealed the scab to consist of erythrocytes embedded within a network of fibrin and fibronectin. In the day two pouch young, two days after surgery, the scab was firm, dry, and proud of the skin surface. In the day 28 pouch young, the scab was present two days after surgery, but had sloughed off the surface by seven days after wounding. In the adult, seven days after wounding, the scab was still present in a deep epithelialized furrow at the wound site (see Fig. 6.5 in color section).

Inflammation

Gross observations of the adult, day 14 and day 28 pouch young wounds revealed a wheal one day after surgery: a similar swelling was not present in the day two pouch young at any time.

The microscopic appearance of the day two pouch young one day after surgery showed a minimal inflammatory response characterized by occasional neutrophils, a few monocytes, lymphocytes, and macrophages (Table 6.3). Two days after wounding, the number of inflammatory cells at the injury site had decreased markedly with only a few macrophages being evident (Table 6.3). Thereafter, the density of inflammatory cells, including macrophages, was similar to the surrounding tissue.

TABLE 6.3 The Total Number of Leukocytes and Macrophages in Adult and Pouch Young Wounds Identified by Immunohistochemistry

Age	Time After Injury (Days)	No. of Leukocytes	Standard Deviation	No. of Macrophages	Standard Deviation
2 Days	1	8	3	3	1
	2	4	3	5	1
28 Days	1	482	23	16	3
	2	1021	41	56	9
	7	28	8	20	4
Adult	1	419	21	13	3
	2	821	31	39	7
	7	26	8	28	6

By contrast, an extensive inflammatory response was evident in both the day 28 pouch young and the adult wounds one day after surgery (Table 6.3). The connective tissue at the wound base was heavily infiltrated by neutrophils, monocytes, and lymphocytes and the subadjacent dermis showed a moderate infiltration by inflammatory cells. Two days after surgery, the number of inflammatory cells at the wound site had increased markedly and macrophages were very evident. By seven days after surgery, the inflammatory infiltrate had largely resolved, although macrophages were still evident. The number of leukocytes within the day 28 pouch young and adult wounds approximately doubles between one and two days after surgery and macrophages become an increasing proportion of the total number of inflammatory cells. If anything, the number of inflammatory cells in the day 28 pouch young wounds exceeds those in the adult. Both have over 200 times the number of inflammatory cells at the wound site, two days after wounding, by comparison with the day two pouch young.

Wound Contraction

Grossly, one day after surgery, the wounds in both the day two and day 14 pouch young gaped and were oval in shape. Two days after surgery, in the day two pouch young, the scab lay proud of the skin surface and the skin around the incision appeared stretched, suggesting that wound contraction had occurred. By comparison, one day after surgery, the day 28 pouch young and adult wounds were open but did not gape; neither did they display any evidence of macroscopic wound contraction until seven days after injury.

Re-epithelialization

Microscopic observations revealed very rapid re-epithelialization of the skin wounds in the day two pouch young by comparison with the day 28 pouch young or adult (Table 6.4). One day after wounding in the day two pouch young, the epithelial cells at the wound edges were thickened, but little cell migration had occurred. After two days, the wounds were completely re-epithelialized, the epithelial cells having migrated across the defect and the scab having been lifted above the level of the skin surface. At the lesion site, the epidermis was approximately eight to nine cell layers thick (Fig. 6.5a). In both the day 28 pouch young

TABLE 6.4 Data on the Time for Complete Re-epithelialization of Wounds in the Adult and Pouch Young Aged 2 and 28 Days

Age	Time After Injury (Days)	% Re-epithelialization	Standard Deviation
2 Days	2	100	—
28 Days	1	15.6	1.2
	2	29.6	3.3
	7	100	—
Adult	1	16.4	2.8
	2	33.9	2.3
	7	100	—

and the adult wounds, there was little evidence of epithelial cell thickening or proliferation at the wound margins. Rather, single epithelial cells were evident, migrating between the nonviable tissue and the underlying connective tissue, one to two days after wounding. Seven days after wounding, the day 28 pouch young and adult wounds were completely re-epithelialized. The epidermis covering the wound was thicker than that of the adjacent intact skin and lacked rete pegs (Fig. 6.5b and c). In the day 28 pouch young, the epidermis covering the wound was at a similar level to that of the adjacent intact skin, by comparison to the deep re-epithelialized furrow present in the adult wounds seven days after surgery (Fig. 6.5).

Extracellular Matrix Molecules

Fibronectin

Normally, fibronectin is more abundant in the day two pouch young dermis (Figure 6.6a) than in the older pouch young or adult skin (Fig. 6.6b and c). In the day two pouch young skin, fibronectin is diffusely distributed throughout the dermis (Fig. 6.6a) whereas in the later pouch young and adult skin, as the dermal papillae form, fibronectin is associated with the collagen fibrils in the papillary dermis and to a lesser extent with those in the reticular dermis (Figs. 6.6b and c). Fibronectin is prominent at the epidermal-dermal junction and in the basement membranes of the hair follicles and blood vessels. The epidermis stains negative for fibronectin, but there is cross reactivity with the secondary antibody, probably due to maternal immunoglobulins in the epithelium (Fig. 6.6h). In the day two pouch young wounds, fibronectin was evident within the fibrin clot in the newly formed wound. It further accumulated at the wound site during the first day after surgery and its accumulation paralleled the recruitment of mesenchymal cells to the wound site (Fig. 6.6d). By two days after wounding, in the day two pouch young, the fibronectin had a similar pattern of distribution (Fig. 6.6e) to the normal skin (Fig. 6.6a), although the staining was slightly more intense and was additionally present in the fibrin of the scab. In the day 28 pouch young and adult wounds, fibronectin was absent from the wound site, except for its appearance in the fibrin clot, until two days after surgery. By seven days after surgery, the wound site was clearly stained for fibronectin (Figs. 6.6f and g). This fibronectin persisted longer, and moreover, was abnormally orientated by comparison with the day two pouch young. It lay essentially at right angles to the epidermal-dermal junction in keeping with the alignment of the scar tissue collagen fibrils.

Laminin

Laminin is normally localized to the basement membranes of the epidermis, hair follicles, and blood vessels (Figs. 6.7a and b). In all wounds, the basement membrane reformed after re-epithelialization of the defect. Laminin, by marking the basement membranes of the vascular endothelium, illustrated the virtual absence of angiogenesis in the day two pouch young wounds by comparison with the extensive angiogenesis in the day 28 pouch young and adult wounds (Fig. 6.7c). Twenty-eight days after wounding in the day 28 pouch young and adult wounds, these capillaries showed some regression to the normal pattern and there was evidence of limited new hair follicle formation.

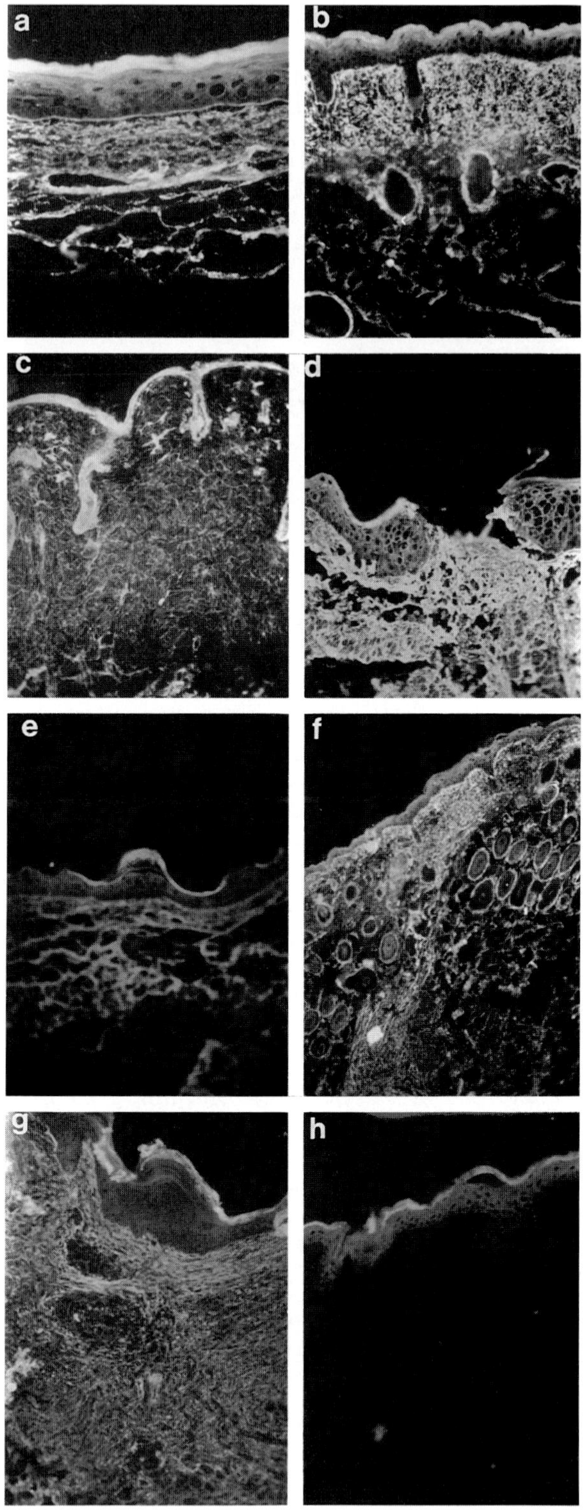

Figure 6.6 Distribution of fibronectin in the intact skin of (a) day 3 pouch young (b) day 16 pouch young (c) adult *Monodelphis domestica*. (d) Fibronectin staining throughout the wound one day postoperatively in a day 2 pouch young. (e) Normal pattern of fibronectin staining 2 days postoperatively in a day 2 pouch young wound. (f) Fibronectin staining throughout the wound in a day 28 pouch young, seven days postoperatively. Note the abnormal orientation of the fibronectin, perpendicular to the basement membrane. (g) Abnormal distribution of fibronectin throughout the entire wound in an adult *Monodelphis domestica* 7 days postoperatively. (h) Control staining with secondary antibody alone, illustrating cross reactivity with the epithelium.

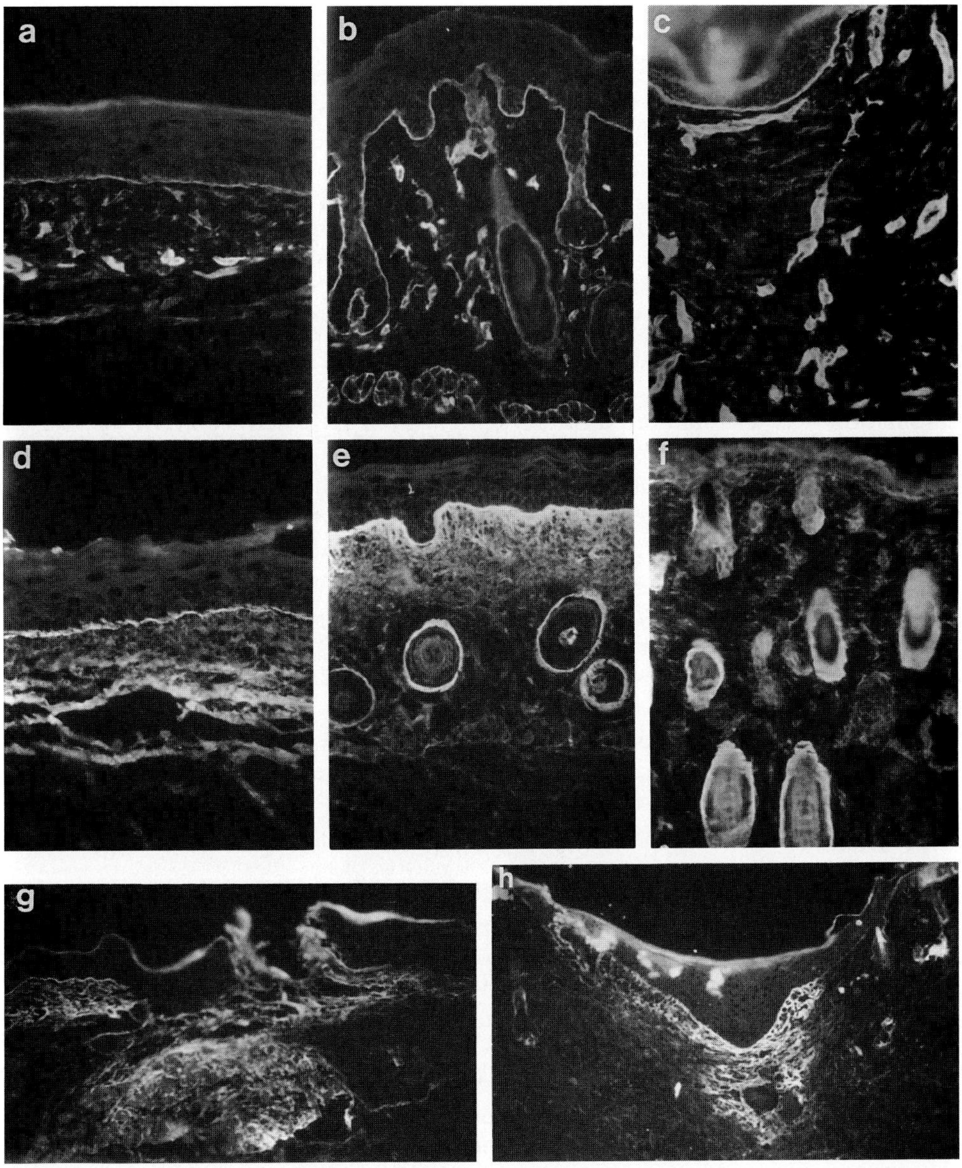

Figure 6.7 (a) Laminin distribution in the basement membrane and dermis of the normal skin of a day 4 pouch young. (b) Laminin distribution in the basement membrane of the epidermis, hair follicles, and capillaries in a day 15 pouch young. (c) Laminin staining in an adult dermal wound seven days postoperatively, illustrating extensive angiogenesis as evidenced by staining in the basement membranes of newly formed capillaries. (d) Distribution of tenascin in the normal dermis and basement membrane of day 4 pouch young skin. (e) Distribution of tenascin in the intact skin of a day 14 pouch young. Note the increased staining in the future papillary dermis, epidermal, and hair follicle basement membranes. (f) Distribution of tenascin in the intact skin of a day 28 pouch young, illustrating its restriction to the basement membranes of the epidermis, hair follicles, and some capillaries. (g) Day 2 pouch young wound stained for tenascin on the first day postoperatively, illustrating accumulation at the wound margins, and in the dermis beneath the wound. (h) Adult wound 7 days postoperatively stained for tenascin, showing an abnormal accumulation in the epidermal basement membrane and subadjacent dermis of the re-epithelialized wound site.

Tenascin

In day two pouch young, tenascin is normally located in the basement membrane and dermis of the normal skin (Fig. 6.7d). This pattern persists during the expansion of the dermis in the first two weeks of pouch life, and staining is particularly intense around the developing hair follicles, dermal appendages, and capillaries (Fig. 6.7e). In the day 28 pouch young and adult, tenascin is almost completely confined to the basement membrane of the dermal-epidermal junction, capillaries, and hair follicles (Figure 6.7f). The distribution of tenascin in all healing wounds was similar, but its time course of appearance and disappearance was markedly different. In the day two pouch young wounds, tenascin was abundant within the wound area and extended some distances from the wound margins, one day after surgery (Fig. 6.7g). However, by two days after surgery, this accumulation was less marked and the skin showed its normal pattern (as in Fig. 6.7d). Tenascin did not appear in the day 14 pouch young wounds until one day after surgery and in the day 28 pouch young and adult wounds until two days after surgery. At those times, tenascin staining was intense at the wound surface and in the dermis at the wound edge below the migrating epithelium. In the day 28 pouch young wounds, tenascin had reverted to its normal location at the dermal-epidermal junction seven days after wounding but staining was more intense in this region while the newly formed blood vessels in the granulation tissue, identified by laminin staining, were negative. By contrast, adult wounds seven days after wounding showed a continued widespread accumulation of tenascin throughout the granulation tissue beneath the reformed epidermis (Fig. 6.7h), the normal distribution not being restored until some 28 days after wounding.

Type I Collagen

Type I collagen was evenly distributed throughout the normal dermis of the day 2 pouch young (as in Fig. 6.8b). However, as the dermal appendages begin to form, type I collagen staining becomes more extensive in the reticular dermis compared to the papillary dermis, a pattern that persists into adulthood (Fig. 6.8a).

In the day two pouch young, collagen I fibrils were sparse at the wound site one day after surgery. However, by two days after surgery, both the pattern and distribution of type I collagen fibers were identical to those in the adjacent normal skin (Fig. 6.8b). In the day 28 pouch young and adult wounds, collagen type I did not appear until seven days after wounding. In these re-epithelialized wounds, the type I collagen fibers were orientated perpendicular to the wound axis and there was an increased intensity of type I collagen staining compared to the adjacent normal skin (Fig. 6.8c), by contrast to the day two pouch young. This abnormal accumulation and orientation of type I collagen fibers persisted.

Type III Collagen

In general, the distribution of type III collagen in the normal skin and within the healing wounds was similar to that of type I collagen, except that type III collagen appeared earlier. In the day two pouch young wounds, type III collagen was present in the wound area one day after surgery. Fibrils had a reticular basket weave orientation being particularly prominent along the wound edges. By two days after surgery, the type III collagen fibrils were parallel to the reformed epidermis and the distribution and intensity of type III collagen were identical to that of the normal adjacent skin (Fig. 6.8d). By contrast, type III collagen was

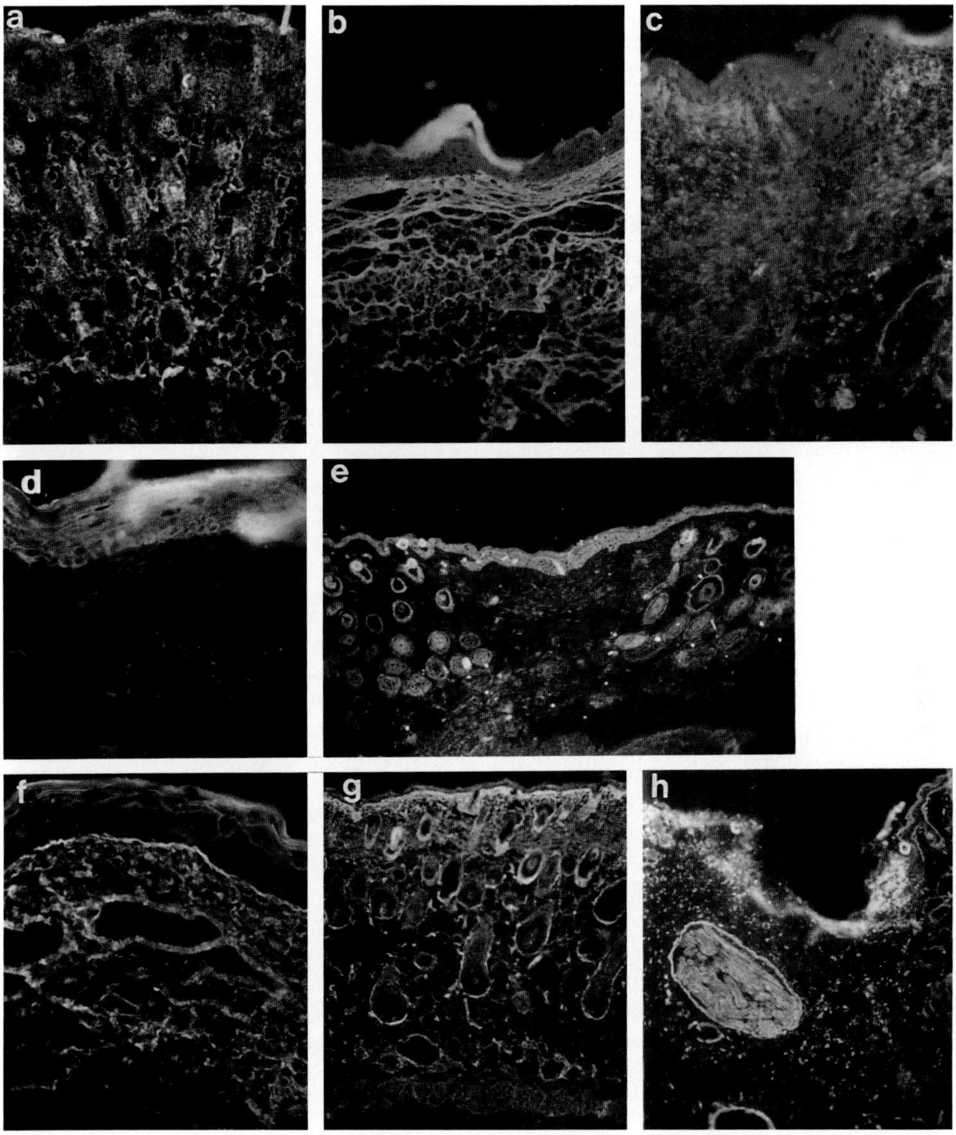

Figure 6.8 (a) Distribution of type I collagen in the intact skin of an adult *Monodelphis domestica*, illustrating the basketweave appearance in the dermis and the honeycomb appearance in the subcutaneous tissues. (b) Day 2 pouch young wound, two days postoperatively, showing a restitution of the normal pattern of type I collagen staining in the dermis and subcutaneous tissues. Note the scab above the wound site which auto-fluoresces. (c) Day 28 pouch young wound, seven days postoperatively, stained for type I collagen, illustrating deposition at the wound margins and in the wound site in an abnormal orientation perpendicular to the basement membrane. (d) Day 2 pouch young wound, two days postoperatively stained for collagen type III and co-stained with a pan cytokeratin antibody. Note the normal distribution of type III collagen in a horizontal lattice, parallel to the basement membrane. (e) Adult wound seven days postoperatively stained for type III collagen and co-stained with a pan cytokeratin antibody. Note the accumulation of type III collagen at the wound site and the loss of hair follicles. (f) Distribution of collagen type VI in the intact skin of a day 3 pouch young Monodelphis. Note the localization in the basement membrane and dermis. (g) Distribution of collagen type VI in the intact skin of a day 28 pouch young, illustrating its localization at the epidermal junction, and in the basement membrane, surrounding the hair follicles. (h) Adult wound one day postoperatively stained for collagen type VI. Note the accumulation at the wound margin and the speckled appearance within the body of the wound.

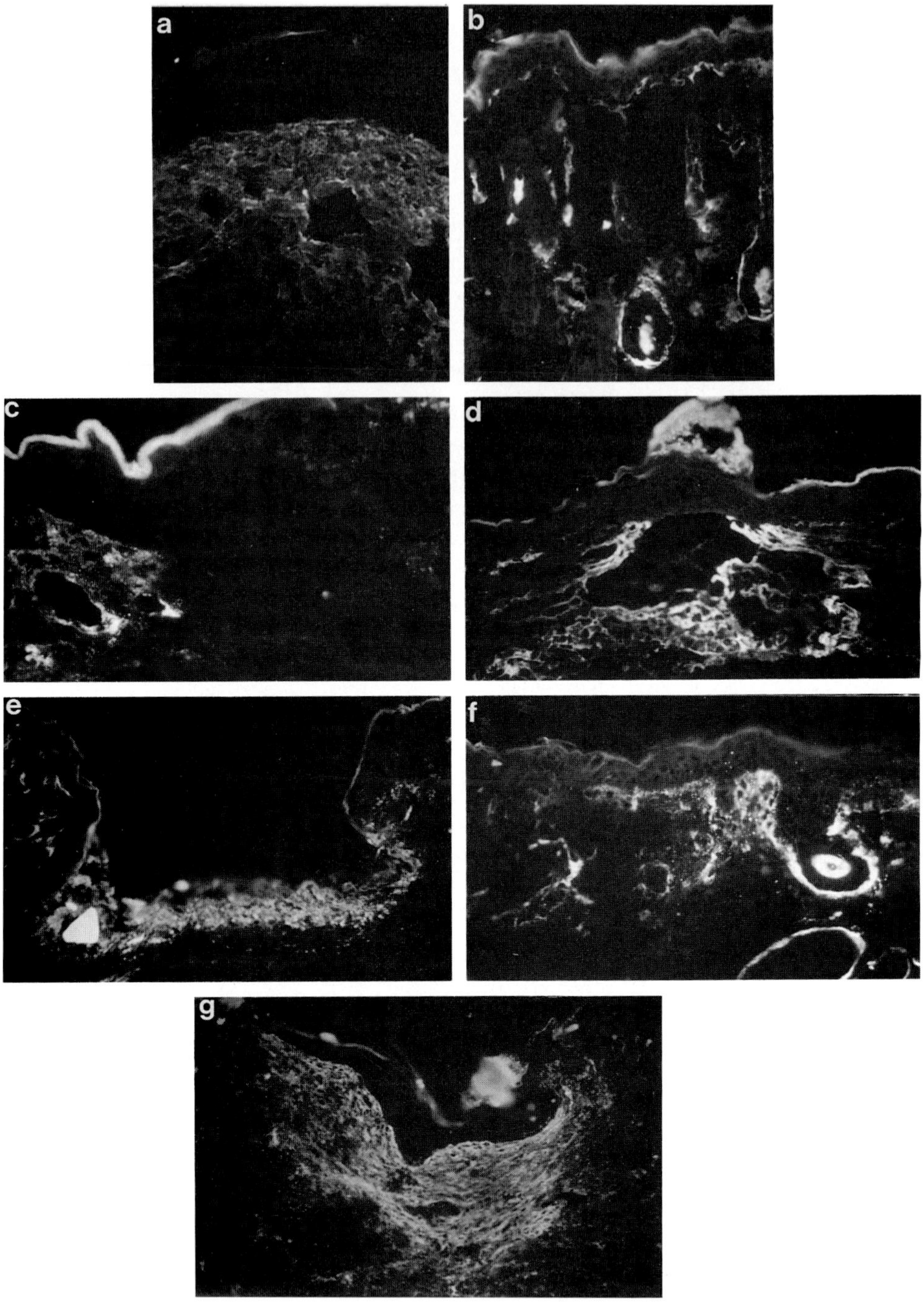

Figure 6.9 (a) Distribution of chondroitin sulphate in the intact skin of a day 3 pouch young, illustrating its localization in the dermis. (b) Distribution of chondroitin sulphate in the intact skin of a day 28 pouch young, illustrating its restriction to the basement membranes of the epidermis hair follicles and some capillaries. (c) Day 2 pouch young wound, one day postoperatively, illustrating chondroitin sulphate accumulation at the wound edges. (d) Day 2 pouch young wound, two days postoperatively, illustrating the accumulation of chondroitin sulphate throughout the wound dermis. (e) Day 28 pouch young wound, one day postoperatively, illustrating the distribution of chondroitin sulphate at the wound margins and the wound base. (f)

not present in the day 28 pouch young or adult wounds until two days after surgery. By seven days after surgery, the type III collagen staining of the wound site was more intense than that of the surrounding skin and the fibrils were orientated in a direction perpendicular to the basement membrane, particularly in the reticular dermis (Fig. 6.7e). By 28 days after wounding, the intensity of type III collagen staining was reduced.

Type VI Collagen

Type VI collagen was normally localized in the dermis of the day two pouch young, predominantly in the papillary dermis of the day 28 pouch young and adult and intensely in the basement membranes of the epidermis and hair follicles at all ages (Figs. 6.8f and g). In all wounds, type VI collagen appeared one day following surgery as faint stipples within the extracellular matrix of the wound site and intensely beneath the dermis of the wound margins and the re-epithelializing epidermal cells (Fig. 6.8h). Despite this similarity of onset, the normal pattern of type VI collagen staining was restored within two days in the day two pouch young wounds, whereas in the day 28 pouch young and adult wounds, an abnormal accumulation of type VI collagen in the developing scar tissue was present at and after 28 days following wounding.

Chondroitin Sulphate

In the day two pouch young, chondroitin sulphate is fairly uniformly distributed throughout the dermis (Fig. 6.9a), whereas, in the day 28 pouch young and adult, it is restricted to the basement membranes of the epidermis, hair follicles, and capillaries (Fig. 6.9b).

In the day two pouch young, chondroitin sulphate is intensely localized at the wound margins in the dermis beneath the epithelium (Fig. 6.9c). Staining also appears in a stippled fashion within the wound matrix. Two days after wounding in the day 2 pouch young, chondroitin sulphate staining was more extensive in the reformed dermis at the wound site compared to the control adjacent skin (Fig. 6.9d).

In the day 28 pouch young and adult wounds, chondroitin sulphate also accumulated at the wound margins and in the stippled fashion within the wound one day after surgery (Fig. 6.9e). In the day 28 pouch young, seven days after wounding, chondroitin sulphate was restricted to the basement membrane of the re-epithelialized wound and adjacent dermis, although the staining pattern and intensity were different from normal (Figs. 6.9b, f). Subsequently, chondroitin sulphate became restricted to the basement membrane regions as per normal (Fig. 6.9b). In the adult wound, chondroitin sulphate remained widely distributed throughout the wound site and the wound margins, seven days after wounding (Fig. 6.9g). After 28 days, the chondroitin sulphate pattern was essentially similar to normal.

←

Day 28 pouch young wound, seven days postoperatively, illustrating the accumulation of chondroitin sulphate at the dermal epidermal junction of the wound site. (g) Adult wound, seven days postoperatively, illustrating the extensive accumulation of chondroitin sulphate at the margins of the wound and in the healing wound matrix.

Scar Formation

Intensity of Collagen Staining

Microscopic observation of re-epithelialized wounds revealed an absence of scarring in the day 2 pouch young wounds, compared with prominent scar tissue formation in the day 28 pouch young and adult wounds (Figs. 6.5a–c). Two days after wounding, in the day two pouch young, there was re-epithelialization, reformation of the basement membrane, while mesenchymal cells were denser toward the epidermis than deeper in the wound, and blood vessels had reformed at the dermal subcutaneous junction (Fig. 6.5a). The connective tissue deposited at the wound site had a similar structure and orientation to that of the normal intact skin. The only remaining indication of the lesion site was the slight thickening of the epidermis and a scab on the wound surface. Microspectrophotometric analysis (Fig. 6.10) showed an absorbancy ratio less than one in the dermal tissues (40% of the cutaneous thickness) indicating that the intensity of collagen at the wound site was still below normal. However, in the subcutaneous tissues, the absorbancy ratio was not significantly different from one, indicating the absence of scar tissue formation and a similar intensity of collagen deposition (Fig. 6.10).

By contrast, microscopic observation of the day 28 pouch young and adult wounds, seven and 28 days after surgery revealed intensive scarring (Figs. 6.9b and c). Seven days after wounding, the scar tissue was characterized by an accumulation of fibroblasts, blood vessels, and a dense collagenous connective tissue matrix. Sweat glands and hair follicles were absent. By 28 days after wounding, fibroblasts and blood vessels were at a similar density to those of the surrounding skin and some hair follicle regeneration had occurred. Sweat glands

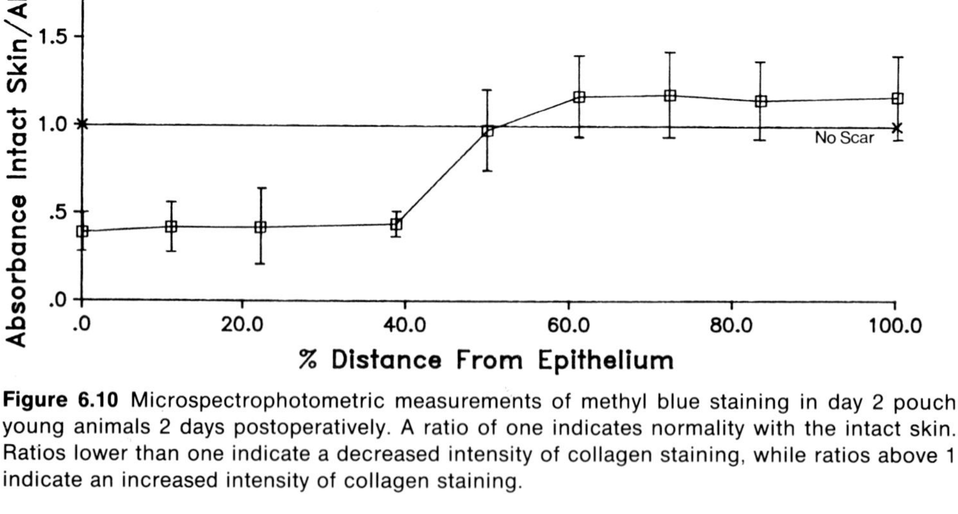

Figure 6.10 Microspectrophotometric measurements of methyl blue staining in day 2 pouch young animals 2 days postoperatively. A ratio of one indicates normality with the intact skin. Ratios lower than one indicate a decreased intensity of collagen staining, while ratios above 1 indicate an increased intensity of collagen staining.

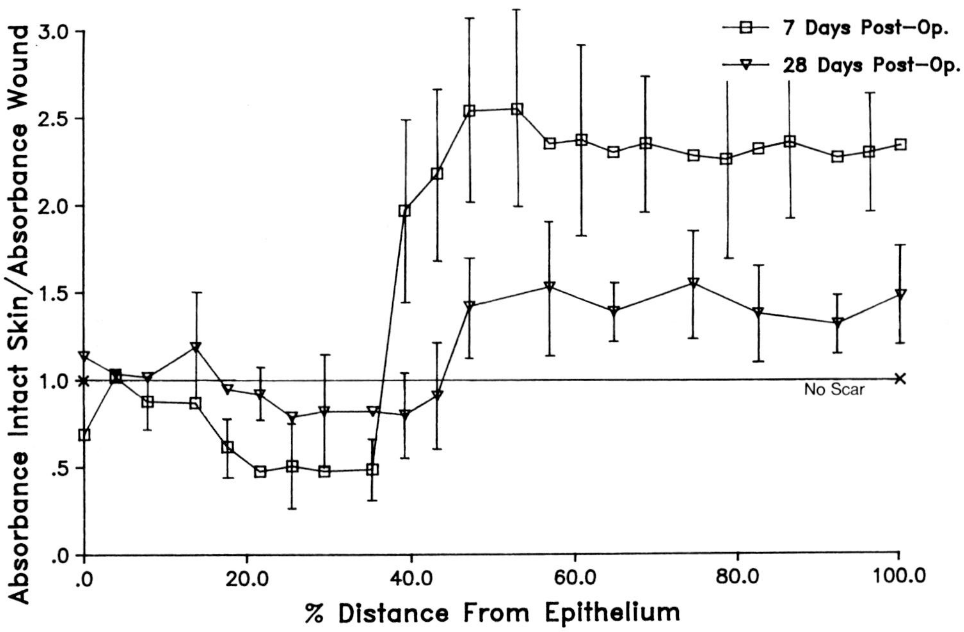

Figure 6.11 Microspectrophotometric measurements of methyl blue staining in day 28 pouch young animals, 7 and 28 days postoperatively. See Figure 6.10.

were absent and the connective tissue matrix was much denser than that of the normal skin, especially in the subcutaneous region of the wound (Figs. 6.5b and c). Microspectrophotometric measurements of the absorbancy ratio showed that at seven days postoperatively, the intensity of collagen staining in the dermal region (approximately 35% of the total cutaneous thickness) was less than normal. However, by 28 days postoperatively, values were closer to unity, indicating a similar intensity of collagen staining in the dermal region (Fig. 6.11). By contrast, at both postoperative times, the intensity of collagen staining in the subcutaneous region was much greater than in the surrounding normal tissue (Fig. 6.11). Although the intensity of staining decreased between seven and 28 days postoperatively, it still remained statistically significantly higher than normal in both the day 28 (Fig. 6.11) and adult (Fig. 6.12) wounds. These tracings confirm the prominent scarring in the subcutaneous regions (Figure 9b) of day 28 pouch young and adult wounds.

Orientation of Collagen

When viewed under polarized light, sections of normal pouch young and adult skin show a basketweave-like arrangement of the collagen fibers in the dermal extracellular matrix (Fig. 6.13a) and a hexagonal arrangement in the subcutaneous tissues (Fig. 6.13b). When polarized light was passed through the dermis and subcutaneous tissues, the emitted light showed an increase in brightness or birefringence, which did not alter when the tissues were rotated through 45°.

Analysis of the day two pouch young wounds, two days after surgery, using polarized light confirmed the absence of scar tissue formation (Fig. 6.13c). The extracellular matrix was identically organized to that of the adjacent intact skin

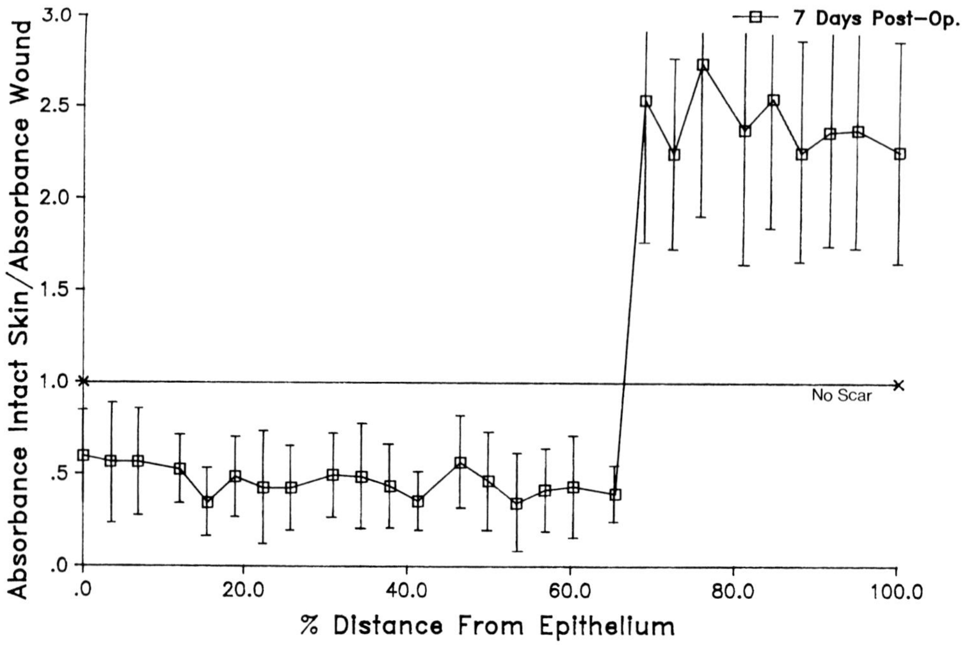

Figure 6.12 Microspectrophotometric measurements of methyl blue staining in an adult wound, seven days postoperatively. See Figure 6.10.

and only the muscle at the base of the wound site showed a change in birefringence as the wound was rotated through 45° (Fig. 6.13c).

By comparison, day 28 pouch young and adult wounds showed considerable differences in both the organization of the extracellular matrix and the birefringence of the wound as it was rotated relative to the plane of polarized light. Seven days after wounding, collagen fibers were present throughout the wound; however, the fibers were larger and more numerous at the wound edges and were arranged perpendicular to the basement membrane (Figs. 6.13d and e). This orientation was confirmed by the birefringence pattern of the wounded tissue, relative to the vibration axis of the polarizer. As the sections were rotated through 45°, the birefringence changed from positive (white fibers—Fig. 6.13d) to negative (dark fibers—Fig. 6.13e); 28 days after surgery in both the day 28 pouch young and adult wounds, the collagen fibers were organized differently from normal (Figs. 6.13f and g). In the dermal region, some basketweave-like organization was evident at the wound site but fine collagen fibers were visible perpendicular to the basement membrane (Figs. 6.13f and g). In the subcutaneous region, the normal hexagonal pattern of organization was completely absent and instead replaced by large parallel bundles of collagen fibers, orientated perpendicular to the basement membrane (Figs. 6.13f and g). These observations confirmed that the orientation and quantity of collagen fibers within the scar were much more abnormal in the deep aspects of the wound, that is, the subcutaneous regions than in the more superficial dermal regions; nonetheless, the entire wounded regions were abnormal by comparison with either the normal skin or the healed wound in the day two pouch young.

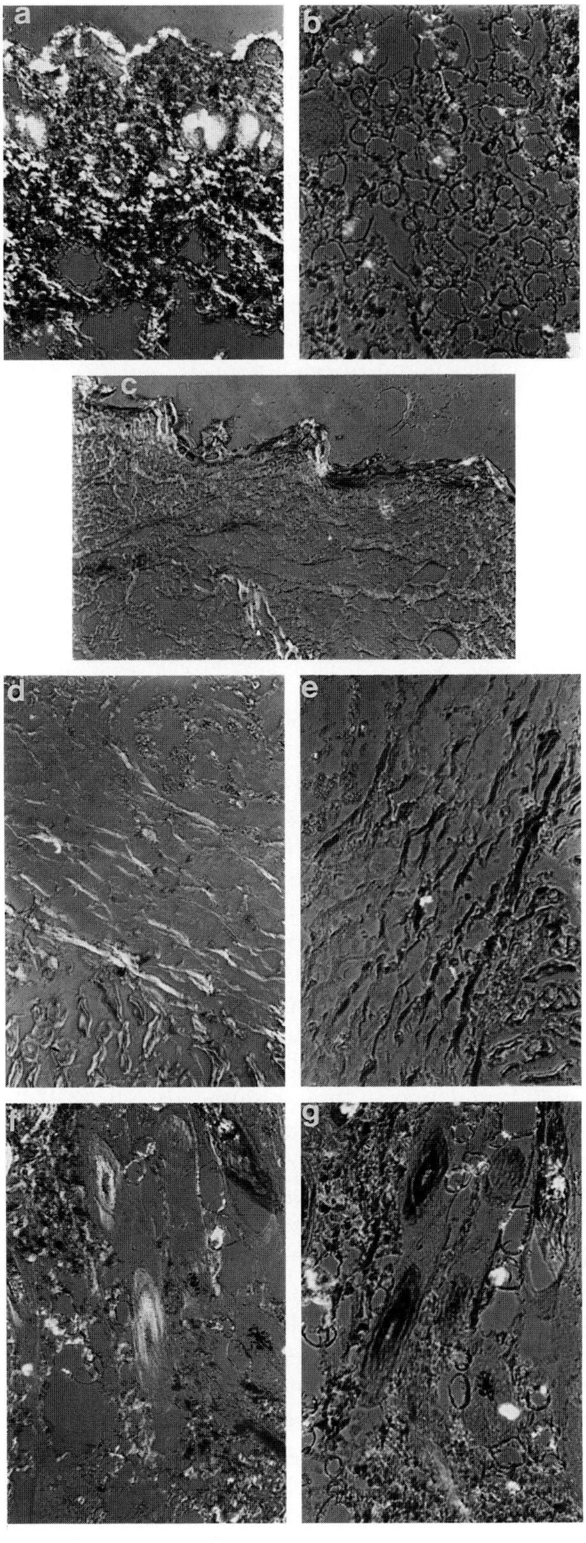

Figure 6.13 Wounded and intact skin images viewed under polarized light. (a) Basketweave appearance of the adult dermis. (b) Hexagonal pattern of the adult subcutaneous tissues. (c) Day 2 pouch young wound two days postoperatively, illustrating that the extracellular matrix of the wound is organized identically to that of the adjacent skin. (d) Adult wound, seven days postoperatively, illustrating parallel bundles of collagen in the scar. (e) Identical section to that in (D), rotated through 45°. The collagen fibrils change from white to black in birefringent appearance. (f) Adult wound 28 days postoperatively, illustrating parallel bundles of collagen fibrils in the dermis and subcutaneous tissues. (g) Same section as (F), rotated through 45°, illustrating the change in the birefringent pattern from white to black. In figures (D) through (G), these parallel bundles of collagen fibrils were perpendicular to the basement membrane.

Discussion

This chapter reports the results of the first investigation into dermal wound healing in pouch young and adult marsupials. The experiments revealed fundamental differences in the wound healing process between the day two pouch young compared with the day 28 pouch young and adult animals. The day two pouch young demonstrated many features of fetal wound healing, namely no scar formation, rapid re-epithelialization and mesenchymal consolidation, poor inflammatory response, minimal angiogenesis, and lack of fibrosis. These fetal-like characteristics of wound healing in day two pouch young *Monodelphis domestica* are comparable to the histological evaluations of embryonic wound healing in a variety of eutherian mammals (summarized in Chapter 10 and in references 28 and 29). Day two pouch young Monodelphis, however, demonstrated scab formation and wound contraction, both features not being uniformly associated with the fetal wound healing pattern seen in eutherian mammals (Tables 1 and 2). The precise transition phase from this fetal-like scar free wound healing pattern of the day two pouch young to the adult like scarring pattern of the day 28 pouch young is unknown. The limited investigations conducted in this study on day 14 pouch young suggested that healing was some way between the fetal and adult patterns with minimal (though not absent) scar tissue formation. Clearly, further experiments are required to accurately delineate the transition phases and events between scar free and scar forming periods.

A major difference between the scar free healing in the day two pouch young and the scar healing in the day 28 pouch young and adult animals was the poor inflammatory response observed in the day two pouch young. All newborn and early pouch young marsupials have very poorly developed immune systems.[19] Precise details are unavailable for *Monodelphis domestica*, but in the closely related *Didelphis virginiana*, at birth, the liver is 50% hematopoietic and there are no lymphocytes in the thymus. Lymphocytes first appear in the thymus at pouch day two, in the blood and lymph nodes at pouch day six to seven, hematopoiesis begins in the spleen at pouch day four, the lymph node rudiments appear, the spleen begins hematopoiesis and Hassals corpuscles appear in the thymus on pouch days five to seven, lymphocytes appear in the bone marrow at pouch days 10–12, in the spleen at pouch days 17–22, while plasma cells and germinal centers appear in the lymph nodes two to three months after birth.[19,30] Adult marsupials possess cell mediated immunity but such responses are completely undeveloped in pouch young.[19] In *Didelphis virginiana*, maternal skin grafts are accepted if transplantation is made before pouch day 12.[19] Moreover, second skin grafts were accepted and remained intact over a three-year period of observation, provided that the recipients were less than pouch day 40 at the time of the first graft.[31]

Equally, adult marsupials make conventional humoral immune responses. At birth, the young marsupial has no humoral responses but develops them throughout pouch life. Marsupials possess immunoglobulins of the IgG, IgM, IgA subclasses and an additional class of 13s embryonic globulins, detected in pouch young around day 20.[19] Experiments injecting antigens (e.g., salmonella flagella antigen) into pouch young of *Didelphis virginiana* showed that animals injected up to and including pouch day seven showed no evidence of antibody formation, those immunized at pouch days 8–15 showed low but detectable titers, while those immunized after pouch day 20 had high antibody titres.[32] This increase in immunocompetence correlates with the appearance of white splenic pulp at pouch days 17–20.

Analysis of the neonatal serum of unsuckled *Didelphis virginiana* failed to detect the presence of any immunoglobulin, suggesting that not only were the pouch young incapable of producing immunoglobulins, but also that there was no prenatal placental transfer of immunoglobulin as is commonly found in eutherian mammals.[33] By contrast, when the serum was analyzed after 12 hours of suckling, high levels of immunoglobulin were detected.[33] This and other marsupial research has confirmed major maternal transfer of immunity, solely via the first secreted milk and movement of immunoglobulin across the pouch young gut wall.[19] When pregnant *Monodelphis domestica* were immunized with sheep red blood cells, antibodies were detected in the maternal milk and transferred to the pouch young, but were completely absent in neonates which had not suckled, suggesting a lack of transplacental transfer.[34]

It therefore appears as if the pouch young marsupial is ill adapted to deal with antigens introduced directly in the early pouch period, without prior sensitization of the mother. In *Didelphis virginiana,* minor wounds of the pouch young resulted in acute, massive, and fatal bacterial invasion without eliciting an inflammatory response.[30] Such results led Block[30] to suggest that the marsupial pouch was an essential shield for the newborn young against noxious influences. Clearly, this conclusion is not supported by the present results in *Monodelphis domestica.* The early pouch young wounds healed without complicating infection, despite their nonsterile external exposure. Indeed, it could be argued that the moist environment of the pouch, containing the excreta of the pouch young and other debris is a microbiologically more hostile environment than the pouchless exposed environment of *Monodelphis domestica.*

The poorly developed immune response to injury of the early pouch young is comparable to the situation in eutherian mammalian fetuses: both rabbit[35] and monkey[36] fetuses are neutropenic with generally lower levels of all circulating leukocytes and a higher percentage of mononuclear cells than the adult. Therefore, the relative absence of inflammatory cells at the early pouch young wound sites is most likely due to the poorly developed immune system. Additionally, those few immune cells that have differentiated may be unresponsive to the chemotactic signals present at the wound site. In adult animals, the emigration of leukocytes from blood vessels is initiated by various chemotactic factors released within the wound, that is, by products of complement activation such as C5A, cell derived factors like leukotriene B4, platelet derived growth factor, kallikrein, fibrinopeptides produced during clot formation and formyl peptides from bacteria.[37] The idea of defective chemotactic ability in the day two pouch young wounds is supported by a demonstration of lower complement activity in newborn compared to adult sheep, and the absence of complement activity in fetal sheep earlier than 123 days of a 150 day gestation period.[38]

There was little accumulation of edema fluid at the lesion site in the day two pouch young wounds, compared to the day 28 pouch young and adult wounds. The immature vascular endothelium of the early *Monodelphis domestica* pouch young may be unresponsive to the various mediators, including bradykinin and histamine that increase the permeability of the microvasculature, allowing exudation of plasma proteins and fluid into the injury site. It may also be a reflection of the low levels of neutrophils present at the wound site in the day two pouch young, as such phagocytic neutrophils normally release proteolytic enzymes that damage endothelial cells, increasing their vascular permeability.[39] Such observations are in keeping with the documented reduction in vascular leakage of plasma proteins, following administration of histamine and bradykinin to both fetal and newborn rhesus monkeys, compared to the response of yearling monkeys.[40] Despite the poor inflammatory response in the day two pouch young wound, phagocytic function appeared normal, presumably the result of local mesenchymal cells removing any cellular debris and infection.[41] As monocytes mature, they differentiate into macrophages with little proliferation of macrophages present in the wounded tissues; therefore, the poor influx of monocytes into the day two pouch young wounds probably explains the subsequent lower numbers of macrophages in such wounds.

The fact that the early pouch young wounds have so few inflammatory cells present is highly suggestive that the growth factor profile of these wounds, that is, the levels of TGF-β isoforms, PDGF, FGFs, etc. will be very different from the later pouch young and adult wounds. The major sources for such growth factors in normal wound healing are from the degranulating platelets, monocytes, neutrophils, and especially macrophages that colonize the wound site. These are in such low numbers in the early pouch young wounds suggesting that the wound environment will have much lower levels of their contained growth factors, as has been documented in eutherian fetal wounds (see Chapter 10). Such low levels of growth factors in both the eutherian fetal and marsupial pouch young wounds may explain the relative lack of fibrosis and angiogenesis in such wounds. Addition of exogenous TGF-β to fetal wounds induces fibrosis.[42] Collectively, these findings support our view that qualitative and quantitative differences in the growth factor profile of healing wounds may be one of the major factors that determines whether the wound heals with or without scarring.

Lower levels of angiogenic factors such as TGFβ or basic FGF in the day two pouch wounds may be responsible for the reduced levels of angiogenesis; in later pouch young and adult wounds, excessive angiogenesis leads to granulation tissue formation, and such excessive angiogenesis doubtlessly reinforces the infiltration of inflammatory cells at the wound site. Certainly, our observations of reduced angiogenesis and low levels of inflammatory cells correlate with the findings of reduced neovascularization as a result of progressive leukocyte depletion in adult mammals.[43]

The findings in day two pouch young *Monodelphis domestica* support the suggestion that the absence of significant inflammation in fetal wound healing is a result of the immaturity of the fetal tissues and not the sterile aqueous environment of the healing wound.[6] Both pouch young wounds and adult wounds healed with scab formation, by contrast to the situation in fetal wound healing.[28] This suggests that absence of scab formation in fetal wound healing may be due to the aqueous environment and the possible fibrinolytic activity of amniotic fluid. Scab formation doubtless prevents wound dehydration in extra uterine environments[2] and its presence or absence appears to be unrelated to the scar free healing phenotype.

The rapid healing of wounds in the day two pouch young compared to the day 28 or adult pouch young reflects the very rapid and sustained growth and turnover of the early tissues and supports previous studies documenting age related differences in the speed of wound healing in adult animals.[1] The rapid re-epithelialization of the day two pouch young wounds may be related to the early deposition of tenascin and fibronectin within the wound environment, comparable to that seen in fetal wound healing (see reference 28 and Chapter 10). This suggests that contact with amniotic fluid, despite its high EGF content[44] may not be responsible for the rapid re-epithelialization of fetal wounds. Equally, the rapid re-epithelialization of the *Monodelphis domestica* pouch young wounds can occur in the presence of advanced epidermal keratinization. In most systems, retinoids suppress the terminal differentiation of stratified squamous epithelial cells and their expression of keratins 1 and 10, whereas, the same retinoids stimulate epithelial cells to express simple keratins[7,8,18,19] together with vimentin.[45] Such changes imply that the retinoid micro-environment of the healing fetal and pouch young Monodelphis wounds are quite different and that such retinoid levels have no major effects on the scar free healing phenotype. This is an important conclusion, given that retinoids can influence the synthesis of TGF-β isoforms that may be important in wound healing and fibrosis.

The early deposition of tenascin within the day two pouch young wounds may correlate with their early contraction. By decreasing adhesive forces within the wound environment, early deposition of tenascin may facilitate movement, that is, contraction by the anchoring phenotypically altered myofibroblasts at the wound margins. By decreasing the ability of fibroblast cells to adhere to the extracellular matrix, tenascin would allow their continued movement, thus generating the forces of wound contraction. The reduced or absent contraction in fetal wound healing may be due to inhibitory effects of amniotic fluid.[2]

The sequence of events related to extracellular matrix molecule deposition within the healing Monodelphis wounds parallels closely the situation in fetal, neonatal, and adult healing dermal wounds of mice (see reference 28 and Chapter 10). In particular, the early deposition of glycosaminoglycans such as chondroitin sulphate within the day two pouch young wounds probably causes formation of a loose wound matrix and enhanced motility of the mesenchymal cells: these cells invade the loose wound matrix, approximately parallel to the basement membrane. By contrast, the absence of such early deposition of glycosaminoglycans within the later pouch young and adult wounds resulted in a dense wound clot and the migration of mesenchymal cells up and down the axis between the wound margin and the clot. This resulted in the deposition of extracellular matrix molecules in an abnormal orientation at right angles to the basement membrane. This was the first sign of scar formation. These fibrils then increased in size, again, perhaps regulated by the extracellular environment: proteoglycans and glycosaminoglycans are known to regulate collagen fibril diameter.[28] As a result, the normal tissue architecture was re-established in the day two pouch young wounds, whereas this was not the case in the later pouch young and adult wounds. It is important to note that scarring results from a different orientation of the collagen fibrils, not merely an increase in collagen content. Interestingly, in the day 28 pouch young and adult wounds, scarring was much more evident in the subcutaneous tissues by comparison with the dermal tissues. This correlates with the slower turnover of the extracellular matrix in the subcutaneous regions compared to the dermis. The pattern is also very similar to that documented for adult dermal wound healing in rodents[45] where the deeper tissues of the reticular dermis and subcutaneous regions demonstrate scarring with rather minimal scarring in the papillary dermis. It should be noted that there are currently no good animal models of dermal scarring outside man.

In summary, *Monodelphis domestica* presents itself as an interesting model system for elucidating the mechanisms responsible for scar free healing. First, it possesses some of the features of the fetal and the adult environment. This means that factors such as presence of amniotic fluid, the absence of a sterile environment, the absence of scab tissue formation and the absence of a highly differentiated epidermis are not responsible for the scar free healing phenotype observed in fetal wound healing as none of these occur in the early pouch young *Monodelphis domestica* that nonetheless, heals without scarring. Interestingly, features common to the healing of fetal wounds and early marsupial wounds include a poor inflammatory response as a result of the immaturity of the immune system, a consequential qualitative and quantitative difference in the growth factor profile of the wounds, a marked reduction in angiogenesis, and an altered wound extracellular matrix profile (as a result of differences in the kinetics, deposition and turnover of matrix molecules in terms of their quantity, type, and orientation) suggesting that these features may be important determinants of the scar free healing phenotype. Clearly, *Monodelphis domestica,* given all of its advantages of accessibility and ease of experimental manipulation, is an ideal model in which to investigate the importance of these factors for scar free healing and their possible experimental modulation.

REFERENCES

1. Holm-Pedersen P, Viidik A, (1972): Tensile properties and morphology of healing wounds in young and old rats. Scand. J. Plast. Reconstr. Surg. 6, 24–35.
2. Somasundaram K, Prathap K, (1972): The effect of exclusion of amniotic fluid on intra-uterine healing of skin wounds in rabbit foetuses. J. Path. 107, 127–130.
3. Jahoda CAB, Oliver RF, (1984): Vibrissa dermal papilla cell aggregative behaviour in vivo and in vitro. J. Embryol. Exp. Morph. 79, 211–224.
4. Jahoda CAB, Oliver RF, (1984): Histological studies of the effects of wounding vibrissa follicles in the hooded rat. J. Embryol. Exp. Morph. 83, 95–108.
5. Tyndale-Biscoe CH, Janssens PA, (eds) (1988): The developing marsupial: models for biomedical research. Springer-Verlag, Berlin.
6. New DAT, Mizell M, (1972): Opossum fetuses grown in culture. Science. 175, 533–536.
7. New DAT, Mizell M, Cockcroft DL (1977): Growth of opossum embryos in vitro during organogenesis. J. Embryol. Exp. Morph. 41, 111–123.
8. Selwood L, (1987): Embryonic development in culture of two dasyurid marsupials, Sminthopsis crassicaudata (Gould) and Sminthopsis macroura (Spencer), during cleavage and blastocyst formation. Gamete Res. 16, 355–370.
9. Selwood L, (1989): Marsupial pre-implantation embryos in vivo and in vitro. In: "Development of Pre-Implantation Embryos and their Environment" New York: Alan R. Liss Inc. 225–236.
10. Cockcroft DL, (1990): Dissection and culture of post-implantation embryos. In: "Postimplantation Mammalian Embryos a Practical Approach". (eds A.J. Copp and D.L. Cockcroft). Oxford University Press, 15–40.
11. Baggott LM, and Moore HDM, (1990): Early embryonic development of the grey short-tailed opossum, Monodelphis domestica, in vivo and in vitro. J. Zool. 222:623–639.
12. Green B, Merchant JC, (1988): The composition of marsupial milk. In: "The Developing Marsupial" (eds C.H. Tyndale-Biscoe and P.A. Janssens). Berlin, Springer-Verlag, 41–54.
13. Nicholas KR, (1988): Control of milk protein synthesis in the marsupial Macropus eugenii: a model system to study prolactin-dependent development. In: "The Developing Marsupial" (eds C.H. Tyndale-Biscoe and P.A. Janssens) Berlin, Springer-Verlag 68–85.
14. Nelson JE, (1988): Growth of the brain. In: "The Developing Marsupial" (eds C.H. Tyndale-Biscoe and P.A. Janssens) Berlin, Springer-Verlag, 86–100.
15. Reynolds ML, Saunders NR, (1988): Differentiation of the Neocortex. In: "The Developing Marsupial" (eds C.H. Tyndale-Biscoe and P.A. Janssens) Berlin, Springer-Verlag, 101–116.
16. Dunlop SA, Coleman LA, Harman AM, Beazley LD, (1988): Development of the marsupial primary visual pathway. In: "The Developing Marsupial" (eds C.H. Tyndale-Biscoe and P.A. Janssens) Berlin, Springer-Verlag, 117–131.
17. Hubbert AJ (1988): Metabolism and the development of endothermy. In: The Developing Marsupial" (eds C.H. Tyndale-Biscoe and P.A. Janssens) Berlin, Springer-Verlag, 141–161.

18. Moore HDM and Thurstan SM (1990): Sexual differentiation in the grey short-tailed opossum Monodelphis domestica and the effect of oestradiol benzoate on development in the male. J. Zool. 221, 639–658.
19. Deane EM, Cooper DW (1988): Immunological development in pouch young marsupials. In: "The Developing Marsupial" (eds C.H. Tyndale-Biscoe and P.A. Janssens), Berlin, Springer-Verlag 190–199.
20. Hall LS, and Hughes RL, (1987): An evolutionary perspective of structural adaptations for environmental perception and utilization by the neonatal marsupials. Trichosurus vulpecula (Phalangeridae) and Didelphis virginiana (Didelphidae). In: "Possums and Opossums: studies in evolution" (ed M. Archer) Sydney, Surrey Beatty & Sons, 257–271.
21. Fadem BH, Trupin GL, Maliniak E, VandeBerg JL, Hayssen V, (1982): Care and breeding of the grey, short-tailed opossum (Monodelphis domestica). Lab. Animal Sci. 32, 405–409.
22. Reig OA, Kirsch JAW, Marshall LG, (1987): Systematic relationships of the living and neocenozoic american "opossum-like" marsupials (suborder Didelphimorphia) with comments on the classification of these and of the cretaceous and palaeogene new world and european metatherians. In: "Possums and Opossums: Studies in Evolution". (ed. M. Archer) Sydney, Surrey Beatty & Sons 1–89.
23. Baggott LM, Davis-Butler S, and Moore HDM (1987): Characterisation of oestrus and timed collection of oocytes in the grey short-tailed opossum, Monodelphis domestica J. Reprod. Fert. 79, 105–114.
24. Trupin GL, Fadam BH, (1982): Sexual behaviour of the grey short-tailed opossum (Monodelphis domestica) J. Mamm. 63, 409–414.
25. Renfree MB, Fletcher TP, Blanden DR, Lewis PR, Shaw G, Gordon K, Short RV, Parer-Cook E, Parer D, (1989): Physiological and behavioural events around the time of birth in macropodid marsupials. In: "Kangaroos, Wallabies and Rat-Kangaroos" (Ed G. Grigg, P. Jarman and I. Hume). Sydney, Surrey Beatty & Sons., 323–337.
26. Winter GD, (1962): Formation of the scab and the rate of epithelialisation of superficial wounds in the skin of the young domestic pig. Nature 200, 377.
27. Derby MA (1978): Analysis of the glycosaminoglycans within the extracellular environments encountered by migrating neural crest cells. Dev. Biol. 66, 321–336.
28. Whitby DJ, Ferguson MWJ (1991): The extracellular matrix of lip wounds in fetal, neonatal and adult mice. Development 112:651–658, 1991.
29. Longaker MT, Whitby DJ, Adzick NS, Crombleholme TM, Langer JC, Duncan BW, Bradley SM, Stern R, Ferguson MWJ, Harrison MR (1990): Studies in fetal wound healing VI second and early third trimester fetal wounds demonstrate rapid collagen deposition without scar formation. J. Pediatr. Surg. 25, 63–69.
30. Block M (1964): The blood forming tissues and blood of the new born opossum (Didelphis Virginiana) 1. Normal Development through about the one hundredth day of life. Ergeb. Anat. Entwicklungsgesh. 37, 237–366.
31. Waring H, Holmes R, Cockson A, Ashman RB, Stanley NF, (1978): Induction of long term tolerance in the quokka (Setonix Brachyurus) by thymus and skin allografts into early pouch young. Aust. J. Exp. Biol. Med. Sci. 56, 597–604.
32. Rowlands DJ jr., La Via MF, Block MH, (1964): The blood forming tissues and blood of the new born opossum (Didelphis virginiana) ii Ontogenesis of antibody formation to flagella of Salmonella typhi. J. Immunol. 93, 157–164.
33. Hindes RD, Mizell M, (1976): The origin of immunoglobulin in opossum "embryos" Dev. Biol. 53, 49–61.
34. Samples NK, VandeBerg JL, Stone WH, (1986): Passively acquired immunity in the new born of a marsupial (Monodelphis domestica). Am. J. Reprod. Immunol. Microbiol. 11, 94–97.
35. Adzick NS, Harrison MR, Glick PL, (1985): Comparison of fetal, newborn, and adult wound healing by histologic, enzyme-histochemical, and hydroxyproline determinations. J. Pediatr. Surg. 20, 315–319.
36. Schwartz LW, Osburn BI, (1974): An ontogenic study of the acute inflammatory reaction in the fetal rhesus monkey. Lab. Invest. 31, 441–453.
37. Williams TJ, (1988): Factors that affect vessel reactivity and leukocyte emigration. In: "The Molecular and Cellular Biology of Wound Repair". (Ed R.A.F. Clark and P.M. Henson). New York, Plenum Press. 115–147.
38. Rice CE, Silverstein AM (1964): Haemolytic complement activity of sera of foctal and new born lambs. Can. J. Comp. Med. Vet. Sci. 28, 34.

39. Wedmore CV, Williams TJ, (1981): Control of vascular permeability by polymorphonuclear leukocytes in inflammation. Nature 289, 646–650.
40. Schwartz LW (1974): Vascular leakage, a deficient response to exogenous histamine, 48/80 and bradykinin in the fetal newborn monkey. Fed. Proc. 33, 604.
41. Thomasson B, Viljanto J, Jarasheldainen A (1973): Enzyme-histochemical observations on the formation of granulation tissue in rabbit fetuses and Does. Acta. Chir. Scand. 139, 327–333.
42. Krummel TM, Michna BA, Thomas BL (1988): Transforming growth factor beta (TGFβ) induces fibrosis in a fetal wound model. J. Pediatr. Surg. 23, 647–652.
43. Sholley MM, Gimbrone MA, Cotran RS, (1978): The effects of leukocyte depletion on corneal neovascularisation. Lab. Invest. 38, 32–40.
44. Haigh R, D'Souza, Micklewright L, (1989): Human amniotic fluid urogastrone (epidermal growth factor) and fetal lung phospholipids. Br. J. Obstet. Gynaecol. 96, 171–178.
45. Stellmach VM, Fuchs E, (1989): Exploring the mechanisms underlying cell type-specific and retinoid-mediated expression of keratins. The New Biologist. 1, 305–317.
46. Levenson SM, Geever EF, Crowley LV, Oates JF, Berard CW, Rosen H, (1965): The healing of rat skin wounds. Ann Surg 161, 293–308.

CHAPTER 7

Fetal Fracture Healing

Brent R. W. Moelleken
Michael T. Longaker
Joseph C. Cheng
David J. Simmons

The first cases of in utero fetal surgery have recently been reported.[1–6] Currently, fetal surgery is only performed on highly selected fetuses with anatomic defects that have predictable and devastating pathophysiologic consequences. These lesions include congenital diaphragmatic hernia, congenital urinary tract obstruction, and congenital tumors. However, the indications for fetal surgery are expanding as prenatal diagnosis improves, experience with fetal treatment grows, and safety of surgery for the mother is demonstrated. The fetus is now considered a patient.[7]

In the large animal fetal sheep model, skin wound healing proceeds expeditiously without scarring at early and midgestational timepoints.[8–11] However, the information from the sheep model has been confined solely to fetal skin. It is unknown whether we can expect other fetal tissues such as the musculoskeletal system to share the unique healing properties of fetal skin.

Bony deformities can now be diagnosed in humans in utero. These include many types of facial clefting, polydactyly, phocomelia, meningomyelocele, craniosynostosis, and a variety of other bony abnormalities.[12] Fetal surgery may be indicated for catastrophic abnormalities. For those anomalies that enjoy a favorable outcome after early postnatal repair, in utero repair might even be more successful in terms of limiting scar formation and disfigurement and increasing the rate of healing. With experience in correcting prenatal defects in animals, it may be feasible to select the skeletal problems that have the best chance for a favorable outcome following in utero repair in humans. More importantly, by studying the in utero process of fracture healing, lessons may be learned about the biology of normal and abnormal bone development. It may be possible to modulate adult or postnatal fracture healing in such difficult cases as nonunion or large bony defects.

This chapter reviews the processes of fetal fracture healing in endochondral long bone of the large animal fetal sheep and compares the data to the literature on fetal and neonatal fracture healing. The responses to mid-shaft transverse incisional and excisional defects were studied by radiographic, magnetic resonance imaging (MRI), and histologic analysis.

FRACTURE MODEL

Fourteen time-dated pregnant ewes at 100 days gestation (term = 145 days) were used. Under general anesthesia, the uterus was exposed through a midline laparotomy. A 10 cm hysterotomy was made with careful attention to secure all layers of the uterine wall and amniotic membranes. Fetal position was manipulated to expose both forelimbs. A 3 cm incision was made on the anterolateral surface of each fetal forelimb. In the right forelimb, an incision was made in the midshaft of the ulna, creating a clean break (Fig. 7.1). In the left forelimb, a 3 mm segment of the mid-shaft ulna (including periosteum) was excised. The size of the defect relative to the cross-sectional area of the ulna was sufficient to prevent spontaneous healing in adult and senescent animals.[13,14] The radii remained intact and served as an internal splint. No other procedures for internal or external fixation were necessary. The skin was then closed and the fetus was returned to the uterus.

Fetuses whose bones had been fractured at 100 days gestation were sacrificed at three, five, 10, 14, 21, 28, and 40 days after surgery (103, 105, 110, 114, 121, 128, and 140 days gestation respectively). The forelimbs were amputated at the mid-humerus level and immediately imaged by high resolution low kilovolt radiographs and MRI. Control tissues were obtained from non-fractured age-matched fetuses. All specimens were fixed in 70% ethanol.

Low Kilovolt Radiography

Low kilovolt radiographs were utilized to enhance the contrast between soft tissue and bone at the fracture margin.[15] Posterior/anterior and lateral views of the fractured and control limbs were obtained using high resolution mammographic technique. The field of view included radius, ulna, and the proximal joint.

MRI scans were performed using T-2 weighted images on all forelimbs. In all cases, the hindlimb of the fetus was used as an unfractured control.

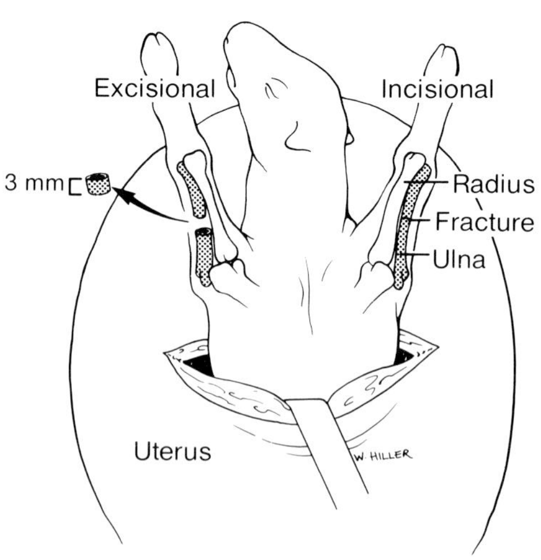

Figure 7.1 Line drawing of fracture model. Following laparotomy and hysterotomy to expose the fetal lamb, an incisional fracture was made on midshaft of the right ulna. A 3 mm excisional section of bone together with periosteum was removed from the midshaft of the left ulna.

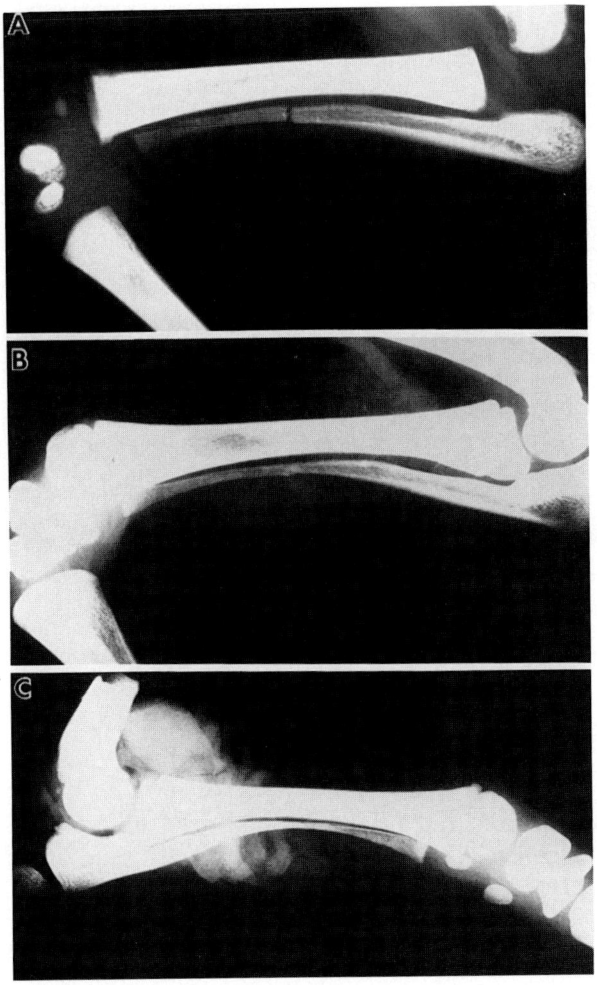

Figure 7.2 Low kilovolt radiographs of incisional fracture in midshaft of ulnae. **(a)** At 3 days postfracture, there is a sharp fracture line with no evidence of healing. **(b)** 14 days postfracture, obliteration of fracture line without callus formation. **(c)** 28 days postfracture, complete healing of fracture, marrow cavity continuous and cortices reformed.

Histology

The ulnae preserved in 70% alcohol were postfixed in 10% neutral formalin, defatted in acetone, and embedded in vacuo with methyl methyacrylate. Serial sections were cut with a microtome, and stained with Hematoxylin, eosin, and Azure II following removal of the embedding medium.

RESULTS

Low Kilovolt Radiography

Incisional Defects

The 3-day incisional fracture is characterized by a sharply defined fracture line without evidence of repair (Fig. 7.2a). The corresponding radiolucency persisted for nearly two weeks postinjury. The first evidence of healing presented at 14 days as a slight periosteal reaction and narrowing of the fracture gap (Fig. 7.2b). Fracture repair progressed to completion in samples later than 21 days postinjury with reformation of the ulnar cortices (Fig. 7.2c).

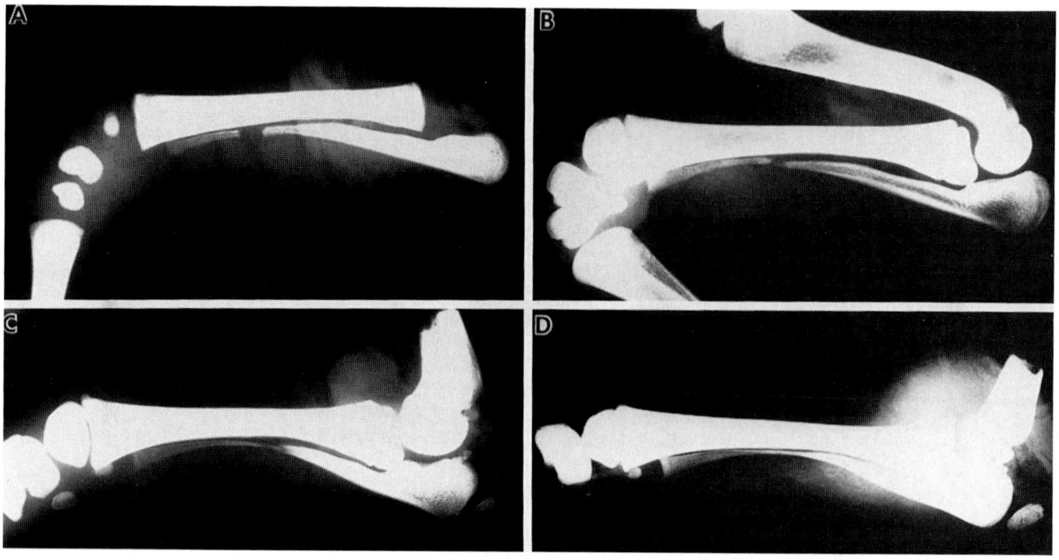

Figure 7.3 Low kilovolt radiographs of excisional fracture in midshaft of ulnae. **(a)** At 5 days postfracture, there is no evidence of healing. **(b)** 14 days postfracture, partial obliteration of the original fracture gap. **(c)** 28 days postfracture, gap is completely bridged with no evidence of callus. **(d)** 40 days postfracture, complete healing of excisional defect with reconstitution of cortices and marrow cavity.

Excisional Defects

The three-day excisional wound demonstrated a large, unbridged defect (Fig. 7.3a). By 14 days postinjury, the defects showed some mineralized tissue filling the gap without evidence of external callus (Fig. 7.3b). At 28 days, the gap was completely bridged without significant external callus (Fig. 7.3c). At 40 days, the fracture site was completely healed, with reconstitution of marrow cavities and cortical bone (Fig. 7.3d).

Magnetic Resonance Imaging

Incisional Defects

The T2 image of the five-day fracture revealed a hypointense region in the ulnae corresponding to the fracture line (Fig. 7.4a). The 10-day fracture demonstrated some high intensity signal within the fracture site indirectly indicating repair with early reconstitution of marrow (fat and water) and corresponding to the fibrocartilaginous union demonstrated on histology (Figs. 7.4b, 7.6c, and 7.6d). In samples obtained later than 21 days postfracture, the dark cortical outline of the ulnae was uniform in intensity indicating complete cortical reformation of the previous fracture gap (Figure 7.4c).

Excisional Defects

The tissue that occupied the fracture gap at five days demonstrated a high intensity signal (Fig. 7.5a). With time, this high intensity signal gradually subsided. The change corresponded to the progressive filling of the gap with new bone (28 days,

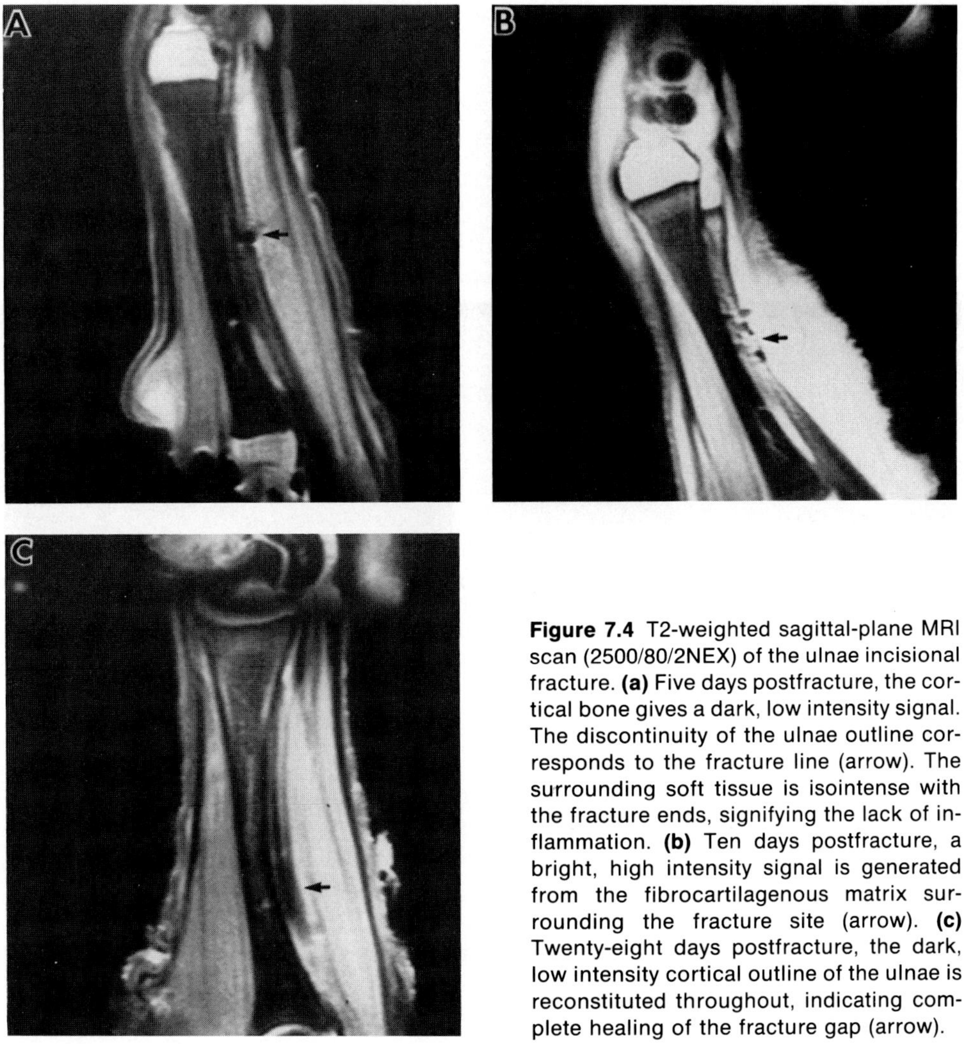

Figure 7.4 T2-weighted sagittal-plane MRI scan (2500/80/2NEX) of the ulnae incisional fracture. **(a)** Five days postfracture, the cortical bone gives a dark, low intensity signal. The discontinuity of the ulnae outline corresponds to the fracture line (arrow). The surrounding soft tissue is isointense with the fracture ends, signifying the lack of inflammation. **(b)** Ten days postfracture, a bright, high intensity signal is generated from the fibrocartilagenous matrix surrounding the fracture site (arrow). **(c)** Twenty-eight days postfracture, the dark, low intensity cortical outline of the ulnae is reconstituted throughout, indicating complete healing of the fracture gap (arrow).

Figs. 7.5b, 7.7a, and 7.7c). By 40 days, the signal from the ulnar cortex was uniform, indicating that the bony defect had been completely restructured with a normal distribution of bone and marrow.

Fracture Histology:

Normal Bone Structure

The fetal sheep ulnar cortex at 100 days gestational age is covered by a thick periosteum and consists of a laminar array of bony trabeculae separated by vascularized connective tissue. The bone surfaces are lined with osteoblasts and a few resorptive lacunae. Most of the thinner newly formed periosteal laminae have a woven architecture (Fig. 7.6a), but the older thicker trabeculae frequently include some lamellar bone (Fig. 7.6e). The endosteal midshaft cortex exhibited some trabeculae that contained cores of cartilage derived from physeal endo-

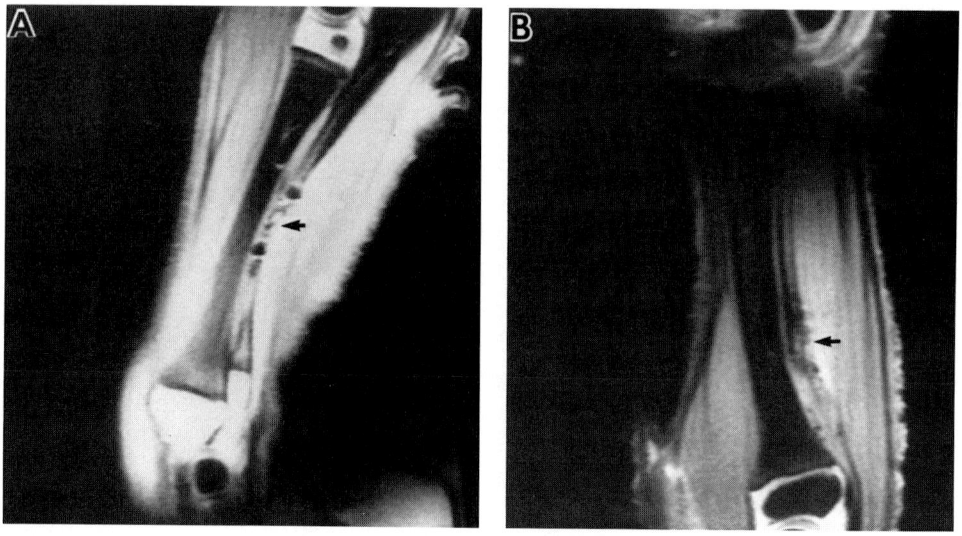

Figure 7.5 T2-weighted sagittal-plane MRI scan (2800/80/2NEX) of the excisional ulnae fracture. **(a)** 5 days postfracture. Bright, high-intensity signal generating within the fracture gap by the fibrocartilagenous matrix laid down during early fracture healing (arrow). **(b)** At 28 days postfracture, some low-intensity signal began to replace the previously high-intensity generating fibrocartilagenous matrix (arrow). This corresponds to calcification of previous laid down fibrocartilaginous material.

chondral bone, but these were absent after 120 days owing to linear growth processes.

Incisional Defects

At three days postfracture, the incision was filled with a fibrin-like material and there was focal thickening of the periosteum. Osteoclast- and macrophage-like cells were apposed to the free cut ends of the trabeculae. Osteocyte death occurred over a 7–8 mm distance from the fracture line, and their lacunae frequently contained pyknotic debris (Fig. 7.6b).

At 10 days postfracture, the fracture site was covered by a very small external periosteal callus. The fracture line had closed and was filled with an admixture of mature fibrocartilage and endochondral bone trabeculae (Fig. 7.6c). Azure II staining cartilage matrix was present only within the forming endochondral trabecular bone (Fig. 7.6d).

At 21 days, there was no longer external or internal evidence of repair tissue. No primary endochondral trabecular bone remained to mark the position of the fracture. The histologic character of the consolidated cortex resembled that of normal fetal sheep bone (Fig. 7.6e).

Excisional Defects

At 5 days, the osteotomy site was largely filled with disorganized connective tissue, but the periosteum was not especially reactive. Osteocyte death was evident at and away from the cut ends of the cortical trabeculae. However, unlike the sequelae to incision, spicules of newly formed bone presented on the cut ends

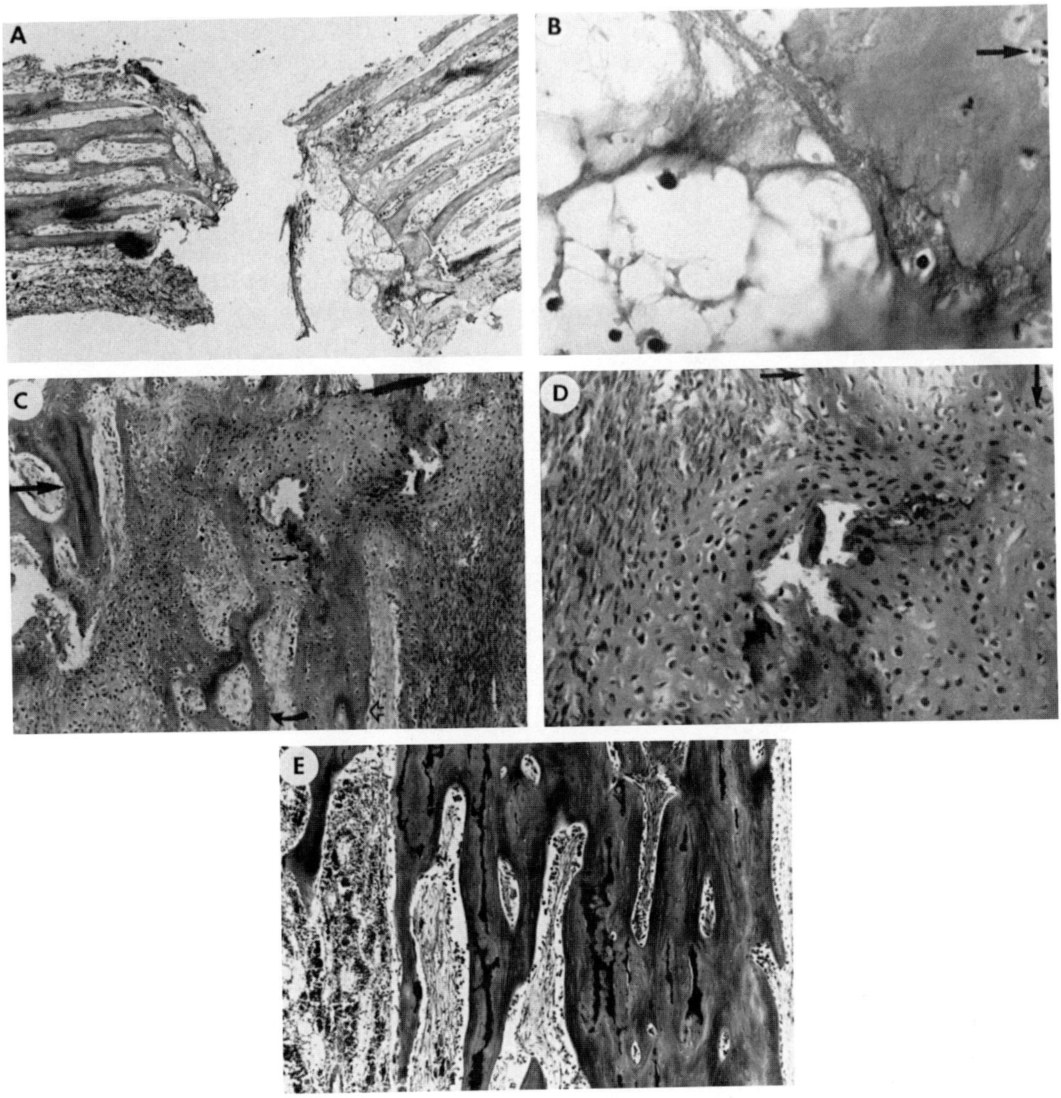

Figure 7.6 Histology of incisional fractures. **(a)** 3 days postfracture. Low power photomicrograph showing incisional fracture line. Note that the periosteum is not thickened and there is no evidence of an external callus (Hematoxylin, eosin and Azure II; Mag 100×). **(b)** 3 days postfracture. High power photomicrograph of fractured end of bone showing bone matrix degradation and fibrin-like strands extending into the fracture line being destroyed by macrophages. The bone contains several osteocytic lacunae with pyknotic nuclei (arrow) (Hematoxylin, eosin and Azure II; Mag 250×). **(c)** 10 days postfracture. Low power photomicrograph of fracture repairing line showing foci of enchondral and endochondral ossification and reactive bone formation. The large black arrow points to the dark-staining core of original (prefracture) bone which is covered by lamellae of newly formed (postfracture) bone. Enchondral ossification with chondrocytic lacunae abutted to and half-included into the dark-stained bone matrix (small black arrow). New thin bony trabeculum have formed via modulation of undifferentiated mesenchymal osteoprogenitor cells (curved arrow). Thickening of original cortical bone laminae by modulation of undifferentiated mesenchymal osteoprogenitor cells is also present (outlined arrow) (Hematoxylin, eosin and Azure II; Mag 150×). **(d)** 10 days postfracture. High power view of endochondral ossification (arrows) (Hematoxylin, eosin and Azure II; Mag 250×). **(e)** 21 days postfracture. Cortical bone consolidation is complete. The fracture line is not visible. Cortex is largely composed of incorporated endochondral trabeculae (shown as dark-staining calcified cartilage remnants (Hematoxylin, eosin and Azure II; Mag 150×).

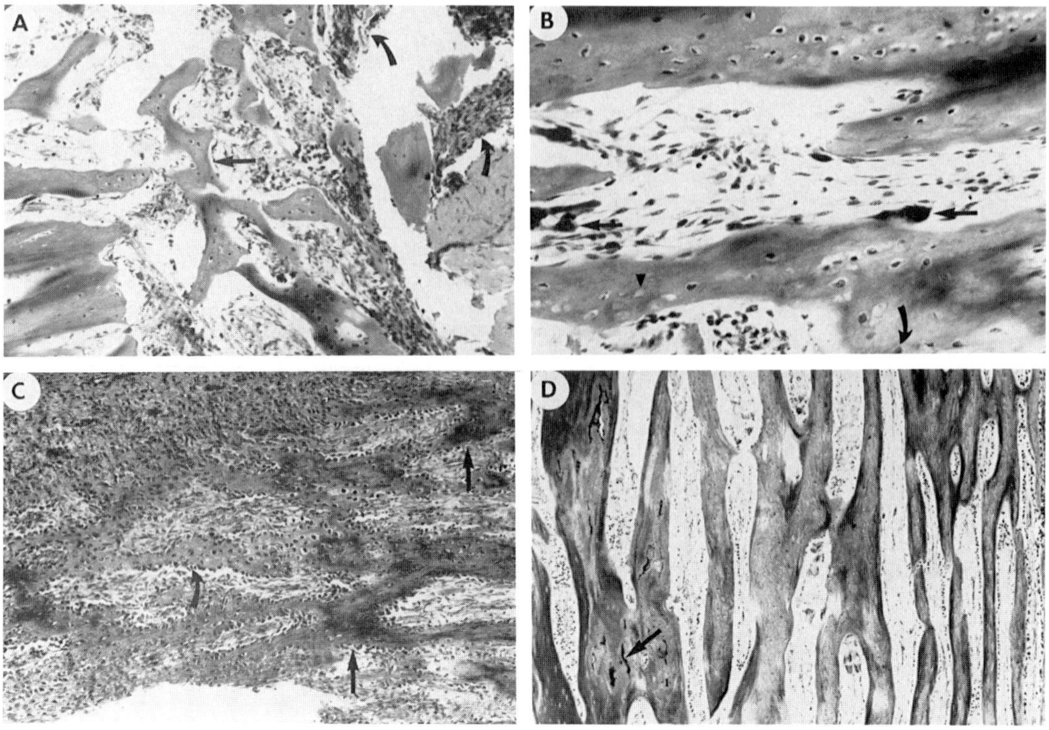

Figure 7.7 Histology of excisional fractures. **(a)** 5 days postfracture. Microphotograph of the cut end of laminar bone covered by newly formed trabeculae (large arrow). A small area of connective tissue (curved arrows) is seen in the excision gap (Hematoxylin, eosin and Azure II; Mag 150×). **(b)** 10 days postfracture. Microphotograph of a longitudinal section of fetal lamb cortex 10 days postfracture showing a transition zone between dead (triangle) and live bone (curved arrow). Note the large number of empty osteocytic lacunae and the osteoclasts recontouring the trabeculae (large black arrows) (Hematoxylin, eosin and Azure II; Mag 250×). **(c)** 28 days postfracture. Photomicrograph showing several areas of endochondral bone (large arrows). In the center of the photograph, the intertrabecular spaces are filled with primitive mesenchymal cells that are modulating to osteoblasts (curved arrow) (Hematoxylin, eosin and Azure II; Mag 150×). **(d)** 40 days postfracture. Photomicrograph showing that consolidation is present and the original fracture line cannot be identified. The area of fracture healing has been modeled to typical cortical bone laminae separated by broad vascular spaces. The endosteal cortex contains a few cartilage rests (arrow) that have been derived from physeal endochondral trabeculae (Hematoxylin, eosin and Azure II; Mag 100×).

of the cortical trabeculae, and they extended a short distance into the osteotomy gap (Fig. 7.7a).

Between five and 10 days postosteotomy, trabecular outgrowth further narrowed the gap (Fig. 7.4b), and the dead cortical bone was being replaced by prominent osteoclastic and osteoblastic activity (Fig. 7.7b).

At 28 days, the periosteum had been completely reconstituted over the osteotomy site, and the gap was filled by thin trabeculae of woven bone oriented parallel to the long bone axis. The bone, in part, exhibited linear patches of Azure II stainable matrix, indicative of a cartilage component during its developmental history.

By 40 days, the osteotomy site could not be identified microscopically, and it appeared that the processes of normal bone modeling had restored the histotypic appearance of the fetal sheep ulna (Fig. 7.7d).

DISCUSSION

The present studies were undertaken to extend our knowledge about the course of fetal wound healing to skeletal tissue. The primary aim was to document the processes attendant to the repair of simple undisplaced fractures or large osteotomy bone gaps. The secondary aim was to try to interpret the observations against a background of experience, largely with skin wounds, in the clinical setting and in the laboratory.

Clinically, fetal skin wounds heal very rapidly without inflammation and scarring, and those outcomes have been supported experimentally in mice,[17] rats,[18] rabbits,[19] sheep,[10] and primates.[20] The results from various animal models do conflict somewhat, but common characteristics include the lack of early inflammation, a wound matrix rich in hyaluronic acid, wound collagen deposited in a highly organized pattern, and the lack of scar formation.

There is no comparable wealth of experience with fetal skeletal tissue repair. In fact, we can only draw upon three studies that may be germane to that general issue. The first dealt with the fate of grafts of quail long bone cartilage rudiments transected after revascularization on the chick chorioallantoic membrane. In this special circumstance, the rudiments healed completely within two to three days, but without an attendant periosteal reaction.[21] In the second study, embryonic chick radii (six to seven day incubation) were fractured in middiaphysis prior to osteogenesis in limb development. The majority of the fractures united within 24–36 hours without typical features involved in fracture healing, namely hematoma or callus formation.[22] The third study followed femoral fracture repair for eight days in the fetal (23–27 days gestation) and newborn rabbit. That work indicated that while the repair processes were similarly sequenced, fetal healing outpaced the newborn animal by several days.[23] In both, the repair processes typically involved distinct stages of hematoma formation, mesenchymal invasion of the fracture site, production of callus cartilage and finally bone formation via endochondral ossification. If points of similarity can be drawn between the short gestation rabbit fracture healing model and fetal soft tissue repair, they are the absence of a significant inflammatory reaction and the early formation of a blastema that effected rapid and firm union. Scarring is not a feature of bone repair in the animal/human fetus or adult.

The present study represents the first study of fetal fracture healing in a large animal model. The authors know of no comparative histologic staging data for fracture healing in adult sheep, but the greater rapidity of fetal lamb bone repair can be inferred from our observations and the fracture literature.[24] While we will consider the incisional and excisional defects as separate issues, they share this common feature of rapid healing.

Incisional Model

Aside from the dramatically faster time course of bone healing and remodeling when compared to adult fracture healing,[25] the most striking result seemed to be the lack of external callus formation in the fetal lamb. The previous study on fetal rabbits involving non-stabilized femur fractures had a large callus that probably reflects motion of the fracture during healing.[23] The lack of callus in this study may be a function of the experimental scheme utilized; the ulnar defect was stabilized by an intact radius. This can be construed as rigid internal fixation for the ulnar fracture, and what we observed was simply primary bone healing. However, previous studies of postnatal fractures in neonatal animals using a similar experimental design to the one used in this study resulted in external callus formation and radio-ulnar synostosis.[26–28] Secondly, close examination of the mineralization process in the fibrocartilagenous tissue of incisional fractures revealed simultaneous enchondral and endochondral ossification. Enchondral ossification has not been previously observed in nonmembranous bone. This seems to be unique and consistent with previous studies in fetal wound repair. The cell lines in the fetus may remain pluripotential and one cell line may be converted directly to another cell line; in this case, a direct modulation of chondroblasts and primitive mesenchymal cells into osteoblasts occurred without the intervening steps of chondroblast hypertrophy and death followed by replacement of osteoprogenitor cells. This activation of mesenchymal cells to osteoprogenitor cells may decrease with increasing age.[29,30]

Excisional Model

In the excisional fracture, we chose a defect (three times bone width including periosteum) that could not be overcome in postnatal animals.[13,14,27,28] Connective tissue matrix was already seen occupying the fracture gap at five days. Repair processes progressed rapidly, and by 28 days, the osteotomy gap was filled with primary bone trabeculae that contained some cartilage rests. Radiographically, the gap was completely bridged.

This involvement of repair via endochondral ossification was common to the healing process in both the incisional and excisional models, but incisional repair alone arose from a cartilaginous growth plate. The complete restitution of normal fetal bone architecture that followed must have also occurred by active osteoclastogenesis from circulating promonocytes and bone resorption, as well as by a number of other modeling processes: enchondral ossification of the chondrocyte lacunae,[31] and the modulation of undifferentiated perivascular mesenchymal cells in the intertrabecular spaces to osteoblasts.[32]

Our findings are relevant to Zadek's[27] demonstration that puppies are better able to heal standardized 3 cm radial defects than either adolescent or skeletally mature mongrel dogs. The defects in puppies were gradually filled with new bone via the multicentric conversion of fibrous connective tissue cells within the osteotomy gap to cartilage and bone cells. In contrast, the defects in adult dogs were only partially filled, and the new bone appeared to form from osteoprogenitor cells that proliferated from the cut ends of the bone. Both of these aspects were common to the repair of the ulnar defects in fetal lambs. It is probable that with age, this species would also exhibit a spectrum of repair mechanisms and declining osteogenic efficiency. The histotypic spectrum for scarless skin healing in the fetal lamb is also age-specific.[33]

This study included the use of MRI to document fetal fracture healing. The role of MRI in fracture healing is largely untested. Fracture of the bone is followed by a definite sequence of repair and the prominent role of soft tissue elements in this sequence suggests that MRI may provide useful information on the progress of fracture healing. MRI provides an excellent degree of contrast between different kinds of soft tissue and provides this information in a number of orientations.[33] Imaging of the intramedullary cavity and peripheral tissues may supply useful information regarding the presence or lack of edema and inflammation that characterize adult fracture healing.

MRI scans of the fetal fractures showed a characteristic pattern compatible with the recognized histomorphometry of fracture repair. The fracture line was demonstrated as a marked decrease in signal intensity and discontinuity in the dark cortical outline. In the soft tissues surrounding the fracture, the signal intensity remained isointense throughout the entire limb, reflecting the lack of inflammation and edema that generate a high intensity signal on the MRI scan. During repair, the fibrocartilagenous matrix appeared as a high intensity region on the subsequent scans. This region gradually developed a granular appearance with embedded low-intensity nodules corresponding to areas of calcification in the fibrocartilagenous matrix seen by histological analysis. The MRI scan of healed fractures all revealed reconstitution of the dark ulnar cortical outline and reconstitution of marrow cavity in both incised and excised models.

In summary, we have described fracture healing in the fetal lamb radiologically and histologically. Prenatal fracture healing in this large animal model demonstrated rapid and complete healing of both incisional and large excisional defects. Fracture healing occurred initially through deposition of a fibrocartilaginous framework with only minimal callus. Endochondral ossification of this cartilagenous matrix as well as enchondral ossification completes this repair process. Normal bony architecture was restored by 21 days in incisional defects and by 40 days in large excisional defects equal to three times cortical width. This is a preliminary study to determine how fetal skeletal elements respond to injury. Further studies examining the biochemical processes regulating this repair process may someday help us to modulate difficult fracture problems such as nonunion in the adult.

REFERENCES

1. Longaker MT, Golbus MS, Filly RA, et al.: Maternal outcome after open fetal surgery: A review of the first 17 human cases. JAMA 265:737–741, 1991.
2. Harrison MR, Adzick NS, Longaker MT, et al.: Successful repair in utero of a fetal diaphragmatic hernia after removal of herniated viscera from the left thorax. New Engl J Med 322:1582, 1990.
3. Crombleholme TM, Harrison MR, Langer JC, et al.: Early experience with open fetal surgery for congenital hydronephrosis. J Pediatr Surg 23:1114, 1988.
4. Harrison MR, Langer JC, Adzick NS, et al.: Correction of congenital diaphragmatic hernia in utero. V. Initial clinical experience. J Pediatr Surg 25:47, 1990.
5. Harrison MR, Adzick NS, Jennings RW, et al.: Antenatal intervention for congenital cystic adenomatoid malformation. Lancet 336:965, 1990.
6. Langer JC, Harrison MR, Schmidt KG, et al.: Fetal hydrops and death from sacrococcygeal teratoma: Rationale for fetal surgery. Am J Obstet Gynecol 160:1145, 1989.
7. Harrison MR, Filly RA, Golbus MS, eds: The Unborn Patient. Philadelphia, WB Saunders, 1990.
8. Longaker MT, Chiu ES, Harrison MR, et al.: Studies in fetal wound healing: IV. Hyaluronic acid stimulating activity distinguishes fetal from adult wound fluid. Ann Surg 210:677, 1989.
9. Longaker MT, Chiu ES, Adzick NS, et al.: Studies in fetal wound healing: V. Prolonged presence of hyaluronic acid characterizes fetal wound fluid. Ann Surg 213:292, 1991.
10. Longaker MT, Whitby DJ, Adzick NS: Studies in fetal wound healing: VI. Second and early third trimester fetal wounds demonstrate rapid collagen deposition without scar formation. J Pediatr Surg 25:63, 1990.
11. Burrington JD: Wound healing in the fetal lamb. J Pediatr Surg 6:523, 1971.
12. Dunne KB, Clarren SK: The origin of prenatal and postnatal deformities. Common orthopedic problems. Ped Clin North Am 33:1277, 1986.
13. Mulholland MC, Pritchard JJ: The fracture gap. J Anat 93:590, 1961.
14. McClements P, Templeton RW, Pritchard JJ. Repair of bone gap. J Anat 95:616, 1961.
15. Fischer E: Low kilovolt radiography. In: Diagnosis of bone and joint disorders. Eds, Resnick G, Niwayama G, WB Saunders, Philadelphia, 1987, pp 108.

16. Hayes CE, Edelstein WA, Schenk JF, et al.: An efficient highly homologous radiofrequency coil for whole body NMR imaging at 1.5 T. J Mag Reson 63:622, 1985.
17. Hallock GG: In utero cleft lip repair in A/J mice. Plast Reconstr Surg 75:785, 1985.
18. Dixon JB: Inflammation in the foetal and neonatal rat: The local reactions to skin burns. J Pathol Bacteriol 80:73, 1960.
19. Krummel TM, Nelson JM, Diegelmann RF, et al.: Fetal response to injury in the rabbit. J Pediatr Surg 22:640, 1987.
20. Sopher D: A study of wound healing in the foetal tissues of the cynomolgus monkey. Lab Anim Handbook 6:327, 1975.
21. Simmons DJ, Kahn AJ: Cell lineage in fracture healing in chimeric bone grafts. Calcif Tissue Int 27:246–253, 1979.
22. McCullagh JJ, Gill P, Wilson DJ: Repair of cartilaginous fractures during chick limb development. J Ortho Res 8:127–131, 1990.
23. Ris MP, Wray JB: A histological study of fracture healing within the uterus of the rabbit. Clin Orthop Rel Res 87:318–321, 1972.
24. Simmons DJ: Comparative physiology of bone. In Bourne G (ed): The Biochemistry and Physiology of Bone, Vol. IV. Academic Press, New York, 1976, pp 445–516.
25. Aegerter and Kirkpatrick: Orthopedic Diseases, 3rd Ed., WB Saunders, Philadelphia, 1969. pp 231.
26. Bolander ME, Balian G: The use of demineralized bone matrix in the repair of segmental defects. JBJS 68-A(8):1264–1274, 1986.
27. Zadek RE, Robinson RA: The healing of osteal-periosteal discontinuity of standard length in skeletally mature and immature canine radii. In: The healing of osseous tissue: a workshop sponsored by the committee on the skeletal system. pp 9–22. Division of medical sciences, National Academy of Science-National Research Council, October 22–23, 1965. Washington D.C., 1967.
28. Anderson KJ, Dingwall JA: The osteogenic repair of long-bone defects in immature and mature cat. In: The healing of osseous tissue: a workshop sponsored by the committee on the skeletal system. pp 23–40. Division of medical sciences, National Academy of Science-National research council, October 22–23, 1965. Washington D.C., 1967.
29. Irving JT, LeBolt SA, Schneider EL: Ectopic bone formation and aging. Clin Ortho Rel Research 154:249–253, 1981.
30. Syftestad GT, Urist MR: Bone aging: Clin Ortho Rel Research 162:288–297, 1982.
31. Kahn AJ, Simmons DJ: Chondrocyte-to-osteocyte transformation in grafts of perichondrium-free epiphyseal cartilage. Clin Orthop & Rel Res 129:299–304, 1977.
32. Krukowski M, Simmons DJ, Kahn AJ. Cell lineage studies: In: Kunin AS and Simmons DJ (eds): Skeletal Research—An Experimental Approach. Academic Press, New York, 1983, pp 89–117.
33. Laasonen EM, Kyro A, Korhola O, Botsman O: Magnetic resonance imaging of tibial shaft fracture repair. Arch Orthop Trauma Surg 108:40–43, 1989.

CHAPTER **8**

Human Fetal Skin: Ontogeny and Repair

H. Peter Lorenz
Michael T. Longaker
N. Scott Adzick

Human fetal skin development progresses in an orderly manner, forming an organ capable of providing a barrier to bacteria and water loss as well as a mechanism for heat regulation. Fully differentiated adult skin is composed of epidermis and dermis. Multiple cell layers comprise the epidermis, which include the basal cell layer, stratum granulosum, stratum spinosum, and stratum corneum. The dermis and epidermis are attached by the basement membrane zone. The dermis is composed of collagenous mesenchymal tissue, ground substance, vessels, nerves, and epidermal appendages.

Despite detailed studies of fetal skin development, our knowledge remains limited to morphology. Although a large body of literature has produced a great deal of morphologic detail in fetal skin ontogeny, the physiology of fetal skin has not been systematically studied. This chapter will provide an overview of human fetal skin development and discuss a novel experimental model for the study of human fetal skin wound healing.

HUMAN EPIDERMAL DEVELOPMENT

A primitive epidermis first appears in the 20 day embryo after the neural groove has invaginated. Four weeks after conception, the epidermis consists of the periderm and the basal cell layer,[1] and these two layers comprise the epidermis during the embryonic period (gestational age <8 weeks). Periderm is the outermost single cell layer of the epidermis and is distinguished by microvilli and blebs, posing some to hypothesize a secretion/absorption function. Through the rest of gestation, the periderm remains a solitary cell layer until it is sloughed off.

The fetal stage of development (gestational age >8 weeks) is characterized initially by an epidermal stratification period from 9–14 weeks gestation.[2] During this stage an intermediate cell layer develops and begins to stratify between the basal cell layer and the periderm layer (Fig. 8.1).

By the 16th week gestation, an adult epidermal pattern is present. The epidermis has progressed to four to five cell layers, including the intermediate cell layer, which is two to three cell layers thick. Basal cells have a minimal content of glycogen, which is by now approaching adult characteristics. Although the replication rate of the basal cell layer is decreasing at this stage, it is still greater than in the adult.[3] Prekeratins are present in the basal cell cytoplasm and are

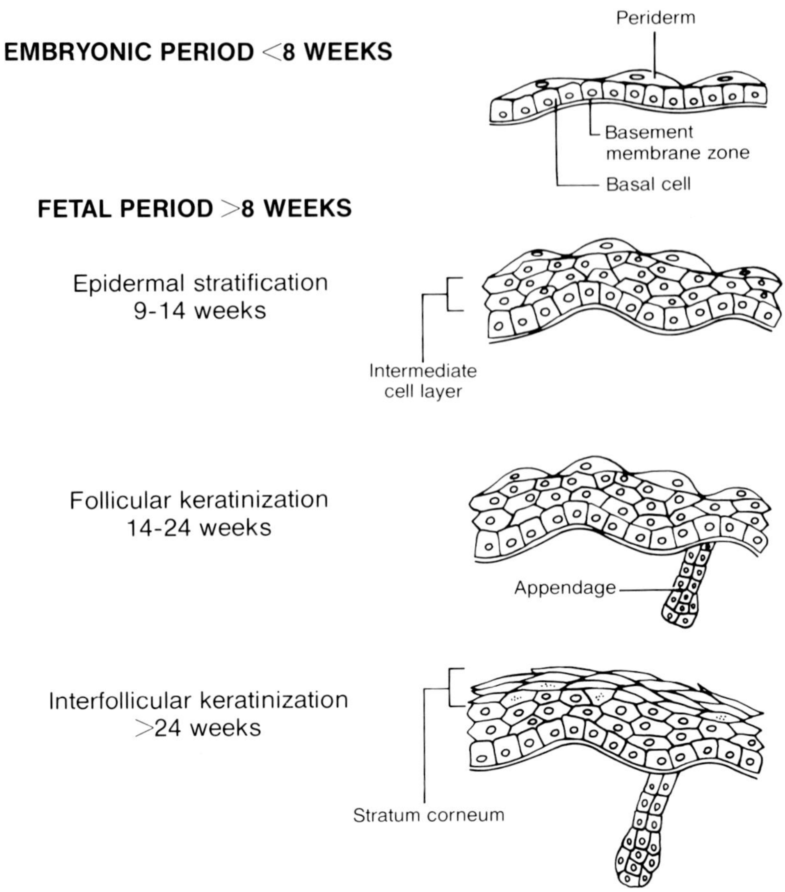

Figure 8.1 Diagram of ontogeny of human fetal epidermal development sequence as proposed by Lane. Used with permission.[2]

associated with desmosomes and hemidesmosomes. Basal cell attachment to the basal lamina is becoming apparent through the developing hemidesmosomes and anchoring filaments.[4] The basement membrane zone (BMZ) separates the epidermis from the dermis. The temporal sequence of development of BMZ antigens has been mapped.[2,5]

The cells of the intermediate layer of the epidermis have large glycogen stores, for which no physiologic significance has yet been determined.[6] One may speculate that the high glycogen content of the fetal epidermis may reflect absorption of nutrients from amniotic fluid through the periderm. Keratin filament bundles are present and the sequence of keratin expression in human fetal epidermis has been well characterized.[7] Multiple monoclonal antibodies against the various cytokeratins show differences in the basal, intermediate, and periderm cell layers.[4]

The periderm at 14–16 weeks gestation continues to be characterized by microvilli and blebs, thus presenting a large surface area for contact with amniotic fluid. Presently, no function of the periderm has been documented.[6,8,9] At this stage the periderm enlarges with the growing fetus by cellular hypertrophy. Periderm cell replication has been shown to occur through 11 weeks gestation.[9] By

19 weeks gestation, the periderm begins to necrose and slough in locations that have become fully keratinized such as the scalp, face, palms, and soles.[10] By week 24 of gestation, periderm is absent in most locations.

Melanocytes are present in the epidermis by 14–16 weeks gestation.[11] Melanin synthesis has been documented at this time and continues throughout gestation.[12,13] The Langerhans cell is present by seven weeks gestation.[14] A third cell-type, the Merkel cell, is present by 19 weeks gestation[6] and appears to arise from epidermal precursor cells.[15] The roles of the fetal Langerhans and Merkel cells remain unknown.

Follicular keratinization occurs during weeks 14–24 of gestation[2] (Figure 1). The intermediate cell layer stratifies and appendages begin to develop from buds in the basal cell layer. Hair follicles begin as hair germs, which are tightly clustered basal epidermal cells, then progress to hair pegs, which are elongated tongues of epidermal cells that project into the dermis.[6] Hair follicle maturation follows a cephalocaudal gradient.[16] Follicles in the scalp are not only present in a greater density but also are in a more differentiated state than those lower on the body. Signs of keratinization in the hair proper and in the canal that forms the intraepidermal hair tract portion of the follicle are seen earlier in the head than elsewhere in the developing skin. Immunohistochemical staining of the interfollicular and follicular epidermis with cytokeratin antibodies also shows pattern changes consistent with a more advanced differentiation of scalp and head hair follicles relative to the trunk and extremities.[4]

The sebaceous gland anlagen and arrector pili attachment site buds subsequently become apparent on the developing follicle. Eccrine sweat glands begin to develop on the palmar and plantar surfaces first, then on the remainder of the body by 20–24 weeks gestation. These developing glands are marked by carcinoembryonic antigen (CEA) in their earliest stages of differentiation.[17]

It is interesting to relate the events of epidermal wound healing to human fetal skin development. During postnatal healing, the surrounding skin appendages have the potential to form normal epidermis at the site of trauma. However, if the appendages are destroyed, then epidermis from the periphery must proliferate and cover the wound. Whereas the basal cell layer during fetal skin development has the ability to form appendages, the basal cell layer cannot be induced to form appendages in postnatal skin.

HUMAN DERMAL DEVELOPMENT

The embryonic (six to eight week gestational age) dermis is quite cellular and consists of loosely arrayed mesenchymal cells with no clear planes within the dermis or between the dermis and subdermal tissue. These early mesenchymal cells are characterized by a stellate appearance, a high nucleus to cytoplasmic volume ratio, and abundant glycogen stores.[18] Immunohistochemistry studies show a small amount of collagen types I and III present throughout the dermal extracellular matrix, but these collagens are somewhat concentrated in a narrow zone underlying the epidermal-dermal junction.[19] Type IV collagen is present in the basement membranes around vessels, while types III and V collagen are present in vascular sheaths. Simple capillary-like vessels first seen in the embryonic period evolve into vessels that are surrounded by matrix and perivascular cells.[20]

The transition from a cellular to a fibrous dermis occurs as collagen deposition accumulates over gestational weeks nine to 12. The diameters of individual collagen fibrils increase and greater numbers of fibrils form bundles.[21] This gradual increase in collagen in the extracellular matrix is associated with a decrease in the density of dermal fetal fibroblasts, eventually resulting in a less cellular appearance of the dermis.

A fibrous dermis becomes apparent at 13–16 weeks gestational age.[21,22] Fetal fibroblasts at this stage of development have produced significant amounts of types I and III collagen. By immunoperoxidase staining, the type I:III ratio is almost 50%, which is unlike the adult ratio of approximately 85:15.[6] This increased ratio of type III to I in fetal skin favors compliance over tensile strength during fetal growth.[18]

Several collagen modification enzymes are present and active including lysyl hydroxylase.[23,24] Collagenase is synthesized in an increased amount by cultured fetal fibroblasts relative to adult fibroblasts.[25] Other studies have shown increased collagen turnover in fetal skin compared to adult.[26] Elastic fibers can be seen throughout the dermis, but the elastin component is not yet present.[27]

By 19 weeks gestation the dermis has thickened and intradermal planes distinguishing the papillary and reticular dermis as well as the subdermal tissue plane become apparent. Over the remainder of gestation, the water content of the dermis decreases as sulfated glycosaminoglycans slowly replace non-sulfated glycosaminoglycans (GAGs), of which hyaluronic acid (HA) is predominant.[28–30] From 24 weeks gestation to term, dermal development is characterized by further maturation of the various elements on a molecular level whereas little morphologic change occurs during this period. By 24 weeks, fetal skin has the pattern of adult skin, albeit miniaturized.

HUMAN FETAL SKIN WOUND HEALING

From the clinical experience in human fetal surgery at the University of California, San Francisco, Dr. Michael Harrison noted that the human fetus appeared to heal skin wounds without scar formation. This observation has led our group and others to document scarless fetal skin wound healing in multiple animal models, including the rabbit, rat, mouse, sheep, and monkey[31–36] (see Chapter 4). Discrepancies between some of the animal models with respect to fetal skin wound healing characteristics have been observed, which makes extrapolation to the human situation difficult. Because no studies of human fetal skin wound healing have been performed due to obvious ethical limitations, we developed a model of wound healing using human fetal skin.

NUDE MOUSE MODEL

The athymic "nude" mouse can be utilized as an in vivo model of human fetal wound repair. It has been established that nude mice maintain lifetime skin grafts from a wide variety of mammals, including man. Grafts of human fetal skin onto nude mice retain all the morphological and ultrastructural features associated with normal fetal skin development.[37,38] Thus, human fetal skin is transplanted into an adult environment since the amniotic fluid effect is removed. With our model, the transplanted skin is then wounded and its wound healing characteristics studied, which includes examination for scar formation.

The experimental technique is straightforward. Human 19 week gestation fetal skin samples from the trunk and extremities are obtained from therapeutic abortion material after obtaining signed consent for the use of this tissue for research purposes under an approved UCSF Committee on Human Research protocol. Gestational age is determined by fetal characteristics and maternal obstetrical history and physical findings. Adult control skin specimens from elective facial cosmetic procedures are similarly obtained. The samples are placed in cooled media and stored at 5°C for one to 18 hours until transplanted.

Nude mice are utilized as the adult recipient because of their lack of cell-mediated xenograft rejection. Two transplant sites are used on the recipient: (1) externally onto a cutaneous site on the dorsal surface where full-thickness native mouse skin has been excised or (2) internally into a subcutaneous pocket where the mouse panniculus carnosus is raised from the underlying fascia in either the left or the right flank (Fig. 8.2). The dorsal site is prepared by removing a 0.5 cm × 0.5 cm area of full-thickness skin. The cutaneous graft is then anchored with

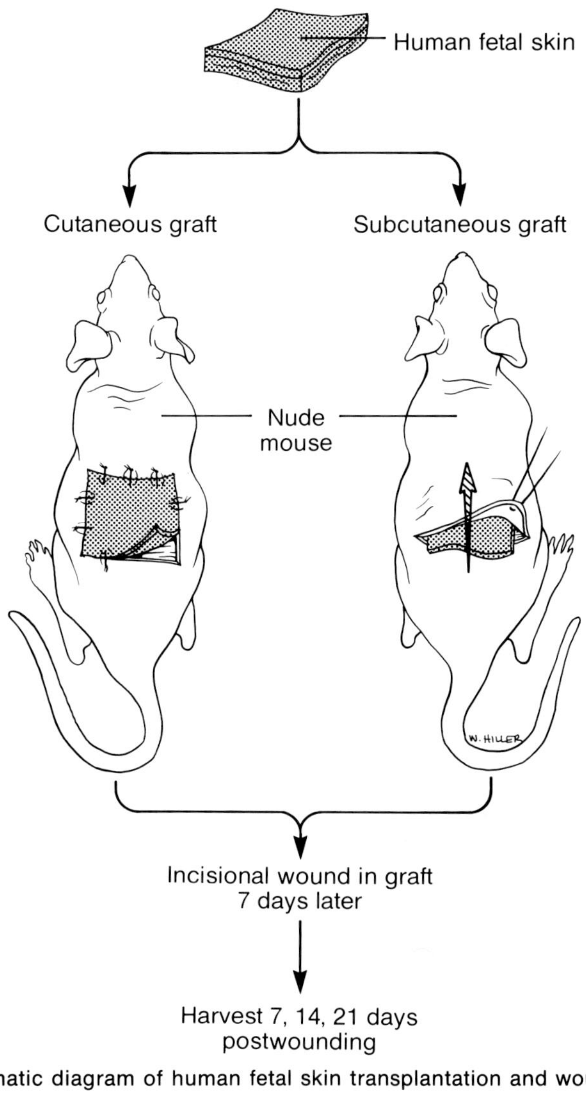

Figure 8.2 Schematic diagram of human fetal skin transplantation and wounding in the nude mouse.

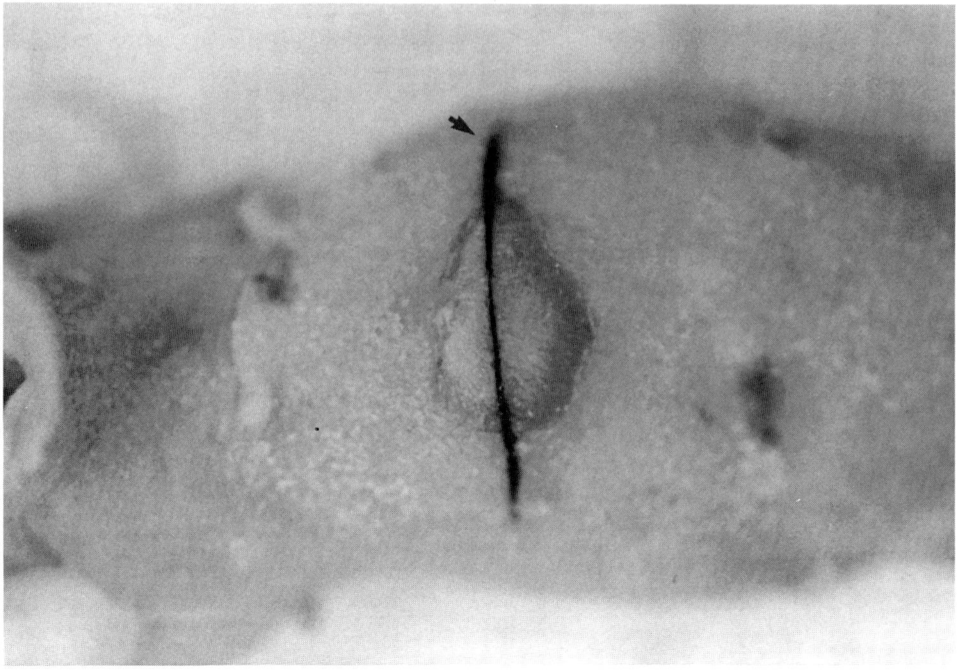

Figure 8.3 Photograph of 19 week gestation human fetal skin cutaneous graft on a nude mouse after making a linear incisional wound through the graft and marking the wound with India ink (arrow).

a dressing and clips. The subcutaneous pocket is created by incising a 1 cm length of skin and panniculus carnosus obliquely along the flank and raising a full-thickness flap to excavate a 1 cm^2 cavity. After the graft is placed inside, the incision is closed with surgical clips and allowed to heal in an airtight fashion. Grafts are positioned such that graft dermis apposes mouse fascia. All procedures are carried out under sterile conditions with general ether anesthesia.

Seven days after transplantation, linear incisions are made through the graft. In the case of cutaneous grafts, a 5 mm extension into murine skin on either graft side is made for experimental mouse controls. India ink is used to mark the wound location (Fig. 8.3). The subcutaneous pockets are reopened through a separate incision and the grafts exposed prior to wounding. The pockets are then reclosed with clips subsequent to wounding.

At days 7, 14, and 21 postwounding, animals are sacrificed. Wounded fetal grafts and murine skin samples are fixed in formalin for either hematoxylin and eosin or trichrome staining.

Results

Cutaneous Grafts

The fetal grafts take readily on their murine fascial bed and are easily distinguished from the surrounding murine skin. Incisional wounds and the graft/donor skin interface in 19 week gestation human fetal skin heal with scar formation as demonstrated by H&E staining (Fig. 8.4). Using Mallory's trichrome stain, a thick

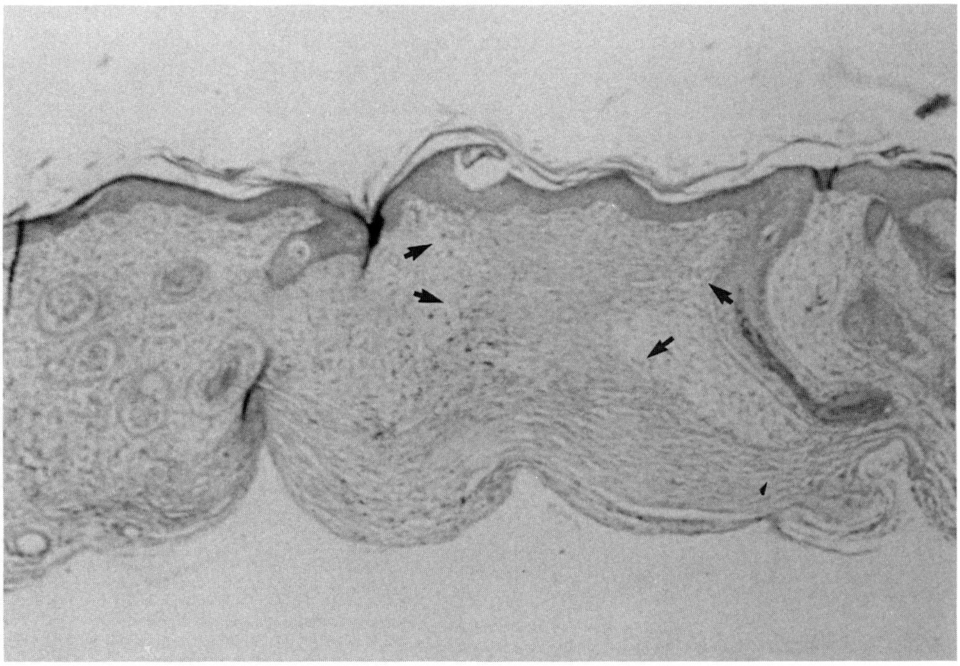

Figure 8.4 Photomicrograph of 19 week gestation human fetal skin cutaneous graft wound, harvested 14 days after wounding and stained with H&E. The scar is outlined by arrows.

collagen scar is quite evident in the incisional wound in both fetal (Fig. 8.5) and adult human grafts. Thickened, parallel collagen bundles comprise the scar. Incisional wounds in the nude mouse skin also heal with scar. Near complete healing by light microscopy is present by seven days, and by 14 days all wounds have healed. At 21 days, scar remains and no graft viability loss is notable.

Subcutaneous Grafts

The fetal skin grafts remain viable and heal their wounds, unlike adult skin grafts that exhibit a low viability rate in the subcutaneous position. The adult grafts' high necrosis rate with inability to heal wounds may relate to inadequate neovascularization to support wound repair at one week post-transplantation. In contrast to cutaneous grafts of 19 week gestational age human fetal skin, subcutaneous grafts of the same gestational age fetal skin heal without a scar (Fig. 8.6).

The India ink wound tattoo makes wound identification possible since regeneration of normal tissue architecture occurs after wounding. Without the presence of India ink in the dermis or epidermis, one has difficulty locating the wound proper. The India ink mark also demonstrates normal appendages present in between the wound edges, which does not occur in a scar (Fig. 8.7). These epidermal appendages may have regenerated within the wound or have been present from the initial time of wounding.

The Mallory's trichrome stained wound shows a normal collagen pattern within the wound when compared to the surrounding unwounded dermis. This more organized collagen deposition in fetal skin wounds compared to adult wounds is the hallmark of scarless repair.

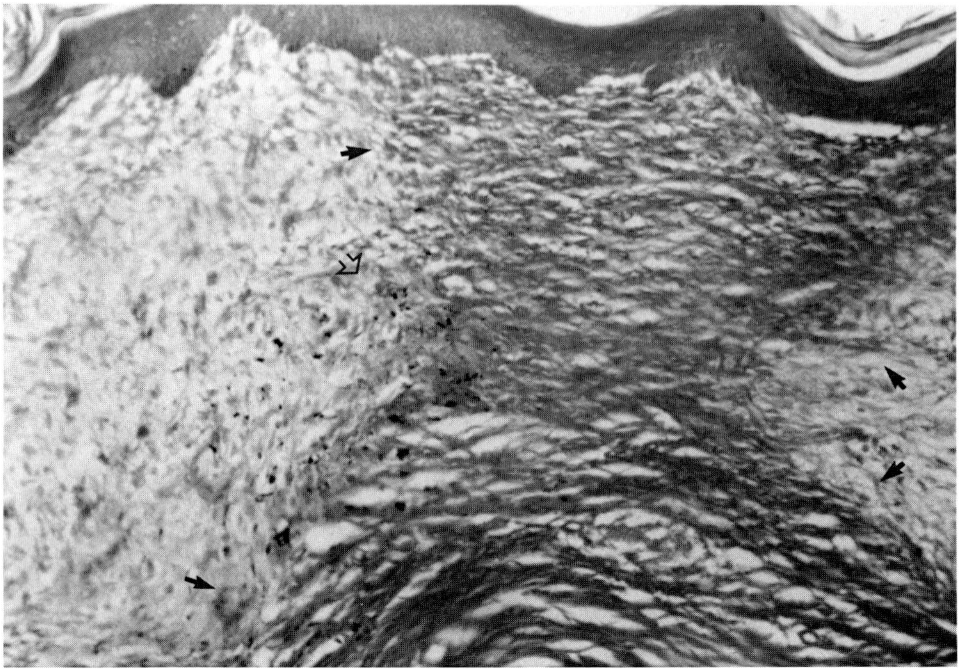

Figure 8.5 Photomicrograph of 19 week gestation human fetal skin cutaneous graft wound, harvested 14 days after wounding and stained by Mallory's trichrome. Thick, parallel bundles of collagen course through the scar (solid arrows). India ink can be seen in the dermis along the left border of the scar (open arrow).

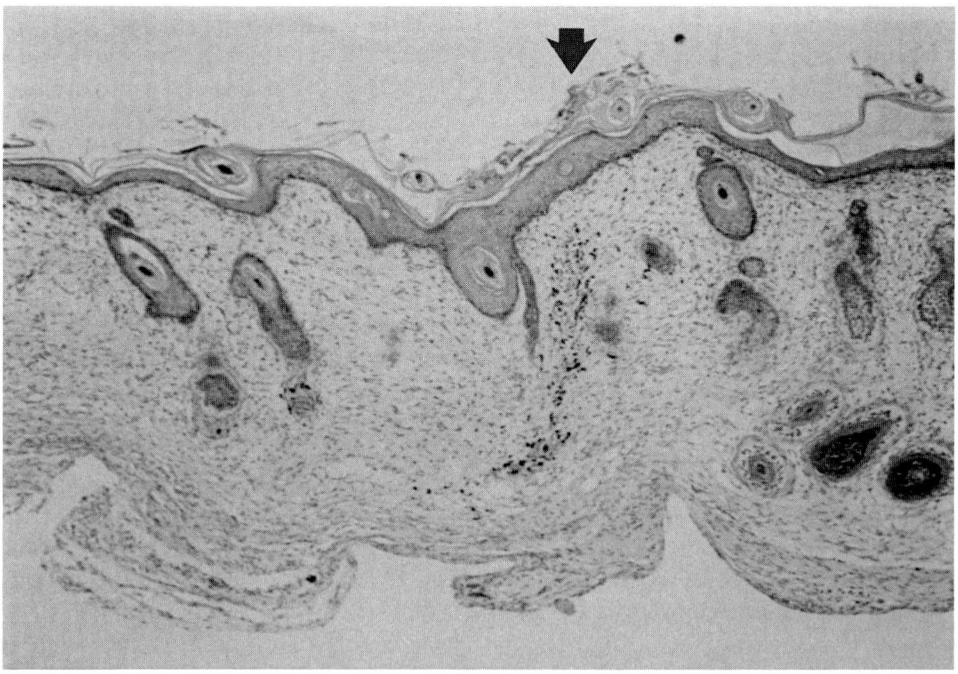

Figure 8.6 Photomicrograph of 19 week gestation human fetal skin subcutaneous graft wound, harvested 14 days after wounding and stained with H&E. India ink marks the wound location (arrow).

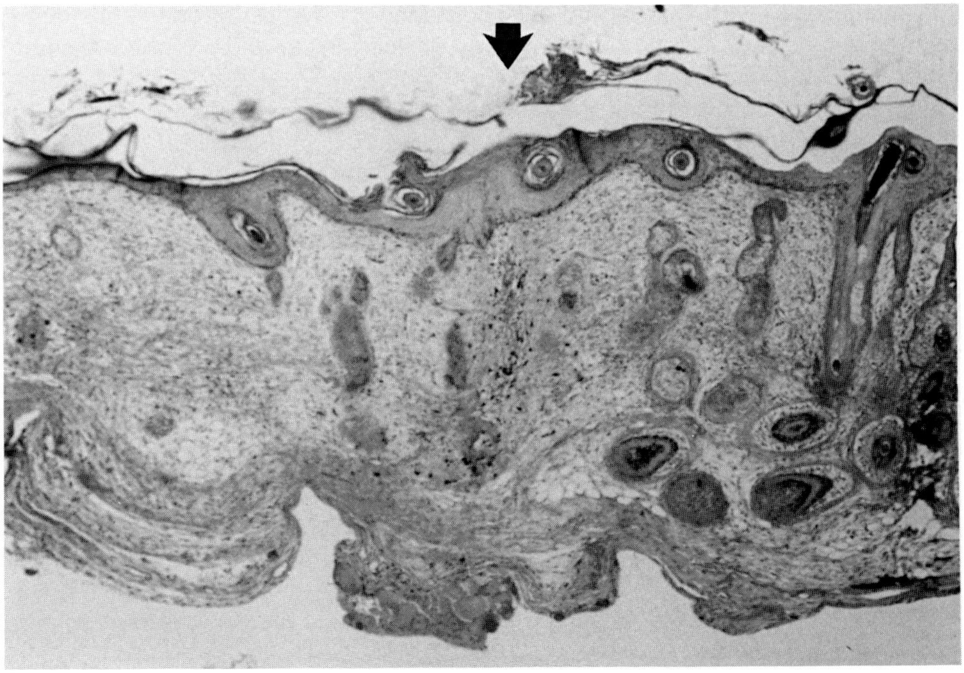

Figure 8.7 Photomicrograph of 19 week gestation human fetal skin subcutaneous graft wound (arrow), harvested 14 days after wounding and stained by Mallory's trichrome. Appendages are present within the wound, which one never sees in scar. The collagen staining pattern is unchanged from the surrounding unwounded skin.

Implications

The biology of human fetal skin wound healing remains relatively unstudied due to the lack of an appropriate model system. We now have a model in which the regulation of scarless human fetal skin repair can be dissected. Not only is there scarless skin repair in the subcutaneous location of the nude mouse, but the same gestational age skin heals with a scar when placed in a cutaneous location. This unique juxtaposition allows for comparison of the mechanisms of skin repair with and without scar formation.

The role of the environment in fetal skin wound healing can be studied. The scarless healing of human fetal skin transplanted into a subcutaneous pocket demonstrates that perfusion by fetal serum and continuous immersion of the wound in amniotic fluid is not essential for scarless fetal repair. Scarless healing appears to be intrinsic to the fetal skin itself, although the location of the human fetal skin graft is crucial. One notable difference is that a subcutaneous pocket is characterized by a sterile, aqueous environment, whereas the cutaneous position is nonsterile and the skin is subject to desiccation.

The environment also affects the rate of fetal skin differentiation. Lane showed that human fetal skin transplanted to a subcutaneous location will differentiate at a rate comparable to in utero. In contrast, human fetal skin transplanted to the surface of nude mice and exposed to air demonstrates an acceleration of development.[38] This more rapid rate of cellular differentiation offers one explanation for why fetal skin of the same initial gestational age may heal scarlessly in one environment and with scar in another environment. Studies in fetal lambs demonstrate a spectrum of fetal healing with a switch to scar and adult-like healing late in gestation when the skin is more differentiated.[39] A correlation of differentiation states with wound healing histology is needed.

Another possible etiologic factor causing cutaneous grafts to heal with scar is a more rapid rate of graft neovascularization, which would bring earlier wound perfusion by adult serum and inflammatory cells. The angiogenic and inflammatory mediators present would be in an adult pattern. For example, the earlier presence of adult macrophages and polymorphonuclear leukocytes may preclude scarless repair.

Using this model, experiments can be planned to systematically study the expression of specific growth factors and extracellular matrix components in both the buried and exposed grafts. In addition, wounded buried and exposed grafts can be manipulated on the nude mouse through the use of topical dressings and growth factor exposure. Notable differences may provide insights into the mechanisms of scarless repair.

The scarless repair of human fetal skin demonstrates that regeneration of normal tissue architecture after trauma is possible in an organ where regeneration does not occur postnatally. The nude mouse model of human fetal skin wound healing provides a promising new system for the study of human fetal skin repair.

REFERENCES

1. Serri FF, Montagna W, Mescon H: Studies of the skin of the fetus and the child. J Invest Dermatol 39:199–217,1962.
2. Lane AL: Human fetal skin development. Pediatr Dermatol 3(6):487–491,1986.
3. Stern IB: The uptake of tritiated thymidine by human fetal epidermis. J Invest Dermatol 63:268–272,1974.
4. Moll R, Moll I, Wiest W: Changes in the pattern of cytokeratin polypeptides in epidermis and hair follicles during skin development in human fetuses. Differentiation 23:170–178,1982.
5. Fine JD, Smith LT, Holbrook KA, et al.: The appearance of four basement zone antigens in developing human fetal skin. J Invest Dermatol 83:66–69,1984.
6. Holbrook KA: The biology of human fetal skin at ages related to prenatal diagnosis. Pediatr Dermatol 1(2):97–111,1983.
7. Dale BA, Holbrook KA, Kimball JR, et al.: Expression of epidermal keratins and filaggrin during human fetal skin development. J Cell Biol 101:1257–1269,1985.
8. Holbrook KA, Odland GF: The fine structure of developing human epidermis: light, scanning and transmission electron microscopy of the periderm. J Invest Dermatol 65:16–38,1975.
9. Hoyes AP: Electron microscopy of the surface layer (periderm) of human fetal skin. J Anat 103:321–326, 1968.
10. Holbrook KA, Odland GF: Regional development of the human epidermis in the first trimester embryo and second trimester fetus (ages related to the timing of amniocentesis and fetal biopsy). J Invest Dermatol 74:161–168,1980.
11. Varelzidis A, Tosca A, Coumantakis E, et al.: Immunohistochemical studies on 70 human embryos concerning the epidermal binding of pemphigus and pemphigoid antibodies. Acta Dermatoverner 60:129–133,1980.
12. Breathnach AS, Wyllie LM: Electron microscopy of melanocytes and Langerhans cells in human fetal dermis at 14 weeks. J Invest Dermatol 44:51–60,1965.
13. Mishima Y, Widlan S: Embryonic development of melanocytes in human hair and epidermis. J Invest Dermatol 46:263–277,1966.
14. Foster CA, Holbrook KA: Ontogeny of Langerhans cells in human and fetal skin: Cell densities and phenotypic expression relative to epidermal growth. Am J Anat 184:157–164,1989.
15. Moll I, Lane AT, Franke WW, et al.: Intraepidermal formation of Merkel cells in xenografts of human fetal skin. J Invest Dermatol 94(3):359–364, 1990.

16. Pinkus H: Embroyology of hair. In: Montagna W, Ellis RA eds. Hair Growth. New York, Academic Press, pp. 1–32,1958.
17. Penneys NS, Kott R, Buck B: Eccrine gland development in fetal skin: An immunohistochemical study with carcinoembryonic antigen (CEA) and S100 protein. J Invest Dermatol 80:338–339A,1983.
18. Smith LT, Holbrook KA: Embryogenesis of the dermis in human fetal skin. Pediatr Dermatol 3(4):271–280,1986.
19. Smith LT, Holbrook KA, Madri JA: Collagen types I, III and V in human embryonic and fetal skin. Am J Anat 175:507–521,1986.
20. Johnson CL, Holbrook KA: Development of human embryonic and fetal dermal vasculature. J Invest Dermatol 93(2)Suppl:10S–17S,1989.
21. Smith LT, Holbrook KA, Byers PH: Structure of the dermal matrix during development and in the adult. J Invest Dermatol 79:935–1045,1982.
22. Smith LT, Holbrook KA: Development of dermal connective tissue in human embryonic and fetal skin. SEM IV:1745–1751, 1982.
23. Anttinen H, Orava S, Ryhanen L, Kivirikko K: Assay of protocollagen lysyl hydroxylase activity in the skin of human subjects and changes in activity with age. Clin Chim Acta 47:289–294,1973.
24. Kirsh E, Weber L, Kreig T, Muller PK: Age dependent variation in the degree of hydroxylation of lysine residues in human skin collagen: possible role in fibril formation. J Invest Dermatol 76:419–420,1981.
25. Widdowson EM: Changes in the extracellular compartment of muscle and skin during normal and retarded development. Bibl Nutr Dieta 13:60–68,1969.
26. Holbrook KA: Structure and function of the developing human skin. In: Goldsmith LA, ed. Biochemistry and physiology of the skin. New York, Oxford University Press, pp. 64–101,1983.
27. Deutsch TA, Esterly NB: Elastic fibers in fetal dermis. J Invest Dermatol 65:320–323,1975.
28. Loewi G, Meyer K: The acid mucopolysaccharides of embryonic skin. Biochem Biophys Acta 27:453–458, 1958.
29. Breen M, Weinstein HG, Johnson RL, et al.: Acid glycosaminoglycans in human skin during fetal development and adult life. Biochem Biophys Acta 201:54–60,1970.
30. Varma RS, Varma R: Glycosaminoglycans and proteoglycans of skin. In: Glycosaminoglycans and proteoglycans in physiological processes of body systems. Basel: Karger 151–164,1982.
31. Burrington JD: Wound healing in the fetal lamb. J Pediatr Surg 6:523–528,1971.
32. Goss AN: The intra-uterine healing of fetal rat oral mucosal, skin, and cartilage wounds. J Oral Pathol 6:35–43, 1977.
33. Krummel TM, Nelson JM, Diegelmann RF, et al.: Fetal response to injury in the rabbit. J Pediatr Surg 22:640–644, 1987.
34. Sopher D: The response of rat fetal membrane to injury. Ann Royal Coll Surg (England) 51:240–245,1972.
35. Block M: Wound healing in the newborn opossum (Didelphis virginianam). Nature 187:340–341,1960.
36. Hallock GG: In utero cleft lip repair in A/J mice. Plast Reconstr Surg 75:785–788,1985.
37. Lane AT, Day KH: Basement membrane zone develpment of human fetal skin tranplanted to the nude mouse. J Invest Dermatol 86:486A,1986.
38. Lane AT, Scott GA, Day KH: Development of human fetal skin transplanted to nude mice. J Invest Dermatol 93:787–791,1989.
39. Longaker MT, Whitby DJ, Adzick NS, et al.: Studies in fetal wound healing: VI. Second and early third trimester fetal wounds demonstrate rapid collagen deposition without scar formation. J Pediatr Surg 25:63–69,1990.

CHAPTER 9

Fetal Wound Contraction

Michael T. Longaker
N. Scott Adzick
H. Paul Ehrlich

FETAL WOUND CONTRACTION

Whether fetal skin wounds actually contract is somewhat controversial and the variability of findings relates to the animal model studied. Almost all of the work has been done in the fetal rabbit and lamb models. This chapter reviews fetal wound contraction studies in fetal rabbits, lambs, and humans.

OVERVIEW OF ADULT WOUND CONTRACTION

The destruction of soft tissue and its eventual repair involves the migration of a number of different cell types into the wound site, leading to the deposition and reorganization of a new connective tissue matrix. Included in the closure of an open defect is the process of wound contraction, whereby the surrounding uninjured skin is pulled over the defect. The appearance of normal skin in the repair site is not due to skin regeneration, but rather the centripetal movement of skin. The newly deposited tissue that occupies the area between skin edges is scar, having no skin appendages and lacking normal dermal fiber structure. The skin that has been pulled over the defect has normal dermal fiber structure and skin appendages. In general, wound contraction is beneficial because there is a reduced area of scar tissue covering the defect.

In contrast to "wound contraction" is "scar contracture," where the contractile process follows the completion of wound closure. Scar contracture can be detrimental to the well-being of the patient, since an established fibrotic tissue undergoes a reduction in surface area that can disrupt the mechanical function of neighboring tissue or structures. For example, scar contracture occurring over a joint will reduce the movement and functioning of that joint. In both contractile processes there appears to be a relationship or cooperation between cellular forces and connective tissue organization.

Cellular Aspects

The mesenchyme-derived cellular component of either granulation tissue or scar connective tissue generates the contractile forces that appear to involve cytoplasmic actin-myosin muscular contractile activity. The dynamic contraction of these cytoplasmic structures produces the force that reorients surrounding connective tissue.

The myofibroblast is histologically characterized by large cable-like actin-rich stress fibers, and this specialized cell is a classic feature of contracting wounds and scars.[1] Consequently, the appearance of myofibroblasts serves as a marker of wound contraction. Myofibroblasts are derived from fibroblasts, but experimental evidence shows that fibroblasts produce the forces of wound contraction.[2] The morphologic change of fibroblasts into myofibroblasts signifies the termination of the active participation of fibroblasts in connective tissue reorganization. It is speculated that myofibroblasts appear in stabilized, organized connective tissue, which may represent a transitional period for the future migration of myofibroblasts from the healed wound.

A model to examine the mechanism of wound contraction is the fibroblast populated collagen lattice (FPCL) introduced by Bell and co-workers.[3] In this model, fibroblasts trapped within a polymerized collagen lattice cause the lattice to contract. The FPCL are manufactured by mixing together collagen, fibroblasts, and serum-containing culture medium. The lattice undergoes a reduction in size by compacting of collagen fibers by resident fibroblasts to a tissue-like structure that resembles dermis.[3] Agents such as cytochalasin B, which disrupt microfilaments, block lattice contraction.[3] Lattice contraction is dependent on cytoplasmic muscle contractile forces.[4] The translation of these cytoplasmic contractile forces into the reorganization of collagen fibrils causes lattice contraction. Resident fibroblasts reorient and compact collagen fibrils, reducing the volume of the tissue. Lattice contraction is expressed as a percent of initial resting area (Fig. 9.1).

The cellular mechanism responsible for the relocation of collagen fibrils has been examined.[2] One hypothesis is that myofibroblasts undergo cell contraction and attached collagen fibrils are moved by this reduction in cellular surface area.[5] Another possibility is that collagen fibrils are pulled over the cell surface by the contraction of individual cytoplasmic microfilaments.[2] The cell surface area is maintained and membrane collagen-attachment sites move over that surface. Experimental evidence supports the latter explanation. Contracted cells are not a characteristic of contracting lattices. Stimulating cell elongation and spreading enhances lattice contraction.

Fibroblasts at the periphery of the FPCL develop a myofibroblast morphology, characterized by a high degree of cell-cell contacts and cytoplasmic cable-like

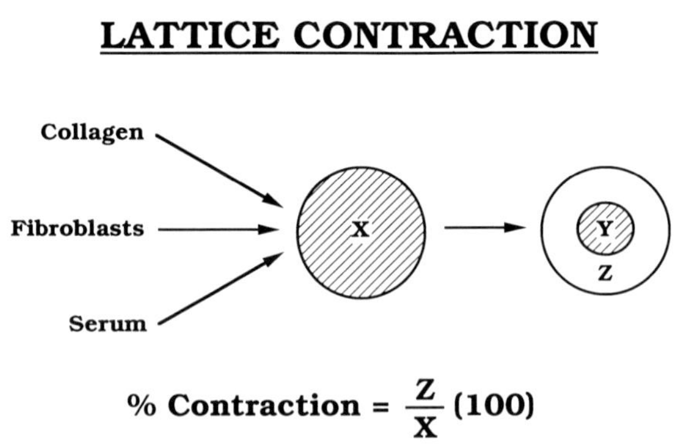

Figure 9.1 Schematic drawing of fibroblast populated collagen lattice. The lattice decreases in size as it contracts and the percent contraction can be calculated using the formula shown.

actin-myosin stress fibers. Cells at the central region of the FPCL retain a fibroblast-like morphology and appear as individual independent cellular units in contact with collagen fibrils along with cytoplasmic fine actin-rich microfilaments. FPCL were cut into equilateral triangular wedges. Some wedges contained the outer edge from the FPCL with a high density of myofibroblasts. Other wedges were cut where central regions from the FPCL made up all edges of the wedge. With time, wedges underwent a reduction in size. The wedges with the myofibroblast-rich edge contracted minimally at the myofibroblast-rich edge, and these wedges developed an asymmetrical isoceles triangular shape. The other wedges contracted uniformly and retained an equilateral triangular shape.[6] The fibroblast-rich region showed maximal contraction and collagen reorganization. Whereas independent fibroblast units with actin filaments organized collagen, multicellular units of myofibroblasts with cytoplasmic stress fibers played only a minimal role in organizing collagen fibers.[2]

In vivo evidence for fibroblasts producing contractile forces has been reported.[1] In contracting open rat wounds, myofibroblasts first appear at seven days, a time when about 50% of wound contraction is completed.[1] One would assume that they would be present before seven days if they were critical for the initiation of wound contraction. Additional evidence is provided by the tight skin mouse model in which open wound closure is delayed for three weeks.[7] Based on actin stress fiber staining, myofibroblasts fill the repair site in these noncontracting wounds. When wound contraction gets underway at four weeks, myofibroblasts with their characteristic actin-staining stress fibers disappear and fibroblasts with fine filamentous actin-staining cytoplasmic microfilaments replace them. When wound contraction is near completion at six weeks, myofibroblasts with cytoplasmic stress fibers reappear. In this model, wound contraction is active when myofibroblasts convert to fibroblasts. The ability of fibroblasts to develop into myofibroblasts and then revert back into fibroblasts supports the postulated transitional nature of the myofibroblast.

Connective Tissue Aspects

There is experimental evidence that the collagen composition of connective tissue can also influence the contractile process. There is a positive relationship between type III collagen concentration and degree of contraction. Healing wounds with granulation tissue that contains a high proportion of type III collagen show wound contraction. Conversely, a mature scar has lower levels of type III collagen and rarely shows contraction. In vitro this relationship can be demonstrated with FPCL. FPCL made with collagen extracted from contracting hypertrophic scar contracts faster and to a greater degree than ones composed of collagen extracted from normal dermis.[2] FPCL composed of type III collagen contract faster and to a greater degree than ones composed of type I collagen.[8]

The mechanism of wound contraction and scar contracture appears to involve the dynamic organization of the connective tissue by the resident fibroblasts—a process that requires cooperation between cells and matrix. There appears to be no specialized contractile cell necessary. Contraction is minimal in mature fibrous scar that has a low cell density and a type III collagen-poor connective tissue matrix. On the other hand, a tissue with a high cell density and an immature matrix rich in type III collagen will readily undergo contraction.

The Fetal Rabbit Model

Somasundaram originally reported that excisional fetal rabbit wounds exposed to amniotic fluid do not contract.[9] However, if excluded from amniotic fluid by a silastic patch, the wounds rapidly healed.[10] Krummel and colleagues recently confirmed these studies.[11] They made incisional wounds on day 24 of gestation (term = 31 days) that were left unsutured and remained exposed to amniotic fluid. The incisional wounds gaped open at term, showing no evidence of contraction. They also examined excisional wound contraction. A 4 mm full-thickness punch wound was created on the back of rabbit fetuses and the wound edges marked with India ink. To control for fetal growth, a circular 4 mm diameter India ink tattoo pattern was placed onto unwounded fetal skin. Wounds were harvested from one hour to six days postwounding. At each time point, there was a significant increase in the wound area when compared to that of the control tattoo pattern. Thus, the wounds not only failed to contract but actually increased in size beyond what could be accounted for by fetal growth. To further document the lack of wound contraction in excisional fetal rabbit wounds, Hayes[12] investigated whether open fetal rabbit wounds contained myofibroblasts, which is a cellular element identifiable in contracting wounds.[1,5,13,14] There was no evidence of myofibroblasts by either myofibroblast-specific anti-muscle actin antibody or electron microscopy. We should note, however, that the presence of myofibroblasts in contracting wounds does not mandate that these cells are essential for wound contraction.[2]

In summary, excisional fetal wounds in rabbits show no evidence of wound contraction but rather enlarge in size beyond that expected by fetal growth. The mechanism for this wound expansion remains unclear.

In Vitro Rabbit Studies

Explanations for the lack of fetal rabbit wound contraction include a defect in fetal fibroblast contractility and/or the presence in amniotic fluid of an inhibitor of wound contraction. To investigate whether there was an intrinsic defect in the ability of fetal fibroblasts to contract, Krummel and coworkers[11] used the FPCL model of in vitro wound contraction.

Actin cytoplasmic filaments were observed with rhodamine-phalloidin staining in both fetal and adult rabbit dermal fibroblasts. Both types of cells undergo cell contraction by adding ATP to monolayer cell preparations. Using the FPCL model, fetal rabbit dermal fibroblasts contracted FPCL composed of either fetal or adult collagen to a significantly greater degree than did adult fibroblasts.[11] Since contractile forces are demonstrated in the FPCL model, the failure of fetal rabbit wounds to close by secondary intention is not due to an inherent defect in either the contractile properties of fetal fibroblasts or in the contractibility of the fetal collagen matrix.

The effect of amniotic fluid on FPCL contraction was then determined by adding amniotic fluid at concentrations from 1% to 100% to identical FPCLs. Interestingly, amniotic fluid concentrations greater than 20% directly inhibited lattice contraction in a dose-dependent fashion. Amniotic fluid was inhibitory with either fetal or adult fibroblasts suggesting that amniotic fluid may contain a wound contraction inhibitor. These in vitro findings may explain Somasundaram's observation that fetal rabbit skin excisional wounds excluded from amniotic fluid by a silastic patch healed within eight days.[10] Whether the silastic patch promoted re-epithelialization by excluding amniotic fluid or functioned as a wound template for regenerating epidermis remains unclear.[15]

The Fetal Lamb Model

Knowledge of fetal wound contraction in large animals is limited. Burrington[16] has stated that excisional fetal lamb wounds do contract, whereas Sopher[17] has suggested that open fetal cynomologous monkey wounds fail to contract. We sought to quantitate contraction of open fetal lamb wounds, delineate the mechanisms underlying this process, and examine the effect of amniotic fluid exposure or exclusion on wound contraction.[18]

There were 9 mm punch biopsy, full-thickness excisional wounds created along the fetal back at 100 days gestation (term = 145 days). A 2-mm-thick silastic patch was sutured over half of the wounds using running 4-0 silk. The remainder of the wounds were left uncovered and thereby were continuously bathed in amniotic fluid (Figs. 9.2 and 9.3). To control for rapid fetal growth, 9 mm circular tattoos were created with India ink onto unwounded fetal skin. The fetus was returned to the uterus and amniotic fluid volume was restored. Full-thickness wounds were also created on the maternal abdomen as adult controls.

Following re-operation three, seven, or 14 days later, the silastic covering was removed from wounds excluded from amniotic fluid, all wounds were photographed, and wound areas were calculated using computerized morphometric analysis. Representative fetal and adult wounds at seven days as well as un-

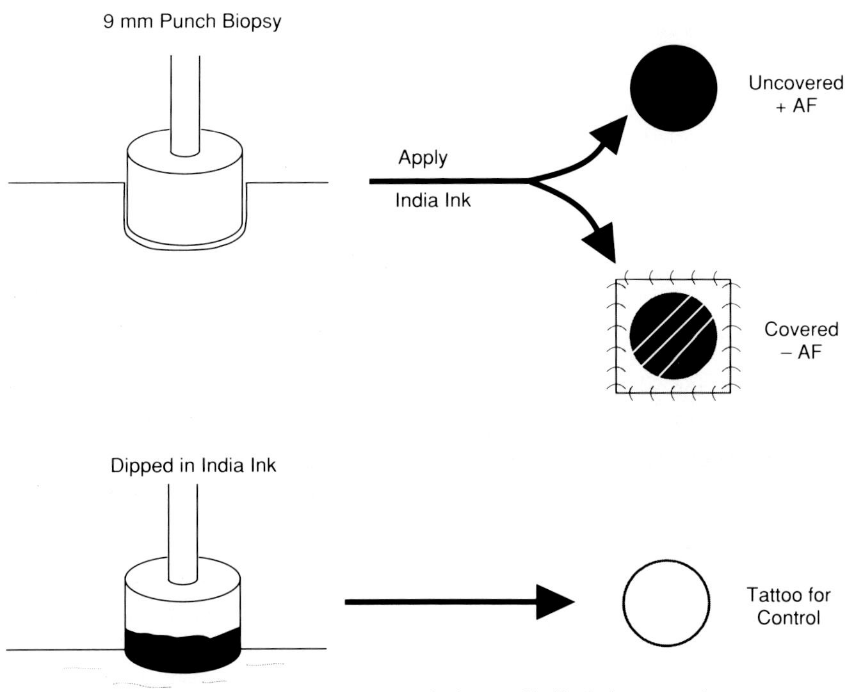

Figure 9.2 Schematic drawing of wounding techniques. Half of the wounds were exposed to amniotic fluid (+AF) and the other half were covered by a silastic patch to exclude amniotic fluid (−AF). To account for rapid fetal growth, circular tattoos were made on the fetus. *Reprinted with permission.*[18]

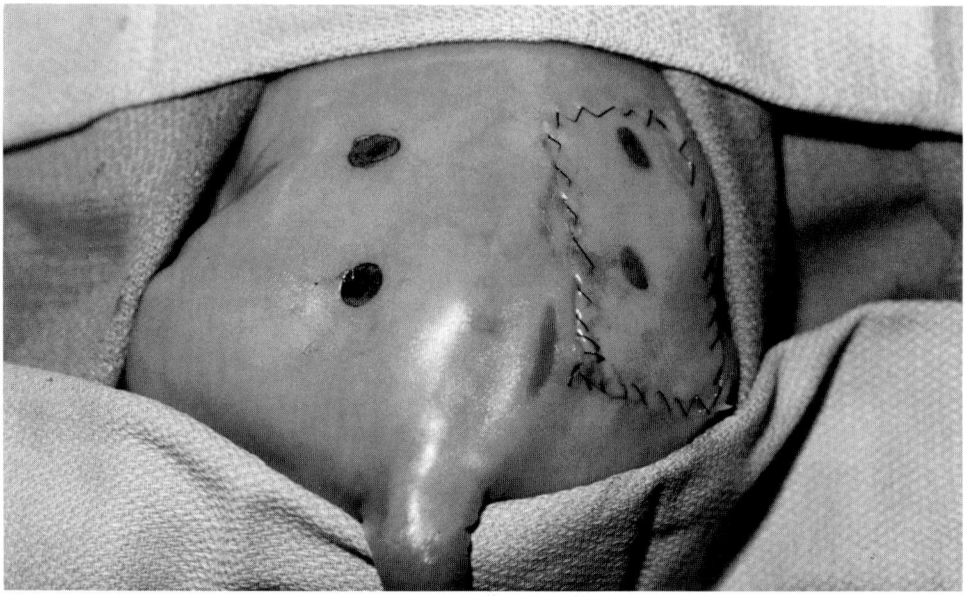

Figure 9.3 Photograph of the back of a 100 day gestation fetal lamb at three day harvest with four excisional wounds marked by India ink. Note the wounds on the right side are covered by a silastic patch and the wounds on the left are exposed to amniotic fluid. *Reprinted with permission.*[18]

wounded fetal and adult skin were analyzed for the presence of myofibroblasts using transmission electron microscopy (TEM) and an anti-muscle actin monoclonal antibody.[19,20]

Initially, the wounds and control tattoo patterns all had an area of 63.6 mm^2. As expected, the tattoo pattern increased in area due to rapid fetal growth (Fig. 9.4). The wounds prevented from direct contact with amniotic fluid rapidly decreased in size over the first week after wounding and were completely closed after 14 days by wound contraction. Interestingly, the wounds directly exposed to amniotic fluid were slightly different. Their closure by wound contraction was retarded to a significant degree ($P < 0.05$) at three days postwounding. The contraction of these exposed wounds quickly caught up to wounds not exposed to amniotic fluid by seven days (Fig. 9.5). They were closed completely by 14 days, identical to the unexposed wounds.

On transmission electron microscopy, myofibroblasts were not identifiable in unwounded fetal or adult skin (Fig. 9.6a). In contrast, myofibroblasts were identifiable in all fetal wounds as well as in adult wounds. They were characterized by: 1) bundles of smooth muscle filaments, which were prominent along the cellular margin of the long axes of the cells (Figs. 9.6b and c); 2) nuclei with irregular borders; 3) well-developed rough endoplasmic reticulum, filled with flocculent material; and 4) secretory vesicles indicating active collagen production. Collagen banding patterns could be seen in the granulation tissue extracellular matrix.

Immunofluorescence studies were performed using the anti-muscle actin monoclonal antibody. This antibody stains the intracellular actin filaments from smooth muscle cells and myofibroblasts but not fibroblasts. These studies demonstrated no myofibroblasts in unwounded fetal or adult skin. In contrast, stained myofibroblasts were present in both fetal and adult wounds at seven days with

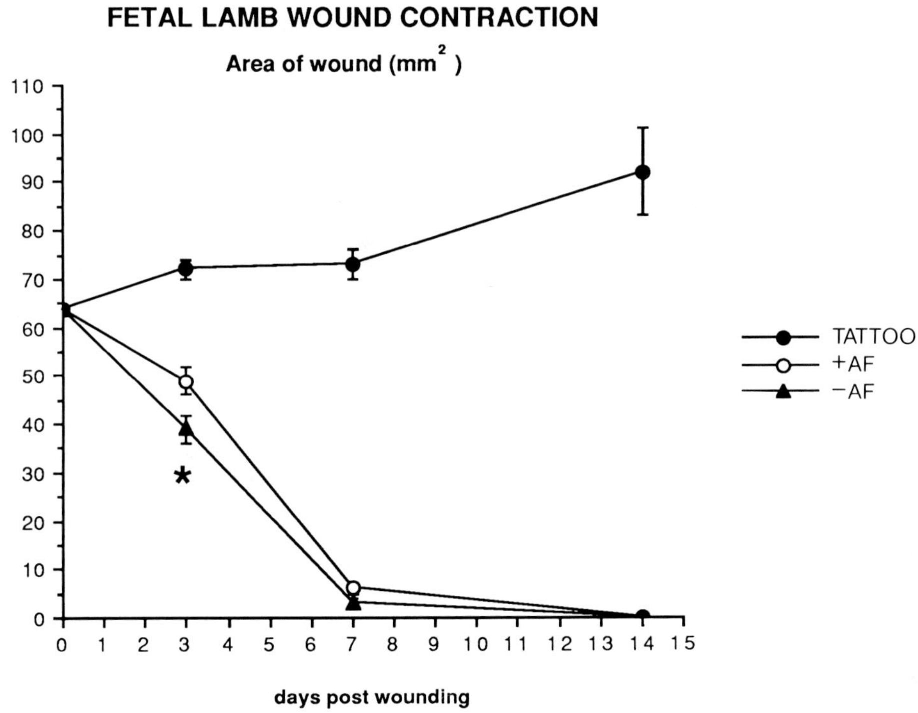

Figure 9.4 Graph of wound areas at 3, 7, and 14 days following wounding. Half of the wounds were exposed to amniotic fluid (+AF) and half were excluded from amniotic fluid using a silastic patch (−AF). At 3 days, the wounds excluded from amniotic fluid were significantly larger than the wounds exposed to amniotic fluid (*$p < 0.05$). However, wounds in both groups were completely contracted and healed by 14 days. As expected, control tattoo areas enlarged as the fetal lambs grew in size. *Reprinted with permission.*[18]

no apparent difference in staining between the wounds exposed and not exposed to amniotic fluid.

Our findings of fetal lamb wound contraction and the presence of myofibroblasts in the wound matrix are in conflict with fetal rabbit studies. The absence of granulation tissue and myofibroblasts in open fetal rabbit wounds suggest that failure of wound contraction in this model may simply be due to the lack of the essential cellular contractile elements in the open wound site. The possible role of amniotic fluid in fetal wound contraction is intriguing. Because wound coverage with a silastic patch had such a dramatic and reproducible effect on fetal rabbit wound contraction, we used this same technique to exclude amniotic fluid in the lamb model. Exposure to amniotic fluid delayed contraction early on, but by seven days both wounds exposed to amniotic fluid and those not exposed to amniotic fluid were contracting equally and by 14 days both had completely contracted and re-epithelialized. Amniotic fluid may contain an inhibitor of contractile elements, which would account for the delay of wound contraction at three days postwounding in the group exposed to amniotic fluid. It is also possible that either the silastic patch did not completely exclude amniotic fluid, or that it only initially excluded it, which may account for the effect of exclusion early on during healing.

Wound contraction may be influenced not only by newly arriving fibroblasts but also by the composition of the wound matrix itself. The matrix of fetal wounds

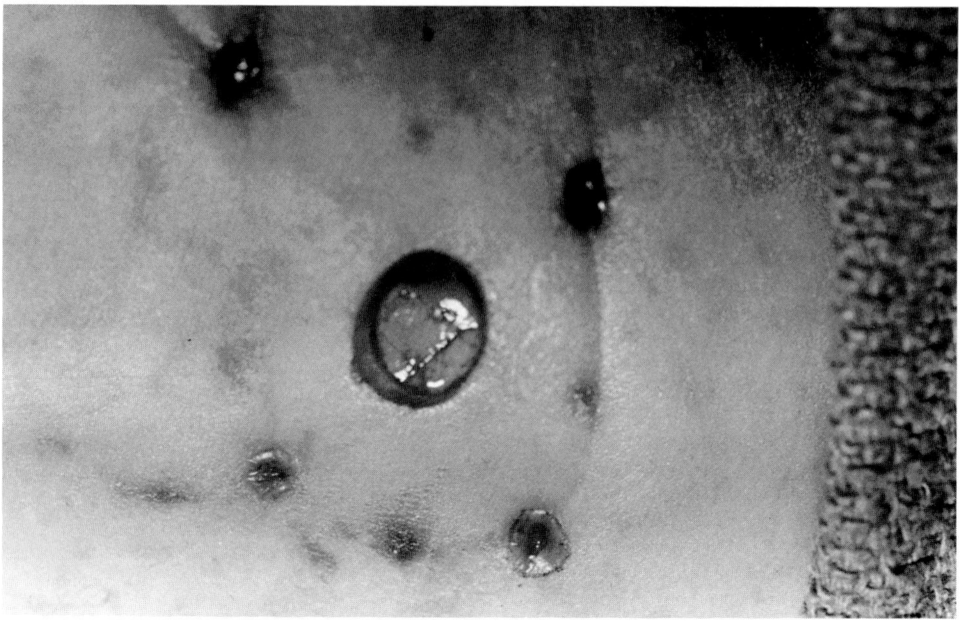

Figure 9.5 Photograph of wounds exposed to amniotic fluid at seven days. Four wounds are seen around a freshly made 9 mm wound for size comparison. Note the small size of the seven day wounds and the surrounding wrinkled skin indicating wound contraction.

is rich in glycosaminoglycans, specifically hyaluronic acid.[21,22] The physical properties of hyaluronic acid, including a large water of hydration, support cell movement within the matrix.[23] The fetal wound matrix may confer a greater degree of organization by resident cellular forces. For a detailed description of fetal lamb wound matrix histology and immunohistochemistry refer to Chapter 10.

It has been demonstrated using the FPCL that type III collagen, which is abundant in the fetal wound matrix, contracts faster and to a greater degree than FPCL composed of type I collagen.[8] It is postulated that type III collagen can be pulled together or that fibroblasts are better at rearranging this collagen type. This finding may provide an explanation for the highly organized fetal wound collagen staining pattern. We have shown that mid-gestational fetal lamb incisional skin wounds stained with collagen type specific antibodies have a pattern indistinguishable from unwounded fetal skin by 14 days following wounding.[24] This high degree of connective tissue organization in the dermis is lost halfway through the last trimester. A narrow band of scar is formed at the wound site during this period. The decreased amount of type III collagen in late gestation fetal skin may explain the decreased organization of collagen in late gestation wounds.

The data demonstrate that fetal lamb excisional wounds contract in utero. Myofibroblasts were present by transmission electron and immunofluorescence microscopy. Amniotic fluid exposure retarded wound contraction early on, but all wounds were closed by 14 days by wound contraction.

In Vitro Lamb Studies

To further delineate the effect of sheep amniotic fluid on wound contraction, Burd and coworkers also utilized the FPCL model.[25] They made lattices from a com-

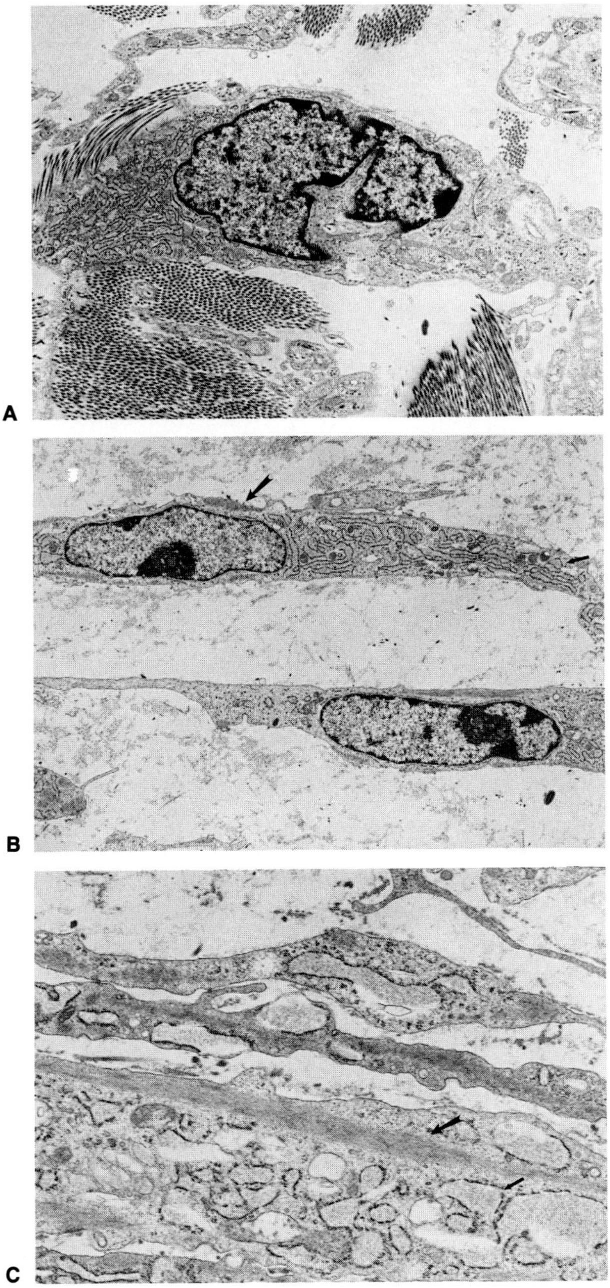

Figure 9.6 Transmission electron microscopy. **(a)** Normal unwounded fetal skin (7200×). This fibroblast has no features of a myofibroblast. **(b)** Fetal wound exposed to amniotic fluid at 7 days (6000×). The two cells have typical myofibroblast characteristics. The large arrow points to the intracellular myofilaments. The small arrow indicates the prominent rough endoplasmic reticulum. **(c)** Intracellular myofilaments magnified 19,800× (large arrow). The dark areas represent so-called electron dense bodies of myofibroblast myofilaments. The small arrow indicates the prominent rough endoplasmic reticulum. *Reprinted with permission.*[18]

bination of second and third trimester fetal and adult sheep collagen and fibroblasts. Lattice contraction was assessed by measuring the change in area of the lattice over a 60-hour period.

Both fetal and adult fibroblasts contracted lattices made from adult collagen. Fetal collagen was less well organized by both fetal and adult fibroblasts. They also evaluated the effect of sheep amniotic fluid on lattice contraction. Lattices were made with and without the addition of 5% amniotic fluid obtained from 80–

TABLE 9.1 Third Trimester Fetal Lamb Fibroblasts and Collagen FPCL

Amniotic Fluid	% Reduction in FPCL Size (± SEM) 48 hours	96 hours
0	11 ± 1.7	52 ± 0.6
4	15 ± 0.6	63 ± 2.7
8	13 ± 1.0	69 ± 2.3*
24	12 ± 2.3	84 ± 0.3**
40	18 ± 2.3	85 ± 2.5***

* p = 0.0094
** p = 0.0001
*** p = 0.0025

85 days gestation fetal lambs. The addition of amniotic fluid to a final concentration of 5% resulted in a stimulation of FPCL contraction. Using third trimester fibroblasts, the differences between the size of fetal collagen lattices with and without amniotic fluid were significant at 24 hours for third trimester collagen ($p = 0.002$), and 36 hours with second trimester collagen ($p = 0.02$). By 60 hours, the two collagen groups showed highly significant differences. Amniotic fluid from 4% to 40% was examined in the FPCL model and a significant dose response was found by 96 hours (Table 9.1).

This experiment demonstrates that fetal lamb fibroblasts are effective in the in vitro FPCL model and correlates with the in vivo data showing that fetal lamb excisional wounds contract. Amniotic fluid stimulates this in vitro model contraction process in a dose-dependent manner.

Rittenberg and coworkers[26] have recently characterized a fibroblast contraction stimulating activity in sheep amniotic fluid. A 40 to 47 kD protein factor, termed 40 K-lattice contraction stimulator (40K-LCS) was isolated. This factor is inactivated by proteolytic digestion and heat denaturation. The mechanism by which 40 K-LCS promotes FPCL contraction is unknown. The factor had no effect on: 1) ATP-induced cell contraction of monolayer fibroblasts; 2) cell elongation on glass or in collagen; or 3) fibroblast proliferation in a collagen matrix. Studies are underway to further characterize, purify and delineate the mechanism of action of 40 K-LCS. The isolation of a fibroblast contraction stimulator and/or the development of blocking antibodies directed against this protein may have clinical application for modulating wound contraction and scar contracture.

Human Fetal Wound Contraction

Studies in the fetal rabbit and sheep models have yielded contradictory results with regard to wound contraction and the effect of amniotic fluid on contraction. The obvious question is whether or not human fetal wounds contract. Because of the limitations to studying human fetal wound healing in vivo, Chang and coworkers[27] utilized the FPCL model to study wound contraction in vitro. They used 18 week gestation human fetal and adult fibroblasts in FPCL made with adult human collagen. Fetal or adult fibroblasts contracted the FPCL to less than 25% of their original size by four days. The human fetal FPCL contracted significantly more than FPCL made with adult fibroblasts by 72 hours. The effect of 20 week amniotic fluid on lattice contraction was also studied. Human amniotic fluid inhibited both fetal and adult FPCL in a dose-dependent manner.

This study does not directly answer the question whether human fetal wounds contract. It does, however, demonstrate that human fetal fibroblasts, like their adult counterpart, can generate the forces necessary to compact a collagenous matrix, and that this ability is inhibited by amniotic fluid. In addition to organic compounds contained in fetal urine, amniotic fluid also contains a large variety of other compounds that may inhibit lattice contraction either through toxicity to the fibroblasts and/or interference with the contraction mechanism. The mechanism of human amniotic fluid inhibition of lattice contraction needs to be identified.

SUMMARY

Studies on fetal wound contraction have yielded a variety of results depending on which species is studied. The role of amniotic fluid in fetal wound contraction has not been studied carefully. The in vitro observations of amniotic fluid inhibiting (rabbit and human) or stimulating (lamb) fibroblast populated collagen lattice contraction has clinical application in minimizing or preventing wound contraction and scar contractures. Due to the limitations in studying human fetal wound healing and contraction in vivo, further studies on human fetal wound contraction will be pursued in vitro using skin organ culture and FPCL models. Finally, little is known about the mechanism whereby fetal wound closure occurs in the absence of scar formation.

REFERENCES

1. Gabbiani G, Ryan GB, Majno G: Presence of modified fibroblasts in granulation tissue and their possible role in wound contraction. Experientia 27:549–550, 1971.
2. Ehrlich HP: The role of connective tissue matrix in wound healing. Prog Clin Biol Res 266:243–258, 1988.
3. Bell E, Ivarsson B, Merrill C: Production of a tissue-like structure of collagen lattices by human fibroblasts of different proliferative potential in vitro. PNAS 76:1274, 1979.
4. Allen TD, Schor SL, Schor AM: An ultrastructural review of collagen gels, a model system for cell-matrix, cell-basement membrane and cell-cell interactions. Scanning Electron Microsc 1:375, 1984.
5. Majno G, Gabbiani G, Hirschel BJ, et al.: Contraction of granulation tissue in vitro: Similarity to smooth muscle. Science 173:548–550, 1971.
6. Ehrlich HP, Rajaratnam RBM: Cell locomotion forces versus cell contraction forces for collagen lattice contraction: An in vitro model of wound contraction. Tiss Cell 22:407–417, 1990.
7. Hembry PM, Bernanke DH, Hayakashi K, et al.: Morphological examination of mesenchymal cells in healing wounds of normal and tight skin mice. Am J Pathol 125:81–89, 1986.
8. Ehrlich HP: The modulation of contraction of fibroblast populated collagen lattice by types I, II, and III collagen. Tiss Cell 20:47–50, 1988.
9. Somasundaram K, Prathrap K: Intra-uterine healing of skin wounds in rabbit foetuses. J Path 100: 81–86, 1970.
10. Somasundaram K, Prathrap K: The effect of exclusion of amniotic fluid on intra-uterine healing of skin in rabbit foetuses. J Path 107:127–30, 1972.
11. Krummel TM, Ehrlich HP, Nelson JM, et al.: Fetal wounds do not contract in utero. Surg Forum 40:613–614, 1989.
12. Haynes JH, Krummel TM, Schatzki PF, et al.: Histology of the open fetal rabbit wound. Surg Forum 40:558–560, 1989.

13. Oda D, Gown AM, Vande Berg JS, Stern R: The fibroblast nature of myofibroblasts. Exp and Mol Path 49:316–329, 1988.
14. Vande Berg JS, Rudolph R, Woodward M: Comparative growth dynamics and morphology between cultured myofibroblasts from granulating wounds and dermal fibroblasts. Am J Path 14: 187–200, 1984.
15. Ditesheim JA, Delozier JB, Rees RS, et al.: Covered fetal excisional wounds by tissue regeneration. Surg Forum 40:615, 1989.
16. Burrington JD: Wound healing in the fetal lamb. J Pediatr Surg 6:523–528, 1971.
17. Sopher D: A study of wound healing in the foetal tissues of the cynomologous monkey. Lab. Animals Handbook 6:327–335, 1975.
18. Longaker MT, Burd DAR, Yen TSB, et al.: Mid-gestation fetal lamb wounds contract in utero. J Pediatr Surg
19. Gown AG, Vogel AM: Monoclonal antibodies to intermediate filament proteins of human cells: Distribution of filament proteins in normal human tissue. Am J Pathol 114:309–321, 1984.
20. Tsukada T, Tippens D, Gordon D, et al.: Muscle actin-specific monoclonal antibody. I. Immunocytochemical and biochemical characterization. Am J Pathol 126:57–60, 1987.
21. Krummel TM, Nelson JM, Diegelmann RF, et al.: Fetal response to injury in the rabbit. J Pediatr Surg 22:640–644, 1987.
22. DePalma LR, Krummel TM, Nelson JM, et al.: Fetal wound matrix is composed of proteoglycan rather than collagen. Surg Forum 38:626–628, 1987.
23. Longaker MT, Harrison MR, Langer JC, et al.: Studies in fetal wound healing: I. A factor in fetal serum that stimulates the deposition of hyaluronic acid. J Pediatr Surg 24:789–792, 1989.
24. Longaker MT, Whitby DJ, Adzick NS, et al.: Studies in fetal wound healing: VI. Second and early third trimester fetal wounds demonstrate rapid collagen deposition without scar formation J Pediatr Surg 25:63–69, 1990.
25. Burd DAR, Longaker MT, Rittenberg T, et al.: In vitro fetal wound contraction: The effect of amniotic fluid. Br J Plast Surg 44:302–305, 1991.
26. Rittenberg T, Longaker MT, Adzick NS, Ehrlich HP: Sheep amniotic fluid has a protein factor which stimulates human fibroblast populated collagen lattice contraction. J Cell Physiol (in press)
27. Chang B, Siebert JW, Longaker MT, Adzick NS, Burd DAR: Do human fetal wounds contract? Ann Plast Surg (in press)

CHAPTER **10**

Immunohistochemical Studies of the Extracellular Matrix and Soluble Growth Factors in Fetal and Adult Wound Healing

David J. Whitby
Mark W. J. Ferguson

INTRODUCTION

Scarless fetal skin wound healing was first demonstrated by histological methods in incisional wound models.[1–3] More recently excisional wounds have also been shown histologically to heal without scar formation in mid-gestation fetal sheep.[4] Histological and immunohistochemical techniques have limitations in the study of wound healing, particularly in defining the mechanisms controlling the process. However, they do not alter the process of wound healing and they do provide a qualitative analysis of the elements present within the wound. Studies using wound implants create an artificial wound environment and a non-healing wound. Regeneration of a normal fetal tissue architecture (that is, scarless wound healing) is not seen within these implants. Relating the data from fetal implant studies to incisional fetal wound healing is thus difficult and is one of the reasons why earlier studies produced conflicting reports on the presence or absence of collagen in fetal wound healing. One of the initial aims of these studies was to resolve the question of the nature of the extracellular matrix (ECM) in fetal wounds by carefully documenting the spatial and temporal localization of several components of the ECM, including collagen types I, III, IV, V, VI, fibronectin, tenascin, laminin, chondroitin, and heparan sulfates, during fetal and adult wound healing in mice.[5] Our other major question was the timing and nature of the transition from fetal, scarless, wound healing to adult wound healing with scar formation. Wounds from fetal mice at days 14, 16 and 18 of gestation, as well as from neonatal and adult mice were therefore analyzed.

The ultimate aim of fetal wound healing studies is to manipulate the adult wound so that it heals in a scarless, fetal-like, fashion. Many growth factors are thought to play a role in wound healing and it is possible that altering the growth factor profile of a wound, either by adding growth factors, or by blocking their action, will alter the quality of wound healing. However, little is presently known of the normal growth factor profile of the fetal wound. Our immunohistochemical studies have therefore also included localization of platelet derived growth factor, transforming growth factor beta and basic fibroblast growth factor.[6]

There are several benefits to using the mouse as a model of fetal wound healing. However, relating the results from these studies to longer gestational animals, in particular primates, must be approached with caution. Fetal sheep provide a suitable long gestational model for study and we have been fortunate in being able to repeat some of these studies in sheep through our collaboration with the Fetal Surgery Laboratory at UCSF.[7,8]

MATERIALS AND METHODS

Fetal Mice

At days 16 and 18 of gestation (term = 19 days), time-mated MF1 mice were anesthetized, and under the operating microscope a 2 mm, vertical, full-thickness wound was made in the left upper lip of three fetuses in each pregnant animal, using techniques previously described.[5] For 14 day fetuses, the approach was modified by dividing the myometrium longitudinally and repairing only the fetal membranes, as reported by Muneako et al.[9]

Adult and Neonatal Mice

Under anesthesia, vertical, 3 mm upper lip wounds were made in neonatal mice at six to 12 hours after birth. A single suture was used to appose the wound surfaces. Similar wounds were made in adult mice at age six to eight weeks.

Mouse Wound Harvest and Tissue Preparation

Animals were killed and fetal wounds harvested at one, six, 12, 16, 20, 24, 48, 72 and 120 hours postwounding. Neonatal and adult wounds were harvested one,

TABLE 10.1 Extracellular Matrix and Growth Factor Primary Antibodies

Primary Ab Raised Against	Primary Ab Raised In	Source	Dilution	Secondary Ab (see Table 2)
Type I collagen	Rabbit	Institut Pasteur de Lyon	1:40	1
Type III collagen	Goat	Seralab	1:100	2
Type IV collagen	Rabbit	Institut Pasteur de Lyon	1:80	1
Type V collagen	Goat	Seralab	1:100	2
Type VI collagen	Rabbit	Dr Shirley Ayad, Manchester	1:100	1
Fibronectin	Sheep	Serotec	1:100	3
Tenascin	Rabbit	Dr R Chiquet-Ehrisman, Basel	1:200	1
Laminin	Mouse (IgG) monoclonal	ICN Biomedicals	1:1000	4
Chondroitin Sulphate	Mouse (IgM) monoclonal	ICN Biomedicals	1:400	5
Heparan Sulphate	Rabbit	Dr P Bletchley & Dr J Anderson, Manchester	1:100	1
MF 20 (light meromyosin)	Mouse (IgG) monoclonal	Developmental Biology Hybridoma Bank, Iowa	1:50	4
PDGF (Human platelets)	Goat	British Biotechnology, Oxford (BDA 16)	1:40	2
TGFβ (Porcine platelets) (detects TGFβ1 & β2)	Rabbit	British Biotechnology, Oxford (BDA 5)	1:5	1
bFGF (Bovine brain)	Rabbit	British Biotechnology, Oxford (BDA 4)	1:40	1

TABLE 10.2 FITC-Conjugated Secondary Antibodies

Table 1 Reference	Secondary Ab Raised Against	Secondary Ab Raised In	Source	Dilution
1	Rabbit	Sheep	Serotec	1:160
2	Goat	Rabbit	Northeast Biomedicals	1:40
3	Sheep	Donkey	Serotec	1:40
4	Mouse IgG	Goat	Zymed Laboratories	1:30
5	Mouse IgM	Goat	Zymed Laboratories	1:30

six, 12, 24, 36, 48 and 72 hours, five, seven, 10 and 14 days postwounding. The tissues were snap frozen, embedded and 7 μm cryostat sections cut for indirect immunostaining.

Sheep Wounds

1 cm linear wounds and 9 mm, full-thickness, excisional wounds were made on the trunk of fetal sheep at 75, 100 and 120 days gestation (term = 145 days) using the methods for fetal sheep surgery as described by Harrison et al.[10] Wounds from 100 and 120 day fetuses were harvested at one, four, eight, 12, 24, 48 and 72 hours, seven and 14 days postwounding. Tissue from 75 day fetuses was harvested one, three, seven, and 15 days postwounding. Similar trunk wounds were also made on adult sheep and harvested at the same time points. Cryostat sections were cut from these wounds after processing as just detailed.

Immunohistochemistry

Primary and secondary antibodies used for indirect immunostaining of extracellular matrix components and growth factors are shown in Tables 10.1 and 10.2. Incubation with primary antisera was 1 hour at 20°C for ECM molecules and 24 hours at 4°C for growth factors. This was followed by three rinses in phosphate buffered saline (PBS) and incubation with FITC-conjugated secondary antisera for one hour followed by a further three rinses with PBS. The sections were mounted in a non-fading medium, DABCO (1,4-diazobicyclo-{2,2,2}-octane), and photographed using a Leitz Dialux microscope and Kodak Ektachrome 160 ASA film corrected for tungsten light.

For each primary antibody, and each time point, control sections were stained, substituting PBS for the primary antibody. Antibody specificity was tested by preincubation of the primary antibody with the antigen in question, followed by immunostaining using the same protocol.

Direct immunostaining of endogenous immunoglobulins, as a marker of an inflammatory response within the wound, was also carried out using antibodies against mouse IgG and IgM.

MOUSE RESULTS

The results from the three groups of fetal wounds were essentially similar and will be presented as a single group. As discussed below there was a gradual transition both in the rate and quality of wound healing from fetus to neonate to adult, rather than an abrupt transition.

Epithelialization, Tenascin, and Fibronectin Deposition

The rate at which wound closure occurred decreased from fetus to neonate to adult. Re-epithelialization was complete in the fetus by 20 h postwounding and the mesenchymal defect had closed by 48 h. In the neonate the epithelial wound was closed by 48 h while in the adult a similar sized wound was closed by 72 h. The dermal wounds had closed by 72 and 120 h postwounding respectively. Interestingly, in each group the oral mucosal wound was closed prior to re-epithelialization of the skin wound.

Fibronectin (Fn) was diffusely present in the normal mesenchymal and dermal tissues adjacent to the wound. At 1 h postwounding a layer of Fn was present on the surface of the fetal wound (Fig. 10.1a; see color section for all art in this chapter). In both the neonatal and adult wounds (Fig. 10.1b) Fn was present at the surface of the wound and within the clot filling the wound. There was increased staining for Fn in the region of the wound, which became patchy as wound healing progressed. In the fetal wound by 72 h the staining pattern for Fn at the site of the wound was similar to the normal adjacent tissue both in intensity and pattern. The intensity of staining for Fn was normal in the neonatal and adult wounds by seven days but the pattern of staining reflected the scar formation within the tissue.

Tenascin (Tn) was very limited in its distribution in normal tissues. In the fetus it was present only at the basement membrane of the oral mucosa and epidermis, particularly around hair follicles. A similar pattern was seen in the neonate and adult, although the staining was less intense and discontinuous.

Tn was faintly present at the surface of the fetal wound 1 h post-wounding (Fig. 10.1c). This staining was more intense at 24 h and Tn was also present within the adjacent dermis (Fig. 10.1d). Tn persisted within the dermis at 48 h (Fig. 10.1e) but by 72 h the dermal staining had disappeared and an essentially normal pattern was apparent, apart from an increased intensity of staining at the dermal-epidermal junction at the site of the wound (Fig. 10.1f).

Tn was also present at the wound surface of both neonatal and adult wounds but the time at which it was first seen differed. In the neonate, Tn was first apparent at 12 h postwounding and the staining became more intense and present within the dermis at 24 h and 48h postwounding (Fig. 10.1g). By 72 h the staining within the dermis was patchy and the most intense staining was apparent at the dermal-epidermal junction (Fig. 10.1h). At 5d Tn was no longer seen within the dermis and there was an essentially normal pattern at the basement membranes apart from the loss of hair follicles (Fig. 10.1i). In the adult Tn was first present at the wound surface (but not within the clot) very faintly at 24 h postwounding. In a similar fashion to the fetus and the neonate the staining for Tn became more intense and present within the dermis as wound healing progressed, before the dermal staining became patchy and disappeared (Figs. 10.1j and k). At 12 d in the adult there was still some patchy staining within the dermis and marked staining at the dermal-epidermal junction where there were epithelial projections into the dermis (enhanced rete pegs) (Fig. 10.1l). The pattern of staining for Fn and Tn are summarized in Table 10.3.

The pattern of Fn deposition both spatially and temporally was similar in all three wound groups suggesting that its role may be similar in fetus and adult (although the possibility of different isoforms of Fn being present in fetal and adult wounds is not excluded; see Chapter 19). The pattern of Tn expression was similar in fetus, neonate, and adult, but the time at which it was first present and the length of time it was expressed within the dermis varied. It was initially seen first in the fetal wounds (1 h) then in the neonatal wounds (12 h) and lastly in the adult wounds (24 h). This parallels the rate of wound healing that is complete first in the fetus and is slowest in the adult. Fn has many potential roles in wound healing (for recent review see Clark[11]) including acting as a substrate for cell adhesion and migration through its interaction with integrins. However the distribution of Fn is too widespread to suggest a role in initiating and controlling cell migration.

The distribution of Tn in adult tissues is very limited.[12,13] During development it is expressed by many tissues at times of epithelial-mesenchymal interactions[14–19] and is present in certain carcinomas.[14,20–22] Both Tn and Fn are present in the migratory pathways of neural crest cells during development and the appearance of Tn correlates with the start of cell migration.[23] The integrin mediated attachment of fibroblasts to Fn is inhibited by Tn[24] and mesodermal cell migration during gastrulation is inhibited by the addition of exogenous Tn.[25] Tn is present in adult wounds[26] and may play a role in initiating cell migration into the wound.

In the fetal, neonatal, and adult wounds studied Tn was present at the margins of the wounds prior to cell migration. The rapid healing of fetal wounds may, therefore, be due to the early appearance of Tn.

Interstitial Collagen Deposition and Scar Formation

Collagen types I, III and VI (CI, CIII, CVI) were widely distributed in normal mesenchymal and connective tissues. Collagen type V (CV) showed a similar wide distribution and also localized in epithelial and endothelial basement membranes. All four types of collagen were present in fetal, neonatal, and adult tissues and were present in the respective wounds. The time at which collagen was first present within the wound differed between fetus, neonate, and adult but the time at which each type of collagen was first seen was the same within each wound group.

The wide distribution of CIII in undamaged fetal tissues is seen in Fig. 10.2a. CIII was first, faintly, present in fetal wounds at 48 h postwounding (Fig. 10.2b). At this time the wound had re-epithelialized and cells had filled the mesenchymal defect. By 72 h the reticular pattern of CIII had been restored at the wound and except for an epithelial furrow at the skin surface the site of the wound was now indistinguishable from the surrounding undamaged tissue (Fig. 10.2c). In this figure regenerating myotubules are seen toward the oral aspect of the wound, outlined by the staining of CIII in their connective tissue sheath. Localization of meromyosin also shows continuous myotubules at the site of the wound confirming muscle regeneration in the fetal wounds (data not shown).

Collagen deposition was first apparent at 5 d in the adult wounds (Fig. 10.2d). At 12 d typical scar formation was present with a band of parallel collagen fibers disrupting the normal tissue architecture (Fig. 10.2e). In the neonate collagen was present in the wound at 48 h. On the oral mucosal aspect there was a normal tissue pattern and no scar (Fig. 10.2f). On the skin surface there was loss of hair follicles in the region of the wound but the pattern of collagen was otherwise grossly normal and the parallel bundles of collagen fibers seen in the adult wound were not apparent.

The other collagens studied, types I, V and VI, showed essentially similar patterns to CIII with regeneration of a normal pattern in the fetal wounds, scar formation in the adult, and a mixed pattern in the neonate. The time at which

TABLE 10.3 Epithelialization, Fibronectin (FN), and Tenascin (TN) Deposition in Wound

		1 Hour	6 Hours	12 Hours	24 Hours	48 Hours	72 Hours	5 Days	7 Days	12 Days
FN	fetus					3 Patchy staining at wound site	2 Normal pattern	2	2	2
	neonate	3 Present at wound margins and within wound clot	3	3	3	3	3	3	2 Pattern reflects scar	2
	adult					3	3	3	2 Pattern reflects scar	2
TN	fetus	1 Present at wound margins	1	1	3 Within adjacent dermis 4 At epidermal-dermal junction	3 Patchy staining at wound site	2 Normal pattern	2	2	2
	neonate	0	0	1 Present at wound margins	3 Within adjacent dermis 4 At epidermal-dermal junction	3 Within adjacent dermis 4 At epidermal-dermal junction	3 Patchy within wound site 4 At epidermal-dermal junction	2 Essentially normal pattern—reflecting loss of hair follicles	2	2
	adult	0	0	0	1 Present at wound margins	3 Within adjacent dermis 4 At epidermal-dermal junction	3 Within adjacent dermis 4 At epidermal-dermal junction	3 Within adjacent dermis 4 At epidermal-dermal junction	3 Patchy within wound site 4 At epidermal-dermal junction	3 At epidermal-dermal junction (Absent from dermis)
epithelial-ization					Complete in fetus	Complete in neonate	Complete in adult			

Relative intensity of staining for molecule at wound site in comparison to normal tissue:
0 = absent
1 = < normal
2 = normal (*not* normal pattern)
3 = > normal
4 = ≫ normal

these collagens were first present in the respective wounds was the same as for type III collagen. The critical difference between the fetal and adult wounds is not the presence or absence of collagen, or specific collagen types, but in the degree of organization of the collagen fibrils deposited in the wound.

Collagen fibril formation is a complex process that is only partially understood.[27,28] Processing of propeptides, interactions of different types of collagen, and interactions with other macromolecules may all play a role. Differences in the proteases present in fetal and adult wounds, different proportions of collagen types and variations in other macromolecules, particularly glycosaminoglycans, in fetal and adult wounds may all affect the supramolecular organization of the collagen fibrils deposited in the wound.

Collagen types I, III and V are present within the same collagen fibrils[29–31] and interactions between different collagens will alter collagen fibril size in vitro.[32] Differences in size between collagen types and the presence of non-helical domains may alter lateral aggregation and thus fibril size. Fetal tissues contain a high proportion of type III collagen to type I collagen in comparison with adult tissues.[33,34] Our studies have shown that fetal and adult wounds contain the same types of collagen but the proportions of these collagens within the wound cannot be defined.

The role of glycosaminoglycans in fetal wound healing is intriguing. Proteoglycans will alter collagen fibril size[35,36] and several studies have shown high levels of hyaluronic acid in fetal wounds.[37–39] Addition of hyaluronic acid to an adult tympanic membrane wound showed reduced scar formation and greater organization of the collagen deposited.[40] In our studies chondroitin sulfate (CS) was diffusely present in the fetal mesenchyme but was not initially present in the wound (Fig. 10.2g). However, CS appeared within the wound from 20 h onwards (Fig. 10.2h) and was, therefore, present in the fetal wound during collagen fibril formation. This contrasts with the adult where CS was only localized around the hair follicles and was absent from the wound at all time points (Figure 2.i). These differences in glycosaminoglycans in fetal and adult tissues may affect collagen fibril formation within the wound. Scott and Hughes[41] showed that during development fetal bovine and chick collagen fibrils were small in diameter at a time when hyaluronic acid was abundant and a rapid increase in fibril size during midgestation coincided with a decrease in hyaluronic acid and chondroitin sulfate content. The localization of collagen types I, III, V, and VI and chondroitin sulfate is summarized in Table 10.4.

Collagen Type IV, Laminin, and Heparan Sulfate Deposition

In normal tissues of the fetus, neonate and adult collagen type IV (C IV) localized in endothelial basement membranes and epithelial basement membranes of skin and oral mucosa.

C IV was not present at the epidermal and mucosal wounds until re-epithelialization was complete. In the fetus, staining for C IV was present at the reforming basement membranes from 24 h postwounding. From 72 h postwounding a normal pattern of C IV was present and the site of the wound was indistinguishable from the normal tissues (Fig. 10.3a). In the neonate by 5 d a normal pattern of C IV was present on the oral mucosal aspect of the wound but on the skin side of the wound the loss of hair follicles was apparent (Fig. 10.3b).

In the adult C IV was present in the reforming epithelial basement membranes at 72 h. At 5 d a band of tissue with minimal staining for C IV in endothelial basement membranes was seen at the site of the wound (Fig. 10.3c). The basement membranes of a few newly formed capillaries within this granulation tissue were highlighted by C IV staining. New vessel formation was more obvious at 7 d (Fig. 10.3d) and by 12 d neovascularization was a prominent feature with multiple capillary loops at the site of the wound (Fig. 10.3e). Neovascularization was not a feature of the fetal or neonatal wounds. The localization of type IV collagen is summarized in Table 10.4.

Laminin (Ln) co-localizes with C IV in epithelial basement membranes following re-epithelialization, and in new capillaries in the adult wound and the pattern of staining is therefore essentially the same (data not shown). The absence of neovascularization in the fetal wounds, as demonstrated by both C IV and Ln staining, may be due to either an absence of angiogenic stimuli or a failure of fetal cells to react to these stimuli. The absence of an inflammatory response in the fetal wound and differences in growth factors between fetal and adult wounds (see next) suggests that a lack of angiogenic stimuli may be part of the reason for the absence of neovascularization in the fetal wound.

Heparan sulfate localized in the oral mucosal and skin basement membranes only, where a similar pattern to laminin and type IV collagen was seen, with heparan sulfate appearing in the reformed basement membrane after epithelialization was complete.

Inflammatory Response

Staining for endogenous immunoglobulins showed IgG and IgM present in neonatal and adult wounds from 12 h postwounding. None of the fetal wounds showed any staining for endogenous IgG or IgM confirming the lack of an immune response widely reported in previous studies.

Growth Factors

PDGF was present at the wound surface and within the clot filling the wound 1h postwounding in fetal, neonatal, and adult wounds (Figs. 10.3f and g). This staining persisted until the mesenchymal or dermal wound was infiltrated by cells and the clot disappeared. The clot within the fetal wounds was much less dense than in the adult wounds and PDGF had disappeared from the wound by 48 h. In the neonatal wound there was patchy staining for PDGF until 48 h and PDGF was not present within the wound at 72 h. PDGF persisted within the adult wound until 72 h postwounding.

The polyclonal TGFβ antibody used in this study was raised against TGFβ from porcine platelets and therefore recognizes both β1 and β2 isoforms. In unwounded fetal skin TGFβ (1&2) localized in a pericellular distribution around the basal epidermis (Fig. 10.3h). There was also marked staining of the hair follicles in fetal skin but TGFβ was not present at, or related to, the wound. Both neonatal and adult tissues showed the presence of TGFβ around hair follicles and in the basal epidermis. Additionally at 1 and 6 h TGFβ was also present at the wound surface and within the clot of both neonatal and adult wounds (Fig. 10.3j).

There was bFGF present within the normal fetal tissues, particularly within the muscle of the fetal tongue (Fig. 10.3k), but it was not visualized in relation

TABLE 10.4 Collagen (C) and Chondroitin Sulfate (CS) Deposition at Site of Wound

		1–12 Hours	24 Hours	48 Hours	72 Hours	5 Days	7 Days	12 Days
CI, III, V, VI	fetus	0	0	1 All collagen types present	2 Regeneration of normal tissue architecture	2	2	2
	neonate	0	0	1 All collagen types present	1 All collagen types present	2 Normal pattern at oral mucosa. Minimal scar at skin	2	2
	adult	0	0		0	1 All collagen types present	3 Parallel bundles of collagen within wound	3 Parallel bundles of collagen within wound
CS	fetus	0	1	2 Normal pattern	2	2	2	2
	neonate	0	0	0	0	0	0	0
	adult	0	0	0	0	0	0	0
C IV	fetus	0	2 Present in epithelial basement membrane	2	2	2	2	2
	neonate	0	0	2 Present in epithelial basement membrane	2	2	2	2
	adult	0	0	0	2 Epithelial BM 1 Neovascularization	2 Epithelial BM 3 Neovascularization	2 Epithelial BM 3 Neovascularization	2 Epithelial BM 4 Neovascularization

Relative intensity of staining for molecule at wound site in comparison to normal tissue:
0 = absent
1 = $<$ normal
2 = normal (not normal patern)
3 = $>$ normal
4 = $\gg$ normal

to the fetal wound. In the adult and neonatal wounds at 1 h bFGF was present at the surface of the wound and within the dermis adjacent to the wound (Fig. 10.3l).

PDGF has many potential roles in wound healing through its chemotactic effects on fibroblasts, monocytes, and neutrophils and its mitogenic effect on cells of mesenchymal origin.[42] It is also capable of stimulating collagen synthesis and regulating the relative synthesis of different types of collagen.[43] PDGF is present in the α granules of platelets[44,45] and is released by activated platelets during coagulation at the site of a wound. The presence of PDGF at the surface of the adult and fetal wounds would therefore be anticipated. The persistent staining for PDGF within the wounds may reflect continued release by other cells known to synthesize the factor, such as macrophages or endothelial cells. It may also be due to binding of the highly cationic PDGF to components of the ECM such as glycosaminoglycans. This binding is thought to be one of the reasons for the extremely short half life of circulating PDGF[46] and may prolong the local activity of the factor at the site of the wound. PDGF was also present within fetal wounds demonstrating that the fetal response to wounding has some components in common with the adult, and that fetal platelets are competent to synthesize and release PDGF.

TGFβ is also contained within platelet α granules and is released by activated platelets. The absence of TGFβ from fetal wounds may be due to an inability of fetal platelets to synthesize and release the factor in the fetal wound or to a relative decrease in the number of degranulating platelets at the fetal wound site. Macrophages are a potent source of TGFβ and the reduced level in fetal wounds may reflect an absent or minimal macrophage infiltrate in these wounds. The presence of TGFβ in the adult wound and its absence in the fetal wound correlates with its known effects in vitro and the differences in the ECM between fetal and adult wounds. TGFβ stimulates matrix synthesis,[47–49] including collagen, while inhibiting matrix degradation.[50] The increased production of the ECM seen in an animal model of glomerulonephritis can be suppressed by antiserum against TGFβ[51] and conversely the implantation of polyvinyl alcohol sponge implants containing TGFβ1 in a fetal rabbit produces fibrosis within the implant.[52] The restoration of a normal collagenous architecture in fetal wounds and the relative lack of collagen in the fetal wound, in comparison to the densely packed collagen seen in the adult wound, may thus be due to lower levels of TGFβ in fetal wounds.

bFGF has many biological properties that may play a role in wound healing including stimulation of angiogenesis and matrix production, thereby suggesting a role in the formation of granulation tissue (for review see Fox[53]). It was present for a short period in both adult and neonatal mouse wounds within the dermis adjacent to the wound, presumably due to release by damaged cells as this is the only presently known mechanism of bFGF secretion. The neovascularization seen in the adult wound and its absence from the fetal wounds thus correlate with the angiogenic effect of bFGF, the presence of this factor in adult wounds and its absence from fetal wounds.

SHEEP RESULTS

In the fetal sheep model we have studied incisional,[7,8] and excisional wounds,[5] localizing collagen types I, III, IV, and VI, fibronectin, tenascin and laminin. The results from these studies broadly correlated with our findings from fetal and adult mice.

The rate of wound closure was most rapid in the 100 d fetus and slowest in the adult. This correlated with the time at which Tn was first seen in the respective wounds. Collagen types I, III, IV, and VI were present in fetal and neonatal wounds. 100 d fetal incisional wounds healed without scar formation while 120 d fetal wounds showed some scar formation that was markedly less than the scar seen in the adult sheep. Therefore, a gradual transition in wound healing occurs, from scarless to scar formation, between 100 and 120 days of gestation.

Epithelialization was complete in the 100 d fetus at 24 h, in the 120 d fetus at 48 h and in the adult between 72 h and 7 d. Fibronectin was diffusely present within the mesenchyme and dermis of fetal and adult animals. It was present at the surface of the wound 1 h postwounding and the increased staining in the region of the wound diminished gradually as the wound defect closed and the clot disappeared, in a similar process to the mouse wounds. Tn was seen at the surface of the 100 d fetal wound 4 h postwounding. The intensity of the staining increased and at 24 h Tn was present within the adjacent dermis (Fig. 10.4a). Tn was present within the dermis at 7 d (Fig. 10.4b) but by 14 d a normal pattern of staining was apparent, with Tn limited to the basement membrane of the epidermis and a few dermal capillaries (Fig. 10.4c). In the 120 d fetus Tn was faintly visible at the wound margin at 12 h, with more intense staining present within the dermis and wound from 24 h to 14 d postwounding. Unlike the 100 d fetus, at 14 d in the 120 d fetus Tn was still present within the dermis (Fig. 10.4d). Tn was first seen in the adult wounds at 24 h and persisted with strong dermal staining still present at 14 d postwounding. The time at which epithelialization was complete in these wounds also appears to relate to the time at which Tn was first present within the wound, substantiating our proposal that Tn may play a critical role in the initiation of cell migration.

Collagen types I, III, and VI were widely distributed in normal fetal and adult dermis (Fig. 10.4e). In 100 d fetal wounds these collagens were deposited initially at 72 h, and by 14 d a normal tissue architecture had been restored, without scar formation (Fig. 10.4f). Similarly in the 75 d fetus by 15 d pw a normal tissue pattern was present at the site of the wound (Fig. 10.4g). In the 120 d fetus at 14 d postwounding a narrow band of scar tissue with parallel bundles of collagen was seen (Fig. 10.4h). In the adult, collagen deposition was not seen until 7 d, and at 14 d a broad band of scar tissue was present (Fig. 10.4i). A similar pattern of staining was present for collagen types I, III, and VI with restoration of a normal tissue pattern in the 75 and 100 d fetus, minimal scar in the 120 d fetus and marked scarring in the adult. Collagen type IV demonstrated neovascularization in the adult wounds that was not present in the fetal wounds.

Healing of excisional wounds occurred rapidly in the 75 d fetus and apart from epithelial furrows at the margins of the original wound there was regeneration of a normal tissue pattern at 15 d when stained for collagen types I, III, and VI (Fig. 10.4j). In the 100 d fetus excisional wounds were not re-epithelialized until 7–14 d postwounding and at 14 d a narrow band of scar tissue was present at the site of the wound (Fig. 10.4k). It is therefore apparent that in the fetal sheep relatively large wounds will heal without scar formation but the time during gestation when wounding occurs is critical. Incisional fetal sheep wounds have shown a transition from fetal healing to scar formation between 100 and 120 d of gestation. The 100 d excisional wounds were unhealed until after 107 d gestation and the scar formation may thus be due to the fact that these wounds are still healing at the time of this transition. More likely, the type of wound healing (scar free or scar) depends on the degree of inflammatory response at the wound site and hence on interactions between the gestational age (and thus the maturity of the immune system) and the degree of tissue damage (incisional versus excisional wounds). It may also depend on the species used (fetal rabbit excisional wounds heal poorly,[54,55] probably due to the unusual composition of their amniotic fluid[56]), the tissue injured,[57] and the method of wounding.

SUMMARY

These studies have shown many differences between the ECM of fetal and adult wounds, highlighting the two most striking characteristics of fetal wound healing—the rapidity with which this occurs and the restoration of an apparently normal tissue structure—and suggesting some potentially useful areas for further study.

The rate of healing per se is not of great clinical interest but by altering the kinetics of the process the structure of the ECM (particularly collagen) deposited in the wound may be affected, and thus the quality of wound healing altered. The gross properties of scar tissue (restriction of function and growth) are a reflection of the collagenous structure of the tissue. Elucidating the mechanisms that control collagen fibrillogenesis in the fetal wound, leading to regeneration of a normal dermal structure, are thus central to our aim of manipulating adult wounds so that they heal in a more fetal-like manner. As discussed above, some of the differences in the ECM and growth factors of the fetal wound may influence fibrillogenesis. The initial framework of fibrin and fibronectin laid down in the wound may also have an important influence on collagen fibril orientation. In the fetal wound fibroblasts are able to rapidly migrate into a loose lattice containing relatively high levels of proteoglycans and glycosaminoglycans. By contrast the provisional scaffold laid down in the adult wound seems more resistant to fibroblast infiltration and migration occurs more easily along the wound margins. These initial differences in the migration and orientation of fibroblasts may establish the pattern of collagen fibrils deposited in the respective wounds, with a loose reticular structure in the fetus and a closely packed, parallel, arrangement in the adult.

Finally, these studies have demonstrated that there is no "magic" phase of transition from scar free to scar type wound healing; rather there is a relationship between scar free healing, the degree of tissue damage, and the time of gestation (the greater the damage, the earlier in gestation one must operate for scar free healing). Such considerations are important when considering the timing of human embryonic/fetal surgery if scarring is to be minimized and optimal results achieved.

This gradual transition is one further indication of the multiple and subtle differences between fetal and adult wound healing and these studies suggest many ways to manipulate the adult wound that may reduce scarring: Add exogenous tenascin to enhance cell migration; facilitate cell migration and alter collagen fibril orientation by addition of glycosaminoglycans; change the growth factor profile of the wound by addition of growth factors or neutralizing antibodies; alter the cellular component of the wound by clonally expanding or transplanting (from the oral mucosa) fibroblasts with embryonic characteristics; alter the immune response at the wound site; alter the biomechanical forces at the wound site. However, duplication and redundancy are features of many biological systems and it is possible that altering just a few of these components will reduce or eliminate scarring in the adult wound.

REFERENCES

1. Burrington JD: Wound healing in the fetal lamb. J. Pediatr. Surg. 6, 523–528, 1971.
2. Robinson BW, Goss AN: Intrauterine healing of fetal rat cheek wounds. Cleft Palate J. 18, 251–255, 1981.
3. Rowsell AR: The intra-uterine healing of foetal muscle wounds: experimental study in the rat. Br. J. Plast. Surg. 37, 635–642, 1984.
4. Whitby DJ, Longaker MT, Jennings RW, Duncan BW, Adzick NS, Harrison MR, Ferguson MWJ: Histology and immunohistochemistry of excisional fetal sheep wounds. Presented at 1st Annual Wound Healing Society meeting, Galveston, 1991.
5. Whitby DJ and Ferguson MWJ: The extracellular matrix of lip wounds in fetal, neonatal and adult mice. Development 112:651–668, 1991.
6. Whitby DJ and Ferguson MWF: Immunohistochemical localisation of growth factors in fetal wound healing. Dev. Biol. (in press).
7. Longaker MT, Whitby DJ, Adzick NS, Crombleholme TM, Langer JC, Duncan BW, Stern R, Ferguson MWJ, Harrison MR: Studies in fetal wound healing: VI. Second and early third trimester fetal wounds demonstrate rapid collagen deposition without scar formation. J. Pediatr. Surg. 25, 63–69, 1990.
8. Whitby DJ, Longaker MT, Adzick NS, Harrison MR, Ferguson MWJ: Rapid epithelialization of fetal wounds is due to early deposition of tenascin. J. Cell Sci. (in press).
9. Muneako K, Wanek N, Bryant SV (1986): Mouse embryos develop normally exo utero. J. Exp. Zool. 239, 289–293, 1990.
10. Harrison MR, Jester JA, Ross NA: Correction of diaphragmatic hernia in utero. I. The model: intrathoracic balloon produces fatal pulmonary hypoplasia. Surgery. 88:174–182, 1980.
11. Clark RAF: Potential roles of fibronectin in cutaneous wound repair. Arch. Dermatol. 124, 201–206, 1988.
12. Chiquet-Ehrismann R.: What distinguishes tenascin from fibronectin. FASEB J. 4, 2598–2604, 1990.
13. Erickson HP, Bourdon MA: Tenascin: an extracellular matrix protein prominent in specialised embryonic tissues and tumours. Ann. Rev. Cell Biol. 5, 71–92, 1989.
14. Chiquet-Ehrismann R, Mackie EJ, Pearson CA, Sakakura T: Tenascin: an extracellular matrix protein involved in tissue interactions during fetal development and oncogenesis. Cell 47, 131–139, 1986.
15. Aufderheide E, Chiquet-Ehrismann R, Ekblom P: Epithelial-mesenchymal interactions in the developing kidney lead to expression of tenascin in the mesenchyme. J. Cell Biol. 105, 599–608, 1987.
16. Mackie EJ, Thesleff I, Chiquet-Ehrismann R: Tenascin is associated with chondrogenic and osteogenic differentiation in vivo and promotes chondrogenesis in vitro. J Cell Biol. 105, 2569–2579, 1987.
17. Thesleff I, Mackie E, Vainio S, Chiquet-Ehrismann R: Changes in the distribution of tenascin during tooth development. Development 101, 289–296, 1987.
18. Vainio S, Jalkanen M, Thesleff I: Syndecan and tenascin expression is induced by epithelial-mesenchymal interactions in embryonic tooth mesenchyme. J. Cell Biol. 108, 1945–1954, 1989.
19. Wehrle B, Chiquet M: Tenascin is accumulated along developing peripheral nerves and allows neurite outgrowth in vitro. Development 110, 401–415, 1990.
20. Stamp GWH: Tenascin distribution in basal cell carcinomas. J. Pathol. 159, 225–229, 1989.
21. Ferguson JE, Schor AM, Howell A, Ferguson MWJ: Tenascin distribution in the normal human breast is altered during the menstrual cycle and in carcinoma. Differentiation 42, 199–207, 1990.
22. Vollmer G, Siegal GP, Chiquet-Ehrismann R, Lightner VA, Arnholdt HR: Tenascin expression in the human endometrium and in endometrial adenocarcinomas. Lab. Invest. 62, 725–730, 1990.
23. Mackie EJ, Tucker RP, Halfter W, Chiquet-Ehrismann R: The distribution of tenascin coincides with pathways of neural crest cell migration. Development 102, 237–250, 1988.
24. Chiquet-Ehrismann R, Kalla P, Pearson CA, Beck K, Chiquet M: Tenascin interferes with fibronectin action. Cell 53, 383–390, 1988.
25. Riou JC, Shi DL, Chiquet M, Boucaut JC: Exogenous tenascin inhibits mesodermal cell migration during amphibian gastrulation. Develop. Biol. 137, 305–317, 1990.

26. Mackie EJ, Halfter W, and Liverani D: Induction of tenascin in healing wounds. J. Cell Biol. 107, 2757–2767, 1988.
27. Fleischmajer R: Collagen fibrillogenesis: A mechanism of structural biology. J. Invest. Dermatol. 87, 553–554, 1986.
28. Burgeson RE: New collagens, new concepts. Ann. Rev. Cell Biol. 4, 551–577, 1988.
29. Birk DE, Fitch JM, Barbiaz JP, Linsenmayer TF: Collagen type I and type V are present in the same fibril in the avian corneal stroma. J. Cell Biol. 106, 999–1008, 1988.
30. Burgeson RE: Do banded collagen fibers contain two or more collagen types? In ISI atlas of science: biochemistry. 88–91, 1988.
31. Keene DR, Sakai LY, Bachinger HP, Burgeson RE: Type III collagen can be present on banded collagen fibrils regardless of fibril diameter. J. Cell Biol. 105, 2393–2402, 1987.
32. Birk DE, Fitch JM, Babiarz JP, Doane KJ, Linsenmayer TF: Collagen fibrillogenesis in vitro: interaction of types I and V collagen regulates fibril diameter. J. Cell Sci. 95, 649–657, 1990.
33. Epstein EH: {α 1(III)} human skin collagen. J. Biol. Chem. 249, 3225–3231, 1974.
34. Merkel JR, DiPaolo BR, Hallock GG, Rice DC: Type I and type III collagen content of healing wounds in fetal and adult rats. Proc. Soc. Exp. Biol. Med. 187, 493–497, 1988.
35. Scott JE: Proteoglycan-fibrillar collagen interactions. Biochem. J. 252, 313–323, 1988.
36. Vogel KG, Trotter, JA: The effect of proteoglycans on the morphology of collagen fibrils formed in vitro. Coll. Rel. Res. 7, 105–114, 1987.
37. Krummel TM, Nelson JM, Diegelmann RF, Lindblad WJ, Salzberg AM, Greenfield LJ, Cohen IK: Fetal response to injury in the rabbit. J. Pediatr. Surg. 22, 640–643, 1987.
38. Longaker MT, Chiu ES, Harrison MR, Crombleholme TM, Langer JC, Duncan BW, Adzick NS, Verrier ED, Stern R: Studies in fetal wound healing: IV. Hyaluronic acid stimulating activity of fetal versus adult wound fluid. Ann. Surg. 210, 667–672, 1989.
39. DePalma RL, Krummel TM, Durham LA, Michna BA, Thomas BL, Nelson J, Diegelmann RF: Characterization and quantitation of wound matrix in the fetal rabbit. Matrix 9, 224–231, 1989.
40. Hellstrom S, Laurent C: Hyaluronan and healing of tympanic membrane perforations. An experimental study. Acta. Otolaryngol. (Stockh.) Suppl. 42, 54–61, 1987.
41. Scott JE, Hughes EW: Proteoglycan-collagen relationships in developing chick and bovine tendons. Influence of the physiological environment. Connect. Tiss. Res. 14, 267–278, 1986.
42. Ross R, Raines EW, Bowen-Pope DF: The biology of platelet derived growth factor. Cell 46, 155–169, 1986.
43. Narayana AS, Page RC: Biosynthesis and regulation of type V collagen in diploid human fibroblasts. J. Biol. Chem. 258, 11694–11699, 1983.
44. Kaplan DR, Chao FC, Stiles CD, Antoniades HN, Scher CD: Platelet alpha-granules contain a growth factor for fibroblasts. Blood 53, 1043–1052, 1979.
45. Kaplan DR, Broekman MJ, Chernoff A, Lesznik GR, Drillings M: Platelet alpha-granule proteins: studies on release and subcellular localization. Blood 53, 604–618, 1979.
46. Bowen-Pope DF, Malpass TW, Foster DM, Ross R: Platelet derived growth factor in vivo: levels, activity, and rate of clearance. Blood 64, 458–469, 1984.
47. Ignotz R, Massague J: Transforming growth factor-beta stimulates the expression of fibronectin and collagen and their incorporation into the extracellular matrix. J. Biol. Chem. 261, 4337–4345, 1986.
48. Roberts AB, Sporn MB, Assoian RK, Smith JM, Roche NS, Wakefield LM, Heine UI, Liotta LA, Falanga V, Kehrl JH, Fauci AS: Transforming growth factor-beta: rapid induction of fibrosis and angiogenesis *in vivo* and stimulation of collagen formation *in vitro*. Proc. Natl. Acad. Sci. USA 83, 4167–4171, 1986.
49. Ignotz RA, Endo T, Massague J: Regulation of fibronectin and type I collagen mRNA levels by transforming growth factor-beta. J. Biol. Chem. 262, 6443–6446, 1987.
50. Laiho M, Sakesela O, Andreasen PA, Keski-Oja J: Enhanced production and extracellular deposition of the endothelial-type plasminogen activator inhibitor in cultured human lung fibroblasts by transforming growth factor-beta. J. Cell Biol. 103, 2403–2410, 1986.
51. Border WA, Okuda S, Languino LR, Sporn MB, Ruoslahti E: Suppression of experimental glomerulonephritis by antiserum against transforming growth factor β1. Nature 346, 371–374, 1990.
52. Krummel TM, Michna BA, Thomas BL, Sporn MB, Nelson JM, Salzberg AM, Cohen IK, Diegelmann RF: Transforming growth factor beta induces fibrosis in a fetal wound model. J. Pediatr. Surg. 23, 647–652, 1988.
53. Fox GM: The role of growth factors in tissue repair: III Fibroblast growth factor. In: The molecular and cellular biology of wound repair, pp 265–271. (Clark RAF, and Henson PM eds.). Plenum Press, New York, 1988.

54. Somasundaram K and Prathap K: Intra-uterine healing of skin wounds in rabbit foetuses. J. Path. 100, 81–86, 1970.
55. Somasundaram K and Prathap K: The effects of exclusion of amniotic fluid on intra-uterine healing of skin wounds in rabbit foetuses. J. Path. 107, 127–130, 1972.
56. Wild AE: Protein composition of the rabbit fetal fluids. Proc. R. Soc. B. 163, 90–115, 1965.
57. Longaker MT, Whitby DJ, Adzick NS, Duncan BW, Ferguson MWJ, Harrison MR. Fetal diaphragmatic wounds heal with scar formation. J. Surg. Res. 50:375–385, 1991.

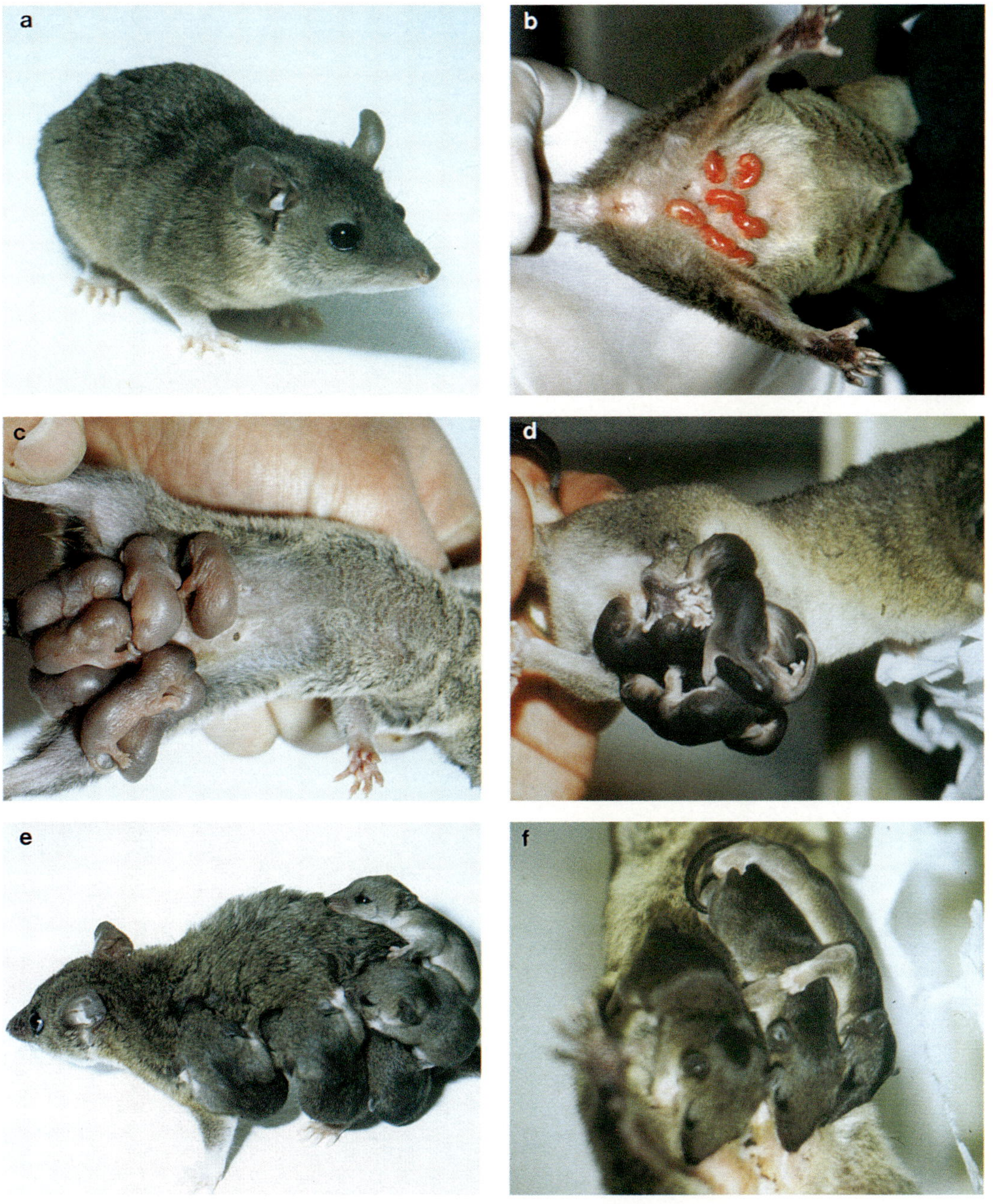

Figure 6.1 **(a)** Adult *Monodelphis domestica.* **(b)** Abdomen of female *Monodelphis domestica,* who has just given birth. Note the small newly emerged pouch young which are attached to the mother's nipple and are bright red, owing to their well developed cutaneous blood supply and transparent skin. **(c)** Day seven *Monodelphis domestica* attached to the nipples on the underside of the abdomen of a female. Note the darker skin, greatly increased size, commencement of eye development and the absence of fur. **(d)** Day 14 *Monodelphis domestica* attached to the nipples on the underside of the mother's abdomen. Note the development of fur. **(e)** Three-and-a-half-week-old *Monodelphis domestica,* clinging to their mother's fur on both the dorsal and ventral aspects of her body. **(f)** Four-week-old suckling *Monodelphis domestica.*

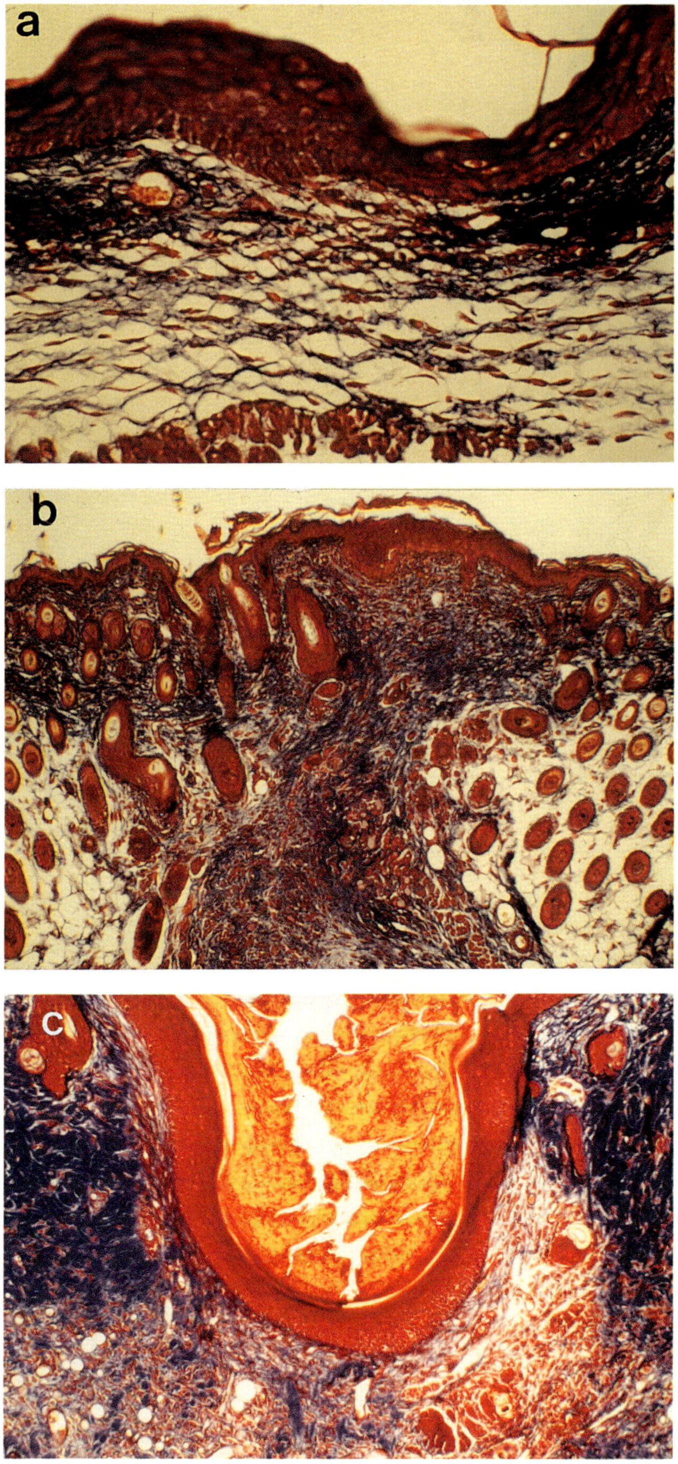

Figure 6.5 (a) Day 2 pouch young wound, two days postoperatively stained with Mallory's trichrome, illustrating an absence of scar tissue formation within the dermis. Note that although collagen deposition has commenced, there is still less collagen at the wound site, marked by a thickened epithelium, compared to the surrounding tissues. **(b)** Day 28 pouch young wound, seven days postoperatively. Note the extensive scarring as evidenced by staining with Mallory's trichrome in the dermal and subcutaneous regions. Note also the abnormal orientation of the collagen fibrils, perpendicular to the basement membrane. **(c)** Adult wound, seven days postoperatively, illustrating extensive scarring and a deep, re-epithelialized furrow with scab.

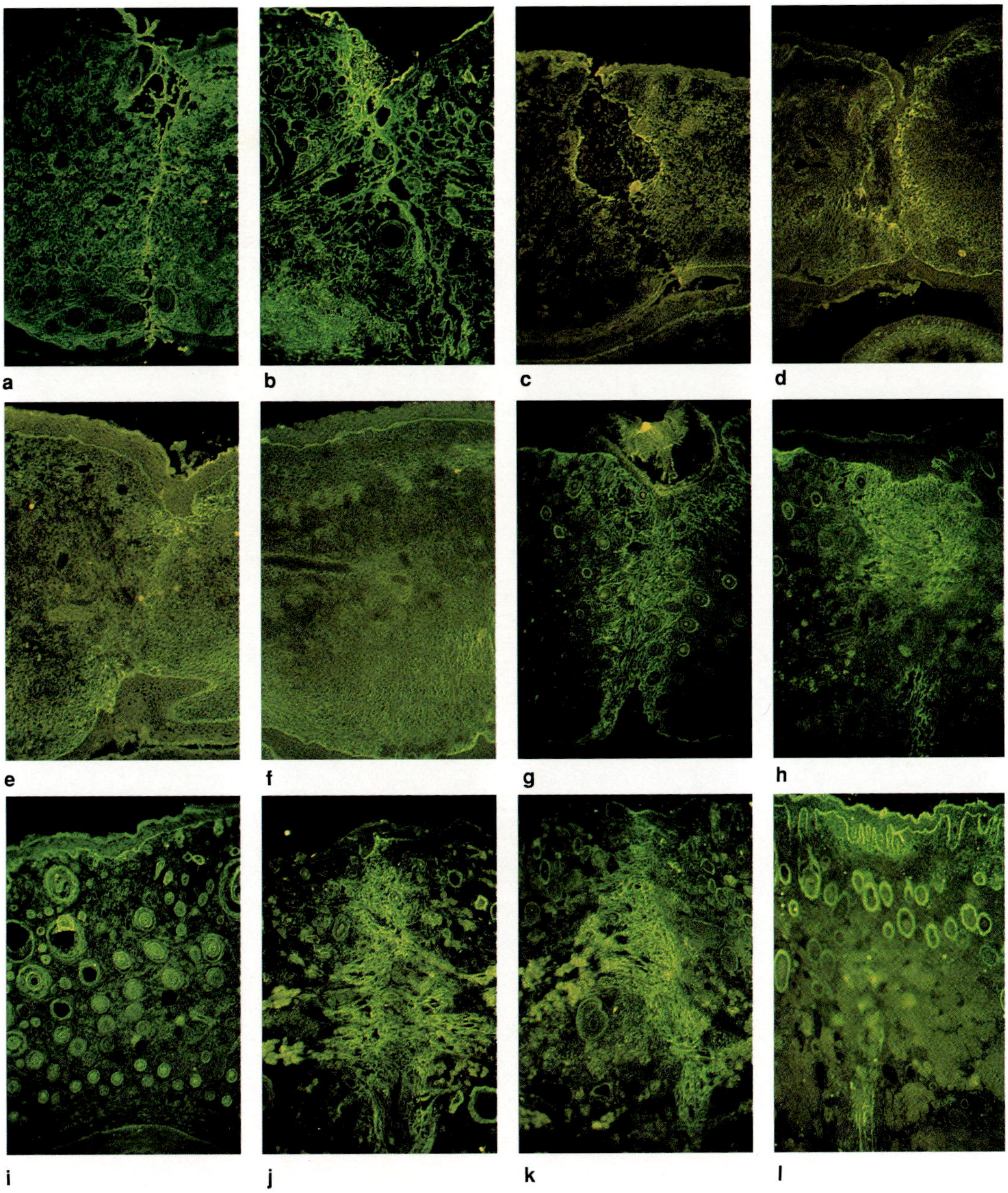

Figure 10.1 Transverse sections, mouse lip. **(a–b)** Stained for fibronectin (Fn). **(a)** 16 d fetus 1 h postwounding (pw). Fn widely distributed in mesenchymal ECM, with linear staining at basement membrane of epidermis and oral mucosa. Layer of Fn seen at wound surface and within clot. **(b)** Adult 1 h pw. Layer of Fn at surface of wound. **(c–l)** stained for tenascin (Tn). **(c)** 16 d fetus 1 h pw. Tn present at the basement membranes of the dermal-epidermal junction and oral mucosa. Tn staining present at surface of wound. **(d)** 16 d fetus 24 h pw. Tn staining present in mesenchyme adjacent to wound, particularly at the interface with the dermal-epidermal junction. **(e)** 16 d fetus 48 h pw. Wound re-epithelialized and mesenchymal defect closed. Staining for tenascin present at site of wound. **(f)** 16 d fetus 72 h pw. Near normal staining pattern for Tn—no staining within wound. **(g)** Neonate 48 h pw. Intense staining for Tn within healing wound. **(h)** Neonate 72 h pw. Patchy staining for Tn largely at dermal-epidermal junction. **(i)** Neonate 5 d pw. Tn staining restricted to epithelial basement membranes—note absence of hair follicles in skin side of wound but normal pattern of staining beneath oral mucosa. **(j)** Adult 5 d pw. Intense staining for Tn within healing wound. **(k)** Adult 7 d pw. Staining for Tn less intense. **(l)** Adult 12 d pw. Increased staining for Tn near basement membrane of epithelial ingrowths at the wound surface. Patchy staining for Tn still present within healing wound. *s*, skin; *m*, oral mucosa; *t*, tongue; *h*, hair follicle; *o*, oral mucosal salivary glands; *b*, basement membrane. Arrow: site of wound. Bar: 100 μm

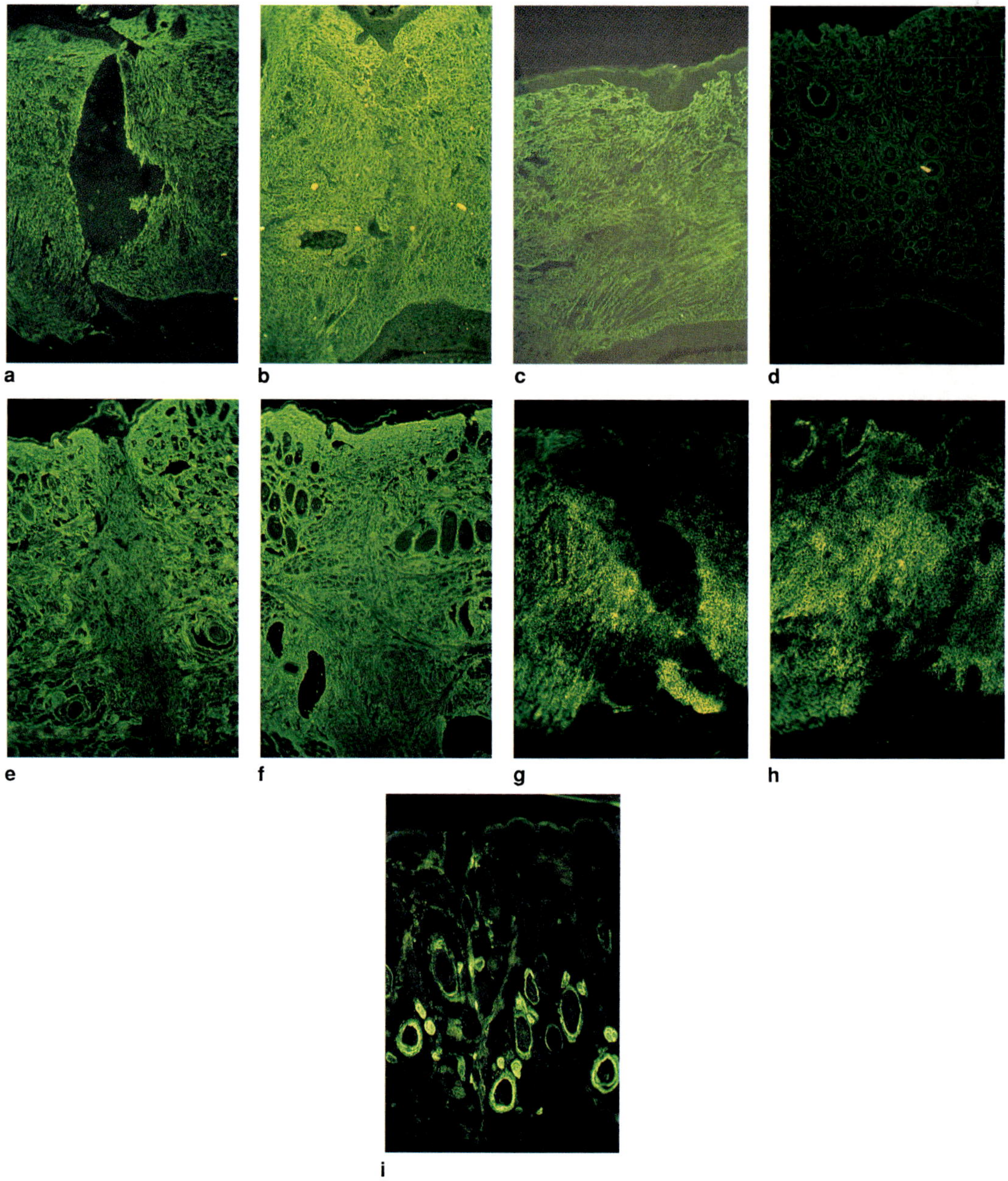

Figure 10.2 Transverse sections, mouse lip. **(a–f)** Stained for type III collagen (C III). **(a)** 16 d fetus 24 h pw. C III widely distributed in ECM of mesenchyme, no staining for C III within wound. **(b)** 16 d fetus 48 h pw. Wound re-epithelialized and C III present within wound. **(c)** 16 d fetus 72 h pw. Normal pattern of C III staining regenerated at site of wound, without scar formation. Epithelial furrow of skin is the only remaining indicator of the original wound. **(d)** Adult 5 d pw. C III present within wound. **(e)** Adult 12 d pw. Parallel bundles of C III forming scar tissue disrupting normal tissue structure. **(f)** Neonate 5 d pw. On the oral side of wound a normal pattern of C III has regenerated. On the skin side of the wound loss of hair follicles is apparent. Apart from this loss the staining for C III appears almost normal and the prominent, parallel bundles of collagen seen in the scar formed in the adult wound (Figure 10.2 **e**) are not seen in the neonatal wound. **(g–i)** stained for chondroitin sulfate (CS). **(g)** 16 d fetus 12 h pw. Diffuse staining for CS in mesenchymal ECM. No staining for CS within wound. Note the blotchy pattern of staining contrasts with the fibrillar pattern seen with collagens and fibronectin. **(h)** 16 d fetus 20 h pw. CS is now present within wound. **(i)** Adult 7 d pw. Staining for CS localized to dermis surrounding hair follicles. CS not present within wound except for a very small area immediately adjacent to the regenerated basement membrane. *s*, skin; *m*, oral mucosa; *t*, tongue; *h*, hair follicle; *o*, oral mucosal salivary glands; *b*, basement membrane. Arrow: site of wound. Bar: 100 μm

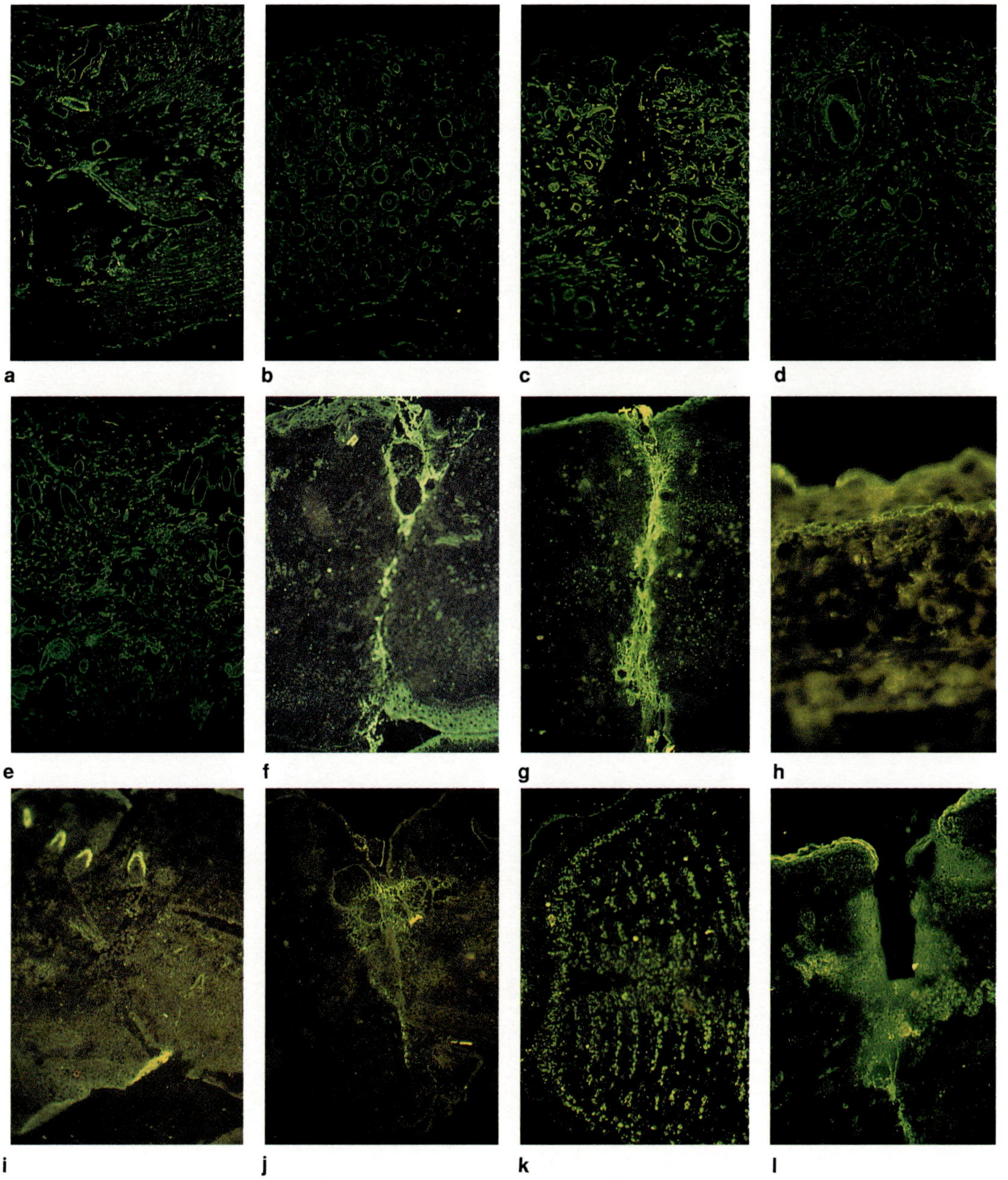

Figure 10.3 Transverse sections mouse lip. **(a–e)** Stained for type IV collagen. **(a)** 16 d fetus 5 d pw. C IV localized in epithelial and endothelial basement membranes. Staining pattern in wound indistinguishable from normal surrounding tissues—no scar formation and no neovascularization. **(b)** Neonate 5 d pw. Regeneration of normal pattern of staining for C IV at oral mucosal aspect of wound. C IV shows loss of hair follicles but normal vascular pattern in skin aspect of wound. **(c)** Adult 5 d pw. Band of scar tissue separating normal tissues. Within scar tissue scanty neovascularization is apparent, with C IV present in the basement membrane of new capillaries. **(d)** Adult 7 d pw. Further new capillary formation present within wound. **(e)** Adult 12 d pw. Profuse neovascularization with multiple capillary loops present in wound site. **(f–g)** stained for PDGF. **(f)** 16 d fetus 1 h pw. PDGF present at surface of wound and within clot. **(g)** Adult 1 h pw. PDGF present at surface of wound and within clot. **(h–j)** stained for TGFβ. **(h)** 16 d fetus, unwounded skin. TGFβ present extracellularly at basal epithelium. **(i)** 16 d fetus 1 h pw. TGFβ present around developing hair follicles, but not present at wound. **(j)** Neonate 6 h pw. TGFβ present at surface of wound and within clot. **(k–l)** stained for bFGF. **(k)** 16 d fetus, transverse section through floor of mouth. bFGF present within muscle bundles of tongue. **(l)** Neonate 1 h pw. bFGF present at surface of wound and within adjacent dermis. (Non-specific staining of epithelium). *s*, skin; *m*, oral mucosa; *t*, tongue; *h*, hair follicle; *o*, oral mucosal salivary glands; *b*, basement membrane. Arrow: site of wound. Bar: 100 μm

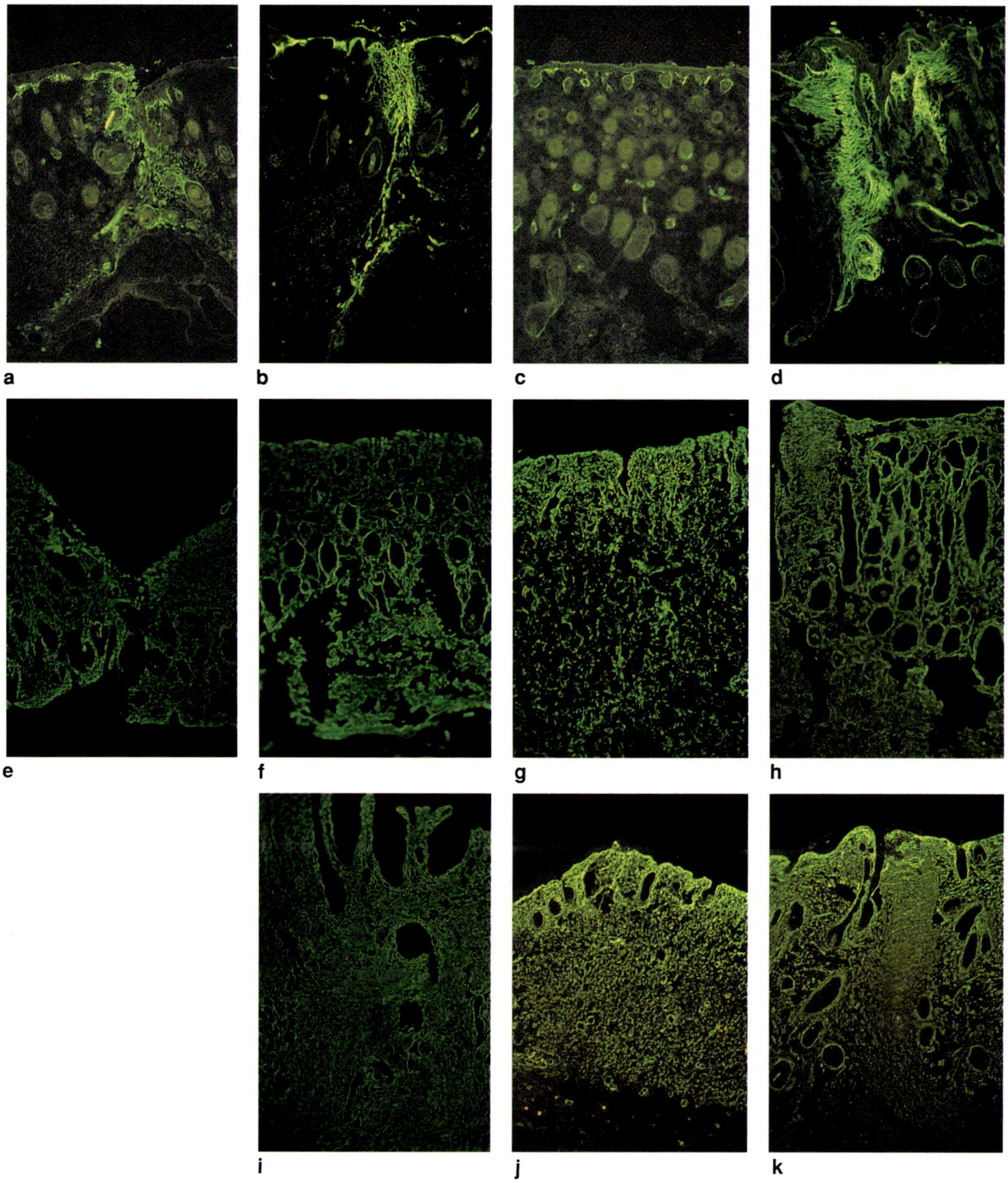

Figure 10.4 Vertical sections, sheep wounds. **(a–d)** Incisional wounds stained for tenascin (Tn). **(a)** 100 d fetus 24 h pw. Tn present at surface of wound and within adjacent dermis. **(b)** 100 d fetus 7 d pw. Wound re-epithelialized and tenascin present at site of dermal wound. **(c)** 100 d fetus 14 d pw. Normal staining pattern for Tn, no scar formation. **(d)** 120 fetus 14 d pw. Tn staining still present at site of wound. **(e–i)** Incisional wounds stained for collagen type VI (C VI). **(e)** 100 d fetus 24 h pw. C VI widely distributed within dermis, absent from wound. **(f)** 100 d fetus 14 d pw. Regeneration of normal tissue architecture, indistinguishable from normal dermis. **(g)** 75 d fetus 15 d pw. Regeneration of normal tissue architecture. **(h)** 120 d fetus 14 d pw. Narrow band of scar tissue at site of wound. **(i)** Adult 14 d pw. Dense, broad band of collagen at site of wound. **(j–k)** Excisional wounds stained for collagen type VI (C VI). **(j)** 75 d fetus 14 d pw. Regeneration of normal reticular pattern of collagen. **(k)** 100 d fetus 21 d pw. Narrow scar at site of excisional wound. *s*, skin; *m*, oral mucosa; *t*, tongue; *h*, hair follicle; *o*, oral mucosal salivary glands; *b*, basement membrane. Arrow: site of wound. Bar: 100 μm

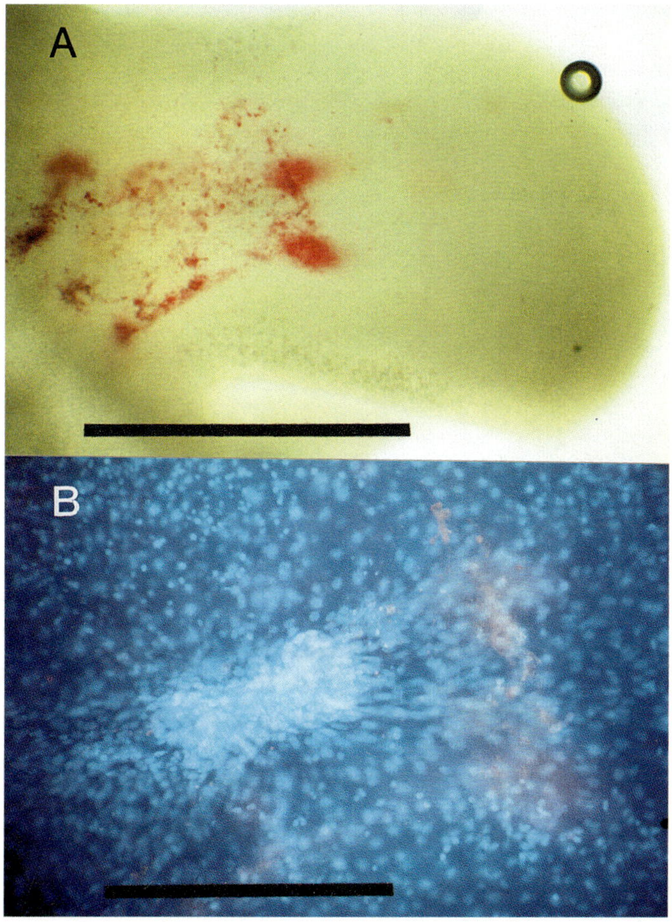

Figure 18.3 A marking experiment demonstrating that the epidermis sweeps in over the exposed mesenchyme during healing of the standard chick limb bud wound. A red dye, DiI, has been applied at the time of wounding (0 hours) to mark the exposed surface mesenchyme cells; the photographs show the result 18 hours later. **a.** Bright-field view of the limb bud as a whole mount, showing a modest contraction of the marked area of mesenchyme. (Scale bar = 1 mm.) **b.** Detail of the same 18-hour specimen, stained additionally after fixation with the fluorescent nuclear dye, DAPI, to show the nuclei of the epidermal cells (blue/white). The epidermis has closed completely over the mesenchyme, forming a typical pimple at the site of closure. (Scale bar = 500 μm.)

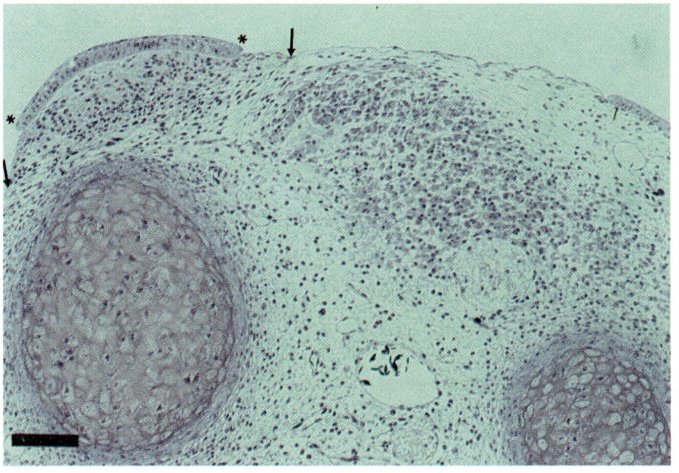

Figure 18.6 Result of the operation diagrammed in Figure 5, 24 hours after the grafting operation. The island of quail epidermis has shrunk back over its own (quail) mesenchyme. Arrows show the boundaries of the quail mesenchyme (determined from an adjacent section stained with Feulgen to reveal the quail nucleolar marker); asterisks show the edges of the quail epidermis. (Toluidine blue stain; scale bar = 100 μm.)

CHAPTER **11**

Collagen Deposition in Fetal Wounds

D. Andrew R. Burd
John Siebert
Michael T. Longaker

When we consider the essential role of collagen in adult wound healing (see Chapter 2) and recognize the structural role of collagen in fetal connective tissue, it is perhaps surprising that there should have been any controversy over the presence of collagen deposition in fetal wound healing. However, small animal studies have led to some conflicting results concerning collagen deposition in fetal wounds.[1–7]

A wound can be defined as a defect in tissue integrity, and healing is the process of restoring that integrity. "Integrity" in the context of these definitions is necessarily an all encompassing term but it does embody function as well as form. For example, the skin is a bilaminar structure consisting of a superficial cell-rich layer, the epidermis, overlying a collagen-rich connective tissue support and strength layer, the dermis. Restoration of the integrity of wounded skin must involve reconstituting an appreciable degree of strength as well as form (cover and support). Collagen is the only macromolecule in the body capable of subserving that function in pre- or postnatal wound repair. Some investigators looking at the biological mechanisms of fetal wound healing using histochemical and biochemical techniques have proposed that collagen deposition was not involved in fetal skin wound healing.[1,3,4,8,9] This conclusion did not come from faulty data but rather the source and interpretation of the data. Conventional histochemical analysis of fetal wounds is not sensitive enough to detect new collagen deposition in small animal models.[1] Biochemical analysis of the content of wound healing models in small animals can similarly suffer from small sample size despite very sensitive analytical techniques. A further complication may arise from the wound healing implant used.

Although Adzick and Krummel came to diametrically opposite conclusions from their studies of collagen deposition in similar fetal rabbit models, they used two different wound implant techniques. Adzick and colleagues reported elevated levels of hydroxyproline, as a measure of collagen deposition,[2] using implanted polytetrafluoroethylene (Gore-tex; W.L. Gore and Associates, Flagstaff, AZ, USA) tubing and an automated amino acid analyzer technique.[10] The Gore-tex tube implant model has been criticized because encapsulation may lead to poor ingrowth of new tissue.[4,11] One observation is that when using the Gore-tex tubing, care must be taken to ensure that the tissue surrounding the tubing is not analyzed with the content of the tubing. Incomplete removal of the connective tissue capsule from the outside of the tube before analysis would contribute to elevated hydroxyproline levels attributed to the tube contents. The silastic/polyvinyl alcohol (PVA) model used by Krummel is purported to overcome this problem by enclosing a PVA sponge within a perforated silastic tube. The tube forms an inert zone between the sponge and the surrounding tissue. Only new tissue will grow into the sponge that can be isolated intact from the surrounding tubing. Krummel reported the absence of hydroxyproline within the enclosed PVA sponges[4] despite using a very sensitive liquid chromatography analytical technique.[12] It is possible that the design of the wound healing implant prevented the deposition of normal wound repair tissue, or that the preparative steps in the technique used to process the PVA sponges resulted in such dilution of the small sample that the lower detection limits may have been reached. The histological events in both wound healing models are reported to be similar to those found in incisional wounds.[2,4]

Collagen deposition in fetal wounds can be investigated in a number of ways using histologic, biochemical, biomechanical, and immunohistochemical techniques (see Chapter 10). In this chapter we will describe our biochemical studies using both small and large fetal animal models that demonstrate that collagen deposition does occur in the fetal wound healing process. Some supportive electron microscopy, histochemistry, and biomechanical analyses are also presented.

COLLAGEN DEPOSITION IN FETAL RABBIT WOUNDS

In our hypothesis of fetal wound healing we assumed that collagen is present and therefore chose to use the Gore-tex tube implant in fetal rabbits. The reported yield of collagen in this model was well within the limits of detection of our microanalytical typing techniques, and our interest lay not so much in the presence of collagen but the type of collagen involved in fetal wound healing.

EXPERIMENTAL DETAILS: RABBIT STUDIES

Wound chambers of 2 cm by 2 mm diameter Gore-tex tubing were surgically implanted subcutaneously in maternal and fetal New Zealand White Rabbits at 23–25 days gestation (term = 31–32 days). Tubing was harvested and analyzed at four, five, six, and seven days in the fetal animals and at four, seven, 10, and 14 days in the adult animals. The tubing has 90 micron pores that permit rapid tissue ingrowth. The implant will fill with sufficient quantities of granulation tissue for histologic and biochemical analysis.

HISTOLOGY

Histologic examination of harvested Gore-tex tubing implants was performed by electron microscopy. Specimens were fixed in 3% phosphate buffered glutaraldehyde pH 7.3 and postfixed in 2% osmium tetroxide. After dehydration in graded alcohols and propylene oxide, they were embedded in Epox 812. Sections of 700 Angstroms were mounted on copper grids and stained with uranyl acetate and lead citrate. Specimens were examined with a JEOL 100-C electron microscope. Banded fibrillar structures were positively identified within the lumen of the implants (Fig. 11.1). The diameter of the fibers measured 27 nm and the banding periodicity was 54 nm. Native collagen does have a banded appearance with a periodicity of 67 nm. The finding of a periodicity of 54 nm does not exclude the

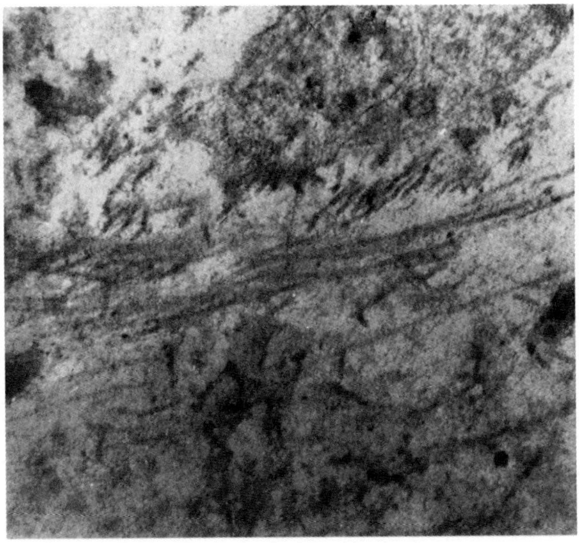

Figure 11.1 Electron micrograph of 700 Angstroms thickness section from Gore-tex tubing implant (×20,000). Banded fibrillar structures are found within the lumen. Fiber diameter is 27 nm and banding periodicity is 54 nm. *Reprinted with permission.*[5]

possibility that this is fibrillar collagen as fixation artifacts can affect the observed periodicity.

COLLAGEN ANALYSIS

Cyanogen Bromide (CNBr) Digestion

Gore-tex tubing implants were cut into 1–2 mm lengths and suspended in oxygen free 70% formic acid. Equal weights of CNBr and sample were combined and the mixture agitated for four hours at 37°C in sealed tubes. The reaction was stopped by diluting with double distilled water. The diluted mixture was frozen and lyophilized. The lyophilate was redissolved in water and relyophilized.

Cation-Exchange FPCL of CNBr Peptides

Lyophilized CNBr samples were taken up (0.5 mg/ml) in starting buffer (20 mM potassium acetate, Ph 4.8). After 30 minutes incubation at 37°C, samples were cleaned by centrifugation. A 200 μl aliquot was loaded onto a Mono S HR 5/5 cation-exchange column (Pharmacia) maintained at 52°C, at a flow rate of 1 ml/min. Following sample loading, the starting buffer was delivered for 5 minutes, then a 30 ml linear gradient was commenced. The gradient was from 0 to 300 Mm lithium chloride in the same acetate buffer. Urea was present in the limiting buffer to maintain a flat baseline. The elution profile was monitored using a Kratos Spectraflowmeter set at 216 nm and changes in optical density recorded with a Hewlett-Packard 3390A Integrator. Cyanogen bromide digest samples as great as 200 μg were run on the Mono S ion exchange column but produced no definitive peptides. Collagen standards as small as 10 μg produced definitive peptides (Fig 11.2). This finding was unexpected as it did not support previous work that involved the use of an identical animal model.[2] A possible explanation for this discrepancy is that we had been very meticulous in ensuring that the tubes contained no encapsulating material before digestion. We were able to demonstrate

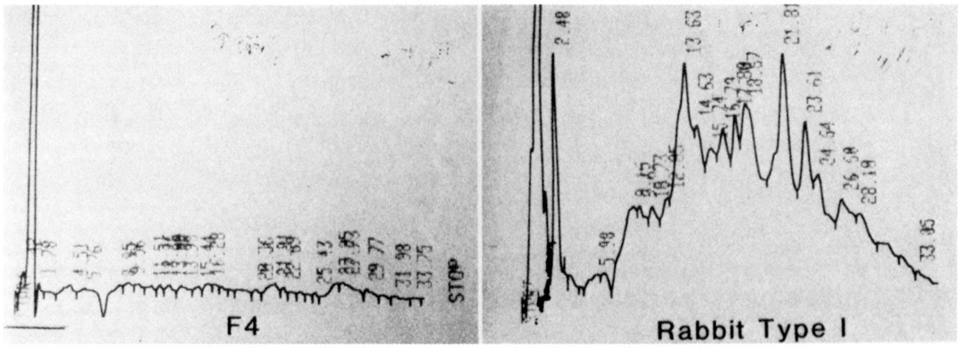

Figure 11.2 Column chromatographs of cyanogen bromide digests. (A) Day 4 fetal tube extracts (200 μg sample), and (B) rabbit type I collagen standard (50 μg sample); the chromatogram of the collagen standard demonstrates the characteristic peaks of cyanogen bromide digest peptides. No definitive peptide peaks are present in the chromatogram of the fetal sample. Subsequent amino acid analysis revealed that this fetal sample contained approximately 820 ng collagen, which is well below the detection limit (10 μg) of this column. *Reprinted with permission.*[5]

collagen peptides in digests of adult tubes so we were not dealing with artifacts from Gore-tex digestion alone.

SDS-Polyacrylamide Gel Electrophoresis (SDS-PAGE) and Enzyme Digestion

Highly purified Clostridial collagenase (Advance Biofactures Corporation) was mixed with the sample in 50 mM Tris. HCl ph 7.6, 100 mM NaCl and 0.1 mM $CaCl_2$. The mixture was incubated for 30 minutes at 37°C and the reaction stopped by freezing. Trypsin, from porcine pancreas (Sigma Chemicals, St. Louis, MO), was used in a concentration of 1 mg/ml and 10 μl was added to the sample at room temperature for 30 minutes. The reaction was stopped by adding SDS and heating to 100°C. CNBr digests with and without prior enzyme digestion were analyzed by 8–20% polyacrylamide gradient gel electrophoresis. Protein bands were stained with Coomassie Brilliant Blue R-250.

Samples of 25, 50, and 100 μg were run on SDS PAGE. Stained bands were evident but they did not correspond either in position or color to bands of the CNBr peptides from Type I and Type III rabbit collagen standards. CNBr collagen peptides stain a reddish-purple color compared to non-collagenous peptides, which stain blue. With the fetal CNBr digested implants only blue bands appeared. CNBr digest of collagen standards treated with bacterial collagenase resulted in a loss of reddish-purple color collagen CNBr digest peptide bands. Collagenase treatment of fetal implant CNBr digest extract produced no loss of the blue staining bands confirming they were not collagenous in nature. Trypsin digestion of implant CNBr extract before electrophoresis showed the loss of stained bands indicating they were composed of protein. Cyanogen bromide digests of adult rabbit collagen, wound fluid, serum, and intact PVA sponge implant were compared to the fetal implant extracts. Identical blue (non-collagenous) peptide banding patterns appeared in all the samples. In addition, the PVA sponge implants from adult rabbits contained a reddish-purple banding pattern indicative of type III collagen. There were no Type I collagen bands evident. Thus the fetal implant extract contained proteins identical to those present in adult wound exudate and serum. It is suggested that the predominant bands are albumin peptides (Fig 11.3).

This section of our studies again failed to demonstrate the presence of collagen in the wound tissue extracts from the fetal rabbit. We have included this information in this chapter since it was the process of investigating the banding patterns of CNBr digests of tissue extracts that led to the discovery of the hyaluronan-collagen-protein association[13] which is described in Chapter 13.

At this stage in our analysis of the extracts from the fetal rabbit wound tissue we were both mystified and concerned. Where we had expected to find abundant collagen deposition we had found none and our original aim, to characterize the collagen, could not be pursued. It was at this stage that we decided to turn over our samples to a third party at the commercially run amino-acid analysis group at the Brigham Hospital, Boston, MA.

Amino Acid Analysis

This was performed using a Beckman 6300 high performance analyzer. Selected samples of CNBr extracts were acid hydrolyzed by adding constant boiling HCl to dry samples in sealed tubes at 108°C and incubating for 18 hours. The values are shown in Table 11.1. Hydroxyproline was identified in all the samples and hydroxylysine was identified in all except for the fetal day four samples. The

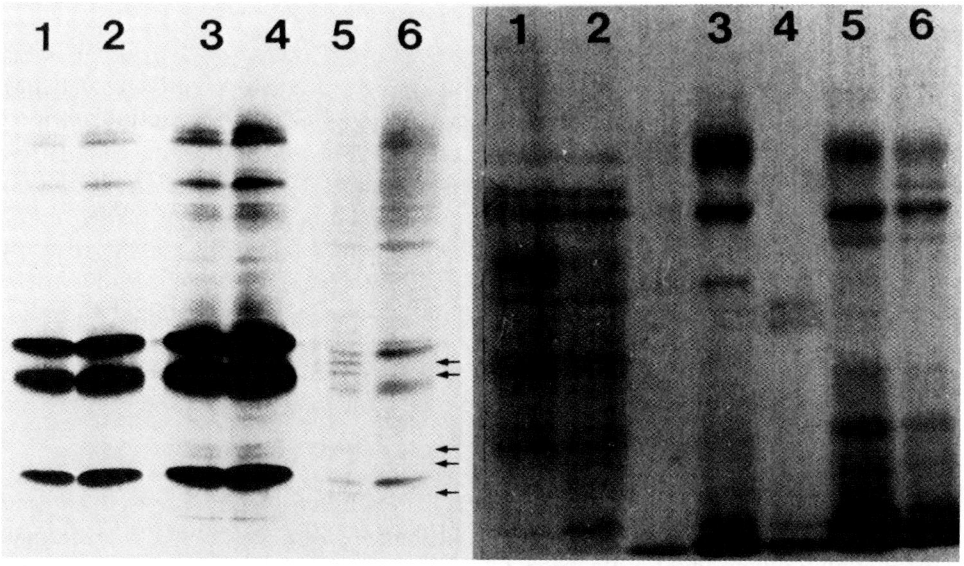

Figure 11.3 A) 12–20% SDS gradient gel of CNBr digests. Lane 1 and 2: Types III and I collagen standards. Lane 3: Fetal day 4 extract. Lane 4, 5, and 6: PVA sponges from 10 week old rabbit following prior digestion with trypsin (lane 4) and collagenase (lane 5). Note the collagenase treated wound peptides have a major matching with the fetal day 4 peptides. Trypsin digestion has eliminated nearly all the bands; the residual bands are most probably trypsin itself. B) 8–20% SDS gradient gel of CNBr digests. Lanes 1 and 2: 25 and 50 μg loadings of adult rabbit wound fluid; lanes 3 and 4: similar loadings of adult rabbit serum. Lanes 5 and 6: PVA sponge extracts from 10 week old rabbit before (lane 5) and after (lane 6) treatment with collagenase. Arrows point to position of bands removed by collagenase leaving bands which correspond to wound fluid and serum samples. *Reprinted with permission.*[5]

TABLE 11.1 Amino Acid Analysis (Residues per 1000; 40-pmol Sensitivity)

	Fetal		Newborn	
	Day 4	Day 7	Day 4	Day 7
HPro	*1*	*4*	*4*	*33*
Asp	89	65	94	77
Thr	52	55	51	41
Ser	54	55	51	46
Glu	116	126	125	109
Pro	57	60	62	78
Gly	67	78	72	160
Ala	99	90	92	92
Val	74	65	69	55
Cys	27	0	32	13
Met	3	12	2	3
Ile	34	37	35	29
Leu	100	90	71	69
Tyr	29	27	30	20
Phe	37	35	34	26
His	28	47	37	28
HLys	*0*	*1*	*4*	*4*
Lys	96	95	91	71
Arg	39	35	45	46
Collagen (ng/tube)	41.5	43.5	198	291
	$n = 22$	$n = 8$	$n = 24$	$n = 24$

amino-acid analysis can detect as little as 40 pmole of hydroxyproline and is more sensitive than the SDS PAGE and column chromatography techniques. Hydroxyproline is commonly used as a marker for collagen but it is not unique to collagen and occurs in other proteins.[14] The combination of hydroxyproline and hydroxylysine, however, strongly supports the presence of collagen.

The combination of the finding of the fibrillar structure on electron microscopy and the amino acid analysis persuaded us that collagen deposition was occurring in the fetal rabbit model. It was apparent though that we were dealing with very small amounts of tissue and, accordingly, we decided to pursue further studies using a large animal model, the sheep.

COLLAGEN DEPOSITION IN FETAL SHEEP WOUNDS

This animal model (Fig 11.4) has been well developed,[15] and we used another well-characterized model of wound healing, the polyvinyl alcohol (PVA) sponge. Histological studies of PVA sponges implanted in adults have demonstrated that the cellular and matrix sequence of events in the sponges reflects the events of incisional wound healing in postnatal skin.[16] In our studies two configurations of PVA sponge discs (12 mm × 3 mm) were implanted subcutaneously. Sponges were either cut in half, and the two halves rejoined by a staple, or an intact sponge was sandwiched between two equal-sized silicone rubber discs. The "sandwiched" sponge allows new tissue deposition to occur only from the periphery of the sponge (Fig 11.5).

Sponges were implanted in the fetuses of eight time-dated pregnant ewes at 75 and 100 days gestation (term = 145 days) and harvested five, 10, 15, and 20 days

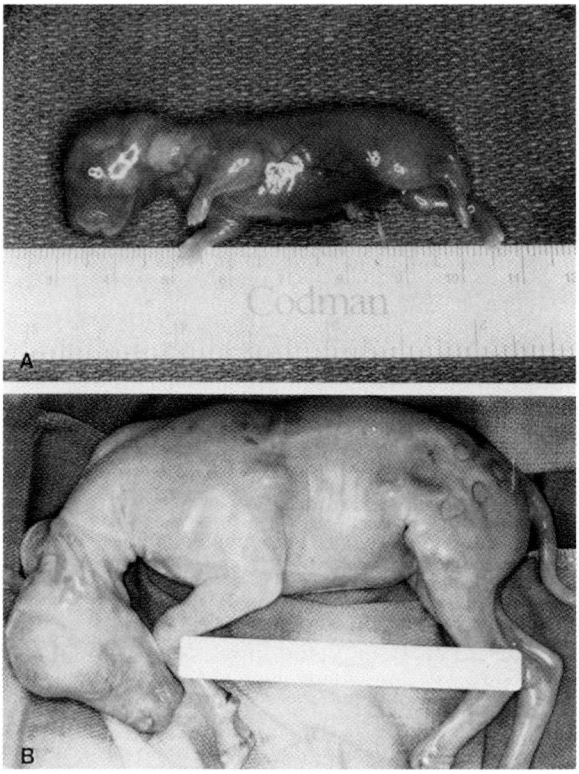

Figure 11.4 A fetal rabbit (A) and fetal sheep (B), both early third trimester. The ruler is 15 cm long. *Reprinted with permission.*[20]

following implantation. Further sponges were implanted in a non-pregnant adult female animal and removed at the same intervals. The sponges were removed "en bloc" with the overlying skin and surrounding tissue intact, snap frozen in liquid nitrogen, and stored at −80°C until analysis.

Biomechanical Analysis

At the time of analysis, the sponges were thawed in a water bath at 24°C and meticulously cleansed of all encapsulating tissue. The reason for this was to ob-

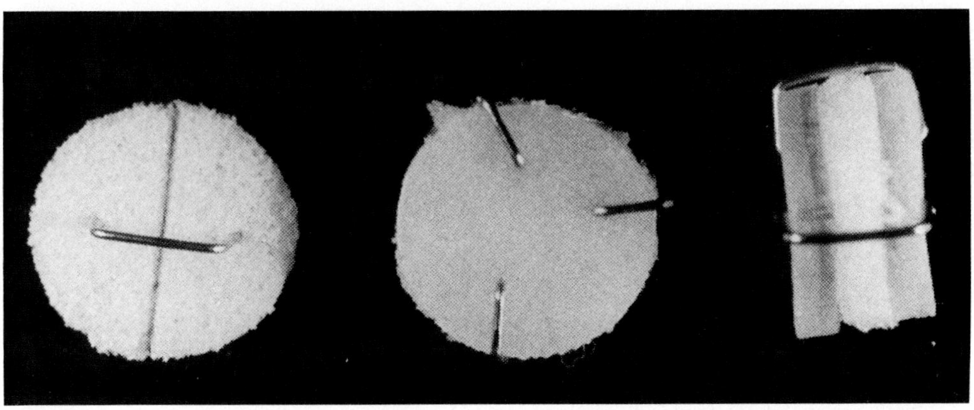

Figure 11.5 The wound healing model showing the bisected and sandwiched sponges.

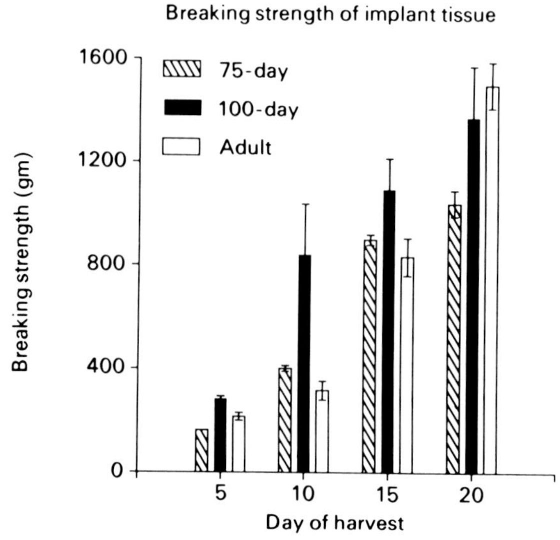

Figure 11.6 Breaking strength of the wound tissue in the sponge implants (error bars ± SEM). *Reprinted with permission.*[20]

viate the criticism previously directed at this wound healing model that the inclusion of encapsulating tissue can give a falsely elevated impression of collagen deposition in the "dead space" of the sponge interstices. The staple was removed so that only newly synthesized tissue between the two halves of the sponge held them together. The force required to separate the sponge halves is the breaking

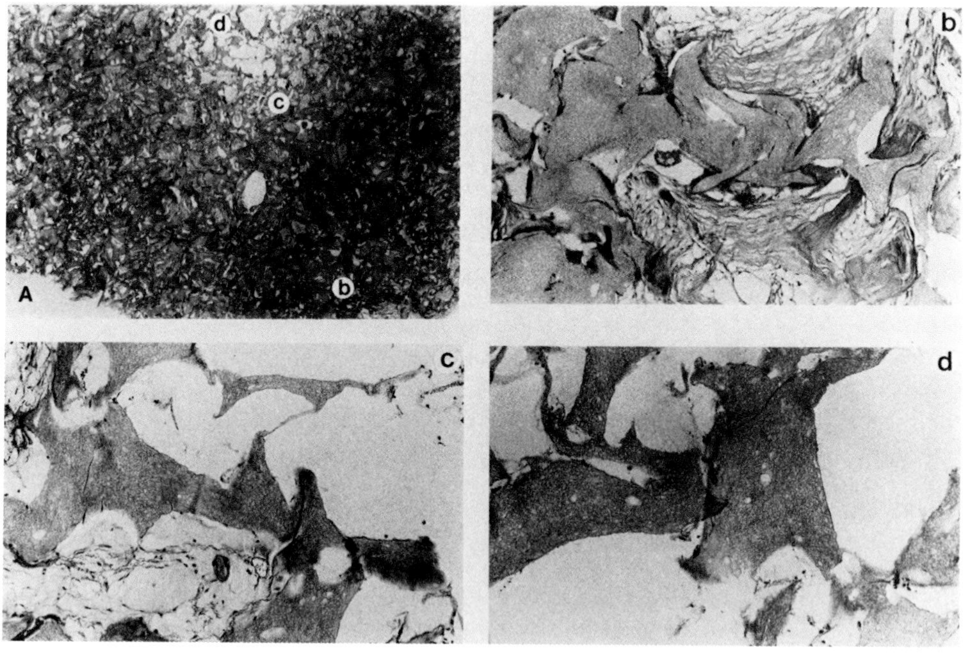

Figure 11.7 Sections of a "sandwiched" sponge implanted for 20 days in a 75 day fetal sheep stained with Trichrome. A) Low power view showing collagen deposition (dark staining) more prominent at the periphery of the sponge. B) High power view of the peripheral region showing fibrillar deposits of dark staining tissue in the interstices of the sponge. C) The deposits become less dense as the center of the sponge is approached. D) There is no tissue deposition within the center of the sponge. *Reprinted with permission.*[20]

strength of this new tissue expressed in grams. The breaking strength (BS) of the tissue deposited in the bisected sponge was determined by clamping the upper half of the sponge in a vertical position. A second clamp was attached to the lower half of the sponge and from this clamp a receptacle was suspended into which water flowed at a constant rate (120 ml/min) until the two halves separated. BS was determined by adding the weight of the lower clamp and receptacle and the volume of water expressed in grams. All testing was performed under uniform environmental conditions.

All three groups (75-day, 100-day, and adult) showed a progressive rise in the breaking strength of the wound tissue. Over the first 10 days, the greatest gain in strength was in the 100-day fetal sponge tissue, but by 20 days the adult sponge tissue exhibited the greatest tensile strength (Fig 11.6).

Histology

Once the silicone rubber discs were removed, the "sandwiched" sponges were fixed in 10% formalin, sectioned, and stained with Trichrome. While we have criticized the use of Trichrome to analyze collagen deposition in small animal models, it was evident that there was abundant collagen deposition in the PVA sponges from all the fetal and adult sponges. The figure demonstrates the appearance of the 75-day fetal sponge implanted for 20 days. Collagen is abundant at the periphery, and deposition has occurred toward the center (Fig 11.7).

Amino Acid Analysis

Amino acid analysis was performed on acid hydrolysates of the halves of three pooled sponges at each time point in each of the three groups. An automated Beckman 6300 Amino Acid Analyzer was used with a citrate buffer system. An increase in both hydroxyproline and hydroxylysine was apparent over the 15-day postimplantation period. Thereafter, the 75- and 100-day fetal levels continued to rise, but the adult levels fell (Fig 11.8).

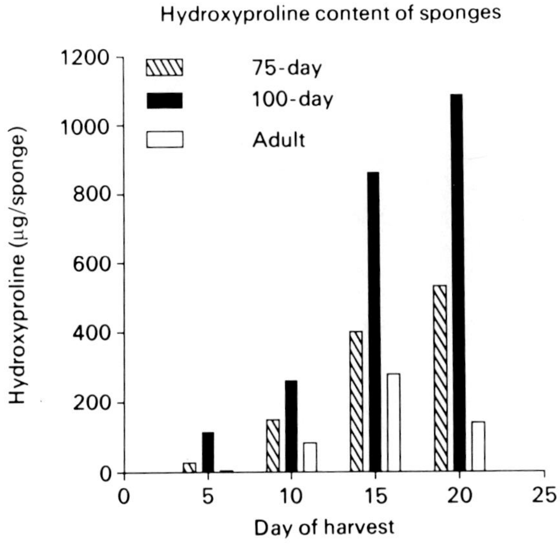

Figure 11.8 Hydroxyproline levels in implants from A) 75-day fetus, B) 100-day fetus, and C) adult. *Reprinted with permission.*[20]

Collagen Extraction

Further analysis was performed on sponges from the 100-day fetal and the adult groups at 10, 15, and 20 days postimplantation. Collagen was extracted using limited pepsin digestion. Type I and III collagens were separated by the differential renaturation method of Chandrarajan,[17] and the collagen purity was confirmed by SDS polyacrylamide gel electrophoresis.[18]

An increase in the proportion of Type I collagen in the implant tissue was found between 10 and 20 days in both the fetal and adult sponges, but by 20 days the total quantity of extracted collagen had decreased in both the fetus and the adult. What is notable is that by 20 days the adult wound was the strongest and yet contained the least collagen, as indicated by both amino acid analysis and direct extraction.

SUMMARY

In summary we have demonstrated that the deposition of collagen occurs in wound healing models in both small and large fetal animal models. The studies described here involve biochemical analysis and complement other immunohistochemical studies (see Chapter 10).[19] There is no longer debate about whether or not collagen is deposited in fetal wounds. The questions that we are now pursuing concern the qualitative analysis of the collagen that is deposited and its subsequent fate in terms of reorganization and remodeling.

REFERENCES

1. Rowsell AR: The intra-uterine healing of foetal muscle wounds: Experimental study in the rat. Brit J Plast Surg 37:635, 1984.
2. Adzick NS, Harrison MR, Glick PL, et al.: Comparison of fetal, newborn, and adult wound healing by histologic, enzyme-histochemical, and hydroxyproline determinations. J Pediatr Surg 20:315, 1985.
3. Hallock GG: In utero cleft lip repair in A/J mice. Plast Reconstr Surg 75:785–788, 1985.
4. Krummel TM, Nelson JM, Dieglemann RF, et al.: Fetal response to injury in the rabbit. J Pediatr Surg 22:640, 1987.
5. Siebert JW, Burd DAR, McCarthy J, et al.: Fetal wound healing: A biochemical study of scarless healing. J Plast Reconstr Surg 85:495, 1990.
6. Merkel JR, DiPaolo BR, Hallock GG, et al.: Type I and type III collagen content of healing wounds in fetal and adult rats. Proceedings of the Society of Experimental Biology and Medicine 187:493, 1988.
7. Hallock GG, Rice DC, Merkel JR, et al.: Analysis of collagen content in the fetal wound. Ann Plast Surg 21:310, 1988.
8. Burrington JD: Wound healing in the fetal lamb. J Pediatr Surg 6:523, 1971.
9. DePalma RL, Krummel TK, Durham LA, et al.: Characterization and quantitation of wound matrix in the fetal rabbit. Matrix 9:224, 1989.
10. Goodson WH, III, and Hunt TK: Development of a new miniature method for the study of wound healing in human subjects. J Surg Res 33:394, 1982.
11. Diegelmann RF, Lindblad WJ, and Cohen IK: A subcutaneous implant for wound healing studies in humans. J Surg Res 40:229–237, 1986.
12. Lindblad WJ and Diegelmann RF: Quantitation of hydroxyproline isomers in acid hydrolysates by high-performance liquid chromatography. Analy Biochem 138:390–395, 1984.
13. Burd DAR, Siebert JW, Ehrlich HP, et al.: Human skin and post burn scar hyaluronan: Demonstration of the association with collagen and other proteins. Matrix 9:322, 1989.
14. Adams E and Frank L: Metabolism of proline and the hydroxyprolines. Ann Rev Biochem 49:1005–1061, 1980.
15. Harrison MR, Jester JA, and Ross NA: Correction of congenital diaphragmatic hernia in utero. I. The model: Intrathoracic balloon produces fatal pulmonary hypoplasia. Surg 88:174, 1980.

16. Schilling JA, Joel W, and Shurley HM: Wound healing: A comparative study of the histochemical changes in granulation tissue contained in stainless steel wire mesh and polyvinyl sponge cylinders. Surg 46:702, 1959.
17. Chandrarajan J: Separation of type III collagen from type I collagen and pepsin by differential denaturation and renaturation. Biochem Biophys Res Comm 83:180, 1978.
18. Laemmli UK: Cleavage of structural proteins during the assembly of the head of bacteriophage T4. Nature 227:680, 1970.
19. Longaker MT, Whitby DJ, Adzick NS, et al.: Studies in fetal wound healing. VI. Second and early third trimester fetal wounds demonstrate rapid collagen deposition without scar formation. J Pediatr Surg 25:63, 1990.
20. Burd DAR, Longaker MT, Adzick NS, et al.: Fetal wound healing in a large animal model: The deposition of collagen is confirmed. Br J Plast Surg 43:571, 1990.

CHAPTER **12**

Hyaluronic Acid and its Modulation in Fetal and Adult Wounds

Michael G. Stern
Michael T. Longaker
Robert Stern

HYALURONIC ACID

Hyaluronic acid (HA) is a high molecular weight glycosaminoglycan (GAG) composed of alternating units of glucuronic acid and N-acetyl glucosamine. It plays a major role in the structure and organization of the extracellular matrix (ECM). Hyaluronic acid is found in high concentrations during embryogenesis and whenever rapid tissue proliferation and regeneration occur.[1] It has been implicated in the detachment process of cells that allow them to move.[2] A burst of HA synthesis occurs just prior to mitosis[3–5] allowing the dividing cell to dissociate from neighboring cells. Hyaluronic acid also inhibits cell differentiation,[6,7] creating an environment that, in some instances, promotes cell proliferation. Because of its highly charged nature, HA can take on a large volume of hydration. This opens up tissue spaces into which inflammatory cells can move, and creates an environment that facilitates fibroblast motility. It is readily apparent that HA is a component of the ECM crucial for wound repair.

HYALURONIC ACID IN ADULT AND FETAL WOUND HEALING

Adult Wound Healing

Studies on excisional wounds in the adult have demonstrated that HA is deposited early, reaches a peak, and then falls in the first few days. The HA is then replaced by sulfated GAGs.[8,9] Studies from this laboratory, in which sterile, wire mesh cylinders were used to obtain wound fluid for HA assay, have confirmed these early observations.[10–12] Aliquots of wound fluid were aspirated from the cylinder at various intervals. Substantial quantities of HA were detectable in the wound fluid within one day of wounding. Levels of HA reached a peak at three days, and then dropped to background levels by seven days (Fig. 12.1).

A similar temporal pattern of HA deposition and degradation can be seen in several normal embryological systems, including the developing chick limb bud, cornea, and kidney.[1] The HA is found consistently early on during the phase of rapid cell movement and proliferation. A particularly well-studied example is that of neural crest cell migration in an HA-rich environment through the body of the

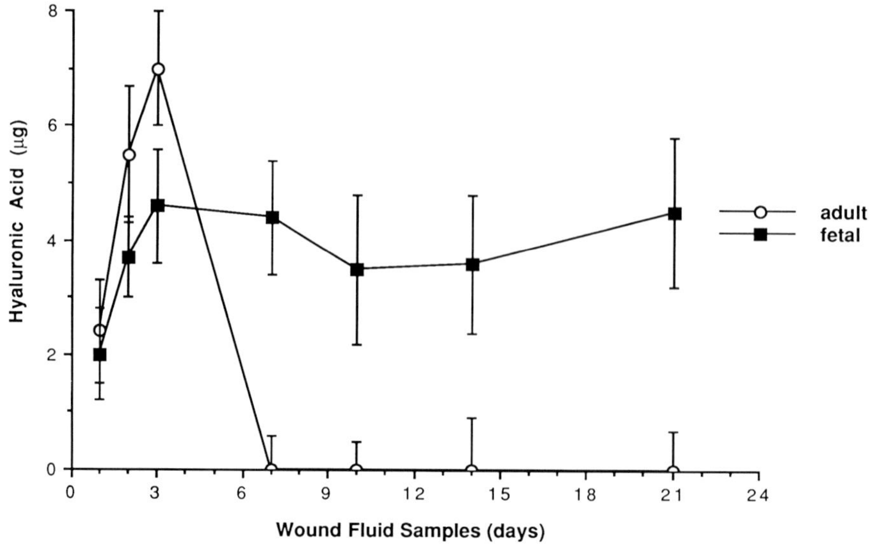

Figure 12.1 HA levels in adult versus fetal sheep wound fluid. Error bars represent the standard deviation of each value run in triplicate.

embryo. When cells reach their destination, hyaluronidase is produced, HA is degraded, cell migration ceases, and cytodifferentiation occurs.[13]

The early stages of wound healing in the adult thus parallels a number of embryological systems with an initial rise in HA. Wound healing in the adult can be construed as a strategic retreat, a temporary reversion to a fetal-like situation. The process of repair then proceeds rapidly through the various stages of ontogeny, until the adult state is again reached and repair is completed.

Fetal Wound Healing

The fetal wound is rich in HA, as was first documented in the rabbit; however, a major limitation of that model is the short gestation time of the pregnant rabbit.[14–16] An animal model of sufficiently long gestation and of sufficient size as to allow surgical manipulation was therefore necessary. The fetal lamb fulfills these criteria. It was first utilized by Burrington[17] and then developed extensively by Harrison and his coworkers.[18–20] The earlier observations in the rabbit were confirmed in this fetal lamb model employing miniaturized Schilling-Hunt wound cylinders.[12] Mid-gestation lambs were exposed by hysterotomy, wound cylinders were inserted into subcutaneous pockets, and wound fluid was withdrawn by percutaneous aspiration. As in the adult, levels of HA rapidly increased until day three. However, elevated levels were maintained for at least 21 days, the period that observations were made (Fig. 12.1). Thus, the first three days of wound healing in the adult and in the fetal lamb are similar, and the "fetal stage" of adult wound healing can be superimposed on that of the fetal process. After day three, an entirely different series of events must be invoked in the fetal situation. The fetal stage is maintained for a prolonged period. It is in this latter stage, from day three on, that the unique properties of fetal wound healing are observed.

The process of wound repair in the fetus becomes adult-like, with inflammation and scarring, by the middle of the third trimester in fetal rats[21] and fetal sheep.[20] Additionally, in cell culture, the fetal fibroblast can undergo a conversion to the adult phenotype after prolonged passage.[22] It would be of intrinsic interest to establish whether the fetal profile of HA deposition converts to the adult pattern during the in utero transition to adult-like wound healing.

SIZE EFFECTS OF HYALURONIC ACID

The degradation products of HA, the small oligosaccharides, have potent angiogenic activities.[23,24] High molecular weight forms of HA have the ability to prevent the formation of new blood vessels.[25] They also exert an inhibitory effect on lymphocytes, macrophages, and neutrophils, as well as on mitogen-induced lymphocyte proliferation.[26] The effect of HA on rates of fibroblast proliferation is also dependent on molecular weight.[22] Variations in molecular size of HA play a major regulatory role in several key steps in wound healing. As HA is processed, the various size species present in both fetal and adult wounds optimally modulate the sequential steps in the wound healing process.

The size distribution of the HA polymers was examined using the material aspirated from wound cylinders. These samples were pretreated with the protease papain to remove the associated HA-binding proteins. It was established that in both the fetal and the adult wound, HA begins as a high molecular weight species that elutes from the excluded volume of a Sepharose CL-2B column. This corresponds to an apparent molecular size of 3×10^6 kDa.[27] In both the adult and in the fetal wound, the HA begins to be degraded within three days, although the short fragments are retained in the fetal wound and do not disappear, as they do in the adult. High molecular weight HA is probably not a critical aspect of fetal wound healing after day three.

STIMULATION OF HYALURONIC ACID DEPOSITION

Despite the obvious importance of HA in basic biological and pathological processes, the regulation of HA deposition is not clearly understood. Modulation of HA synthesis by some low molecular weight compounds has been reported. Insulin,[28] prostaglandins,[29,30] sodium butyrate,[31] and interleukin 1[32] can stimulate HA production. A platelet factor that stimulates HA synthesis has also been identified.[33,34] More recently, fibroblast growth factor has been shown to stimulate HA synthesis in early chick embryo limb buds.[35] PDGF, EGF, bFGF,[36] and particularly TGFβ[37] have also been shown to stimulate HA in fibroblasts.

It has long been recognized that serum is required to support the synthesis of HA by cultured cells, suggesting that a factor in serum stimulates HA synthesis.[38–40] A glycoprotein with 150 kDa molecular-weight was isolated from calf serum by Tomida and coworkers.[38,41]

A tumor-associated HA-stimulating activity (HASA) has been identified[42] and partially purified.[43] We have identified this same HASA using a newly developed assay system for the synthesis of HA in rat fibrosarcoma cells. This cell line produces an abundance of HA and responds to the fetal factor as well as the tumor in a time- and dose-dependent manner.[44,45]

We have demonstrated an HASA in both fetal bovine and sheep serum. The HASA is a glycopeptide factor in the fetal circulation with a peak of activity 40%

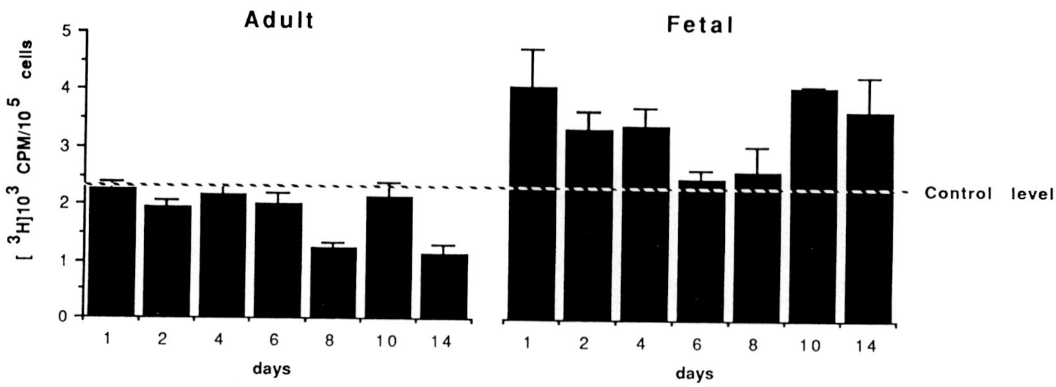

Figure 12.2 HASA levels in adult versus fetal sheep wound fluid. Control level represents culture plates in which no wound fluid was added. Error bars represent the standard deviation of each value run in triplicate.

of the way through gestation, at 120 days (270 days total) in the calf and 60 days gestation (145 days total) in the sheep. Fetal wound fluid also contains high levels of an activity similar to HASA,[46] which may underlie the sustained HA deposition in fetal wounds. No such activity could be detected in the adult wound fluid (Fig. 12.2). Increased levels of HA occur early in the ECM of both fetal and adult wounds, but HA deposition remains elevated for an extended time period only in fetal wounds. We postulate that HASA is the underlying mechanism. Since HASA could not be demonstrated in adult wound fluid at any of the time points examined, even during the first three days when sizable levels of HA do appear, HA deposition must occur in the adult wound by an entirely different mechanism from that in the fetus (Fig. 12.3).

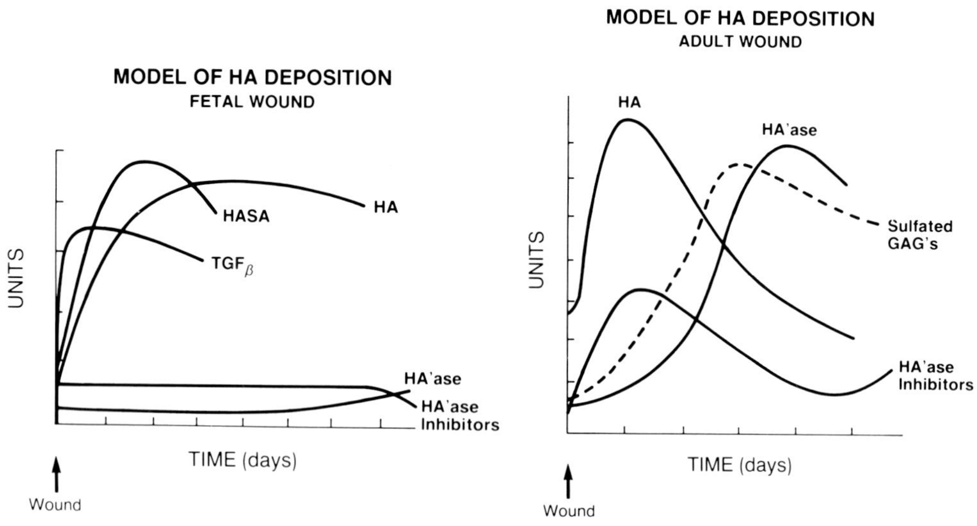

Figure 12.3 Idealized drawing for the mechanism of HA deposition in fetal versus adult wounds. In fetal wounds, HASA rises prior to HA and the prolonged elevation of HASA underlies the prolonged presence of HA. In contrast, HASA is not present in adult wounds at any time. HA is present only initially and is subsequently degraded by hyaluronidase.

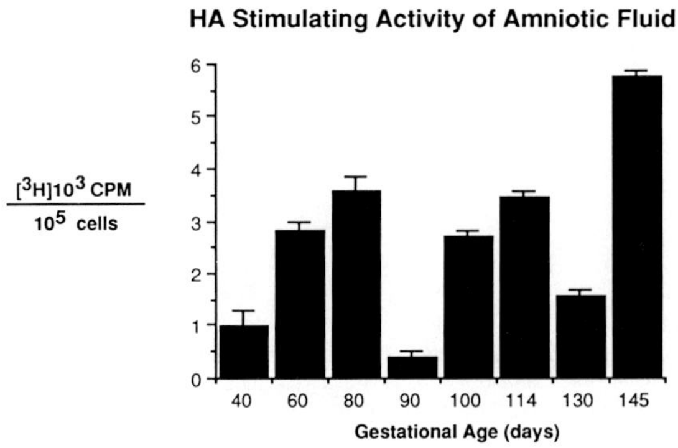

Figure 12.4 HASA levels in sheep amniotic fluid. Error bars represent the standard deviation of each value run in triplicate.

There are a number of intrinsic and extrinsic differences between fetal and adult skin wound repair. One difference lies in the fetal external milieu, amniotic fluid in which fetal skin is continually bathed. The fetus floats in amniotic fluid known to contain growth and trophic factors required for fetal development.[47] Amniotic fluid has been shown to contain high concentrations of HA.[48] Amniotic fluid also has elevated HASA, as measured in sheep amniotic fluid between 40 and 145 days gestation[49] (Fig. 12.4). This may be an additional mechanism by which HA is deposited in the matrix of fetal skin wounds because the wounds are bathed in amniotic fluid that contains both an HASA and HA.

Weigel et al.[50–52] demonstrated that mammalian fibrinogen contains an HA binding site. Fibrinogen is also found in the alpha granules of platelets,[53,54] incorporated into the megakaryocytes from the circulation.[55,56] We postulate that HA in the adult wound is released from the platelet plug, when alpha granule contents are released. Fibrinogen from the circulation may also release their bound HA during this earliest phase of adult wound healing. From some of the factors released by platelets, such as PDGF and TGFβ, stimulation of local production of HA may also occur. These several mechanisms in seriatim may account for the deposition of HA early in adult wound healing, providing the environment that the fetal wound achieves by unrelated mechanisms.

THE ASSOCIATION OF HA AND HASA WITH WILMS' TUMORS

In the process of elucidating the HASA phenomenon, a fortuitous observation was made. A survey of the extracts of fetal bovine organs was performed to identify the source of HASA. A 120-day fetal calf was obtained, corresponding to the gestational age when a peak of circulating HASA occurs. The kidney, of all organs examined, had the highest activity.

There are several reports of increased viscosity of blood in some children with Wilms' tumors. The mysterious mucin in their circulation was subsequently proven to be HA.[57,58] Wilms' tumors are the most common pediatric renal neoplasm and are thought to arise from a rest of fetal kidney, from metanephric renal blastema that persists in the normal kidney postnatally and that subsequently undergoes malignant transformation.

The urine from three patients with Wilms' tumor was shown to have markedly elevated levels of HASA, which fell to normal levels following surgical extirpation of their tumors.[59] The circulating HA in some Wilms' tumor patients results from

TABLE 12.1 Location of HASA Activity

Fetal serum
Fetal plasma
Fetal wound fluid
Fetal kidney extracts*
Fetal urine
Amniotic fluid
Wilms' tumor extracts
Urine of Wilms' tumor patients
Serum of Wilms' tumor patients**
Conditioned media of cultured fetal fibroblasts
Conditioned media of Wilms' tumor cells in primary culture***

* Lesser amounts of activity were present in fetal heart, liver, and placental extracts.

** Levels of HASA in patient serum were not reported since Human Experimentation Committees do not permit drawing blood from children to serve as normal controls.

*** Unpublished observations, Garvin AJ, Longaker MT, and Stern R.

the ability of the malignant tumor to produce a factor that stimulates production of HA, a factor similar to that which the normal fetal kidney produces.

Table 12.1 is a list of biological materials in which an HASA-like activity has been documented. The term "activity" is preferred, rather than "factor." Identity or homology between the various sources of the materials must await sequence determinations.

MECHANISM OF ACTION OF TGFβ AS A MEDIATOR OF HA STIMULATION

In a cell culture system, we have demonstrated that the mechanism of action of TGFβ is through HASA. HASA is secreted into the culture media of fetal fibroblasts in response to increasing levels of TGFβ. At 10 ng/ml TGFβ, synthesis of HASA is increased six- to 10-fold over control levels. HASA may function in both an autocrine and paracrine manner in these fibroblasts. The HASA was

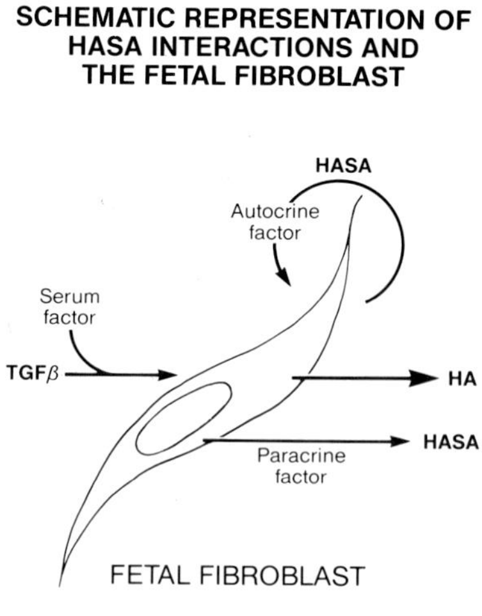

Figure 12.5 Line drawing of HASA interactions with the fetal fibroblast. TGF-β stimulates HA production through HASA. The TGF-β effect has a serum requirement; 0.1% fetal calf serum allows for optimal detection of HASA.

specific for HA synthesis, with relatively little stimulation of other GAGs. A small concentration of fetal serum (0.1%) is necessary for the optimal effect. Further increases in serum do not provide additional enhancement of HASA levels. A schematic diagram demonstrating these interactions is shown (Fig. 12.5).

TGFβ enhances the production of a variety of extracellular matrix components such as collagen and fibronectin in addition to its effect on proteoglycans and HA. It is not known if the other effects of TGFβ on ECM components occur through similar mediators. Also, it would be interesting to establish whether other stimulators of HA synthesis, such as IGF-2 and IL-1, work through an HASA mechanism.

INHIBITION OF HA DEPOSITION

Thyroid hormone and cortisol have been shown to inhibit HA synthesis,[60,61] but to date, no compounds have been identified whose major function is inhibition of HA synthesis. Hyaluronidase activity might be considered an inhibitor of deposition, but a moiety that is actually able to inhibit biosynthesis has not been detected. In the process of adult wound healing, however, such a substance may be produced, to work in concert with hyaluronidase, to account for the decreasing levels of HA observed in wound fluid. The hyaluronidase functions to remove already synthesized polymer, but an actual substance that inhibits HA biosynthesis has not been documented. Elevated levels of HA may themselves be inhibitory of synthesis. Such feedback inhibition would utilize cell surface HA receptors.[62,63] The converse situation, degradation of HA using hyaluronidase, has been documented in cell culture. Lowering HA levels by adding hyaluronidase to cell culture media has the anomalous effect of stimulating HA biosynthesis.[64,65] Incubating cells with hyaluronidase causes an anomalous increase in HA synthetase activity. In fetal wound healing an abeyance of such a mechanism would be invoked. Studies are underway to delineate the role of hyaluronidase and hyaluronidase inhibitors in fetal and adult wounds.

Loss of suppressor genes plays a role in oncogenesis.[66] In considering the many parallels between neoplasia and wound healing, mechanisms that modulate the cessation of adult wound healing are candidates for such tumor suppressor gene products. Inhibitors of HA synthesis would also fit such a model. In fetal wound repair, such a tumor suppression gene mechanism would be held in abeyance, an additional step that may provide a clue to scarless healing.

REFERENCES

1. Toole BP: Glycosaminoglycans in morphogenesis. In: Hay ED (ed), Cell Biology of the Extracellular Matrix. New York, Plenum Press, pp 259–294, 1982.
2. Turley EA, Torrance J: Localization of hyaluronate and hyaluronate-binding protein on motile and non-motile fibroblasts. Exp Cell Res 16:17–28, 1984.
3. Tomida M, Koyama H, Ono T: Hyaluronate acid synthetase in cultured mammalian cells producing hyaluronic acid: Oscillatory change during the growth phase and suppression by 5-bromodeoxyuridine. Biochim Biophys Acta 338:352–363, 1974.
4. Mian N: Analysis of cell-growth-phase-related variations in hyaluronate synthase activity of isolated plasma-membrane fractions from cultured human skin fibroblasts. Biochem J 237:333–342, 1986.
5. Brecht M, Mayer U, Schlosser E, Prehm P: Increased hyaluronate synthesis is required for fibroblast detachment and mitosis. Biochem J 239:445–450, 1986.

6. Kujawa MJ, Pechak DG, Fiszman MY, Caplan AI: Hyaluronic acid bonded to cell culture surfaces inhibits the program of myogenesis. Develop Biol 113:10–16, 1986.
7. Kujawa MJ, Tepperman K: Culturing chick muscle cells on glycosaminoglycan substrates: Attachment and differentiation. Dev Biol 99:277–286, 1983.
8. Dunphy JE, Upuda KN: Chemical and histochemical sequences in the normal healing of wounds. N Engl J Med 253:847–851, 1955.
9. Bently JP: Rate of chondroitin sulfate formation in wound healing. Ann Surg 165:186–191, 1967.
10. Schilling HA, Joel W, Shurley HW: Wound healing: A comparative study of histochemical changes in granulation tissue contained in stainless steel wire mesh and polyvinyl sponge cylinder. Surgery 46:702–710, 1959.
11. Hunt TK, Twomey P, Zederfeldt B, Dunphy JE: Respiratory gas tensions and pH in healing wounds. Am J Surgery 114:302–307, 1967.
12. Longaker MT, Chiu E, Adzick NS, Stern M, Harrison M, Stern R: Studies in fetal wound healing. V. Prolonged presence of hyaluronic acid in fetal wound fluid. Ann Surg 213:290–296, 1991.
13. Pratt RM, Larsen MA, Johnston MC: Migration of cranial neural crest cells in a cell-free hyaluronate-rich matrix. Dev Biol 44:298–305, 1975.
14. Krummel TM, Nelson JM, Dieglemann RF, et al.: Fetal response to injury in the rabbit. J Pediatr Surg 22:640–644, 1987.
15. DePalma RL, Krummel TM, Nelson JM, et al: Fetal wound matrix is composed of proteoglycan rather than collagen. Surg Forum 38:626–628, 1987.
16. DePalma RL, Krummel TM, Durham LA III, et al.: Characterization and quantitation of wound matrix in the fetal rabbit. Matrix 9:224–231, 1989.
17. Burrington JD: Wound healing in the fetal lamb. J Pediatr Surg 6:523–528, 1971.
18. Harrison MR, Jester JA, Ross NA: Correction of congenital diaphragmatic hernia in utero. I. The model: Intrathoracic balloon produces fatal pulmonary hypoplasia. Surgery 88:174–182, 1980.
19. Harrison MR, Bressack MA, Churg AM, et al.: Correction of congenital diaphragmatic hernia in utero. II. Simulated correction permits fetal lung growth with survival at birth. Surgery 88:260–268, 1980.
20. Longaker MT, Whitby DJ, Adzick NS, et al.: Studies in fetal wound healing: VI. Second and early third trimester fetal wounds demonstrate rapid collagen deposition without scar formation. J Pediatr Surg 25:63–69, 1990.
21. Dixon JB: Inflammation in the foetal and neonatal rat: The local reactions to skin burns. J Pathol Bacteriol 80:73–78, 1960.
22. Schor SL, Schor AM, Rushton G, Smith L: Adult, foetal and transformed fibroblasts display different migratory phenotypes on collagen gels: evidence for an isoformic transition during foetal development. J Cell Sci 73:221–234, 1985.
23. West DC, Hampson IN, Arnold F, et al.: Angiogenesis induced by degradation products of hyaluronic acid. Science 228:1324–1326, 1985.
24. West DC, Kumar S: The effect of hyaluronate and its oligosaccharides on endothelial cell proliferation and monolayer integrity. Exp Cell Res 183:179–196, 1989.
25. Feinberg RN, Beebe DC: Hyaluronate in vasculogenesis. Science 220:1177–1179, 1983.
26. Peluso GF, Perbellini A, Tajana GF: The effect of high and low molecular weight hyaluronic acid on mitogen-induced lymphocyte proliferation. Curr Ther Res 47:437–442, 1990.
27. Henrich CJ, Hawkes SP: Molecular weight dependence of hyaluronic acid produced during oncogenic transformation. Cancer Biochem Biophys 10:257–267, 1989.
28. Bashey RI, Fleischmajer R: Increased synthesis of hyaluronic acid by insulin in embryonic chick skin. Proc Soc Exptl Biol Med 145:18–20, 1974.
29. Murota S-I, Abe M, Otsuka K: Stimulatory effect of prostaglandins on the production of hexosamine-containing substances by cultured fibroblasts: (3) Induction of hyaluronic acid synthetase by prostaglandin $F_{2\alpha}$. Prostaglandins, 14:983–991, 1977.
30. Sisson JC, Castor CW, Klavons JA: Connective tissue activation. XVIII. Stimulation of hyaluronic acid synthetase activity. J Lab Clin Med 96:189–197, 1980.
31. Smith TJ: *n*-Butyrate inhibition of hyaluronate synthesis in cultured human fibroblasts. J Clin Invest 79:1493–1497, 1987.
32. Bronson RE, Bertolami CN, Siebert EP: Modulation of fibroblast growth and glycosaminoglycan synthesis by interleukin-1. Collagen Rel Res 7:323–332, 1987.
33. Castor CW, Miller JW, Walz DA: Structural and biological characteristics of connective tissue activating peptide (CTAP-III): A major human platelet derived growth factor. Proc Natl Acad Sci USA 80:765–769, 1983.

34. Myers SL: Canine platelet factors stimulate glycosaminoglycan synthesis by synovial cell and organ cultures. Conn Tiss Res 14:41–49, 1985.
35. Munaim SI, Klagsbrun M, Toole BP: Fibroblast growth factor activity in the early stages of development of chick embryo limb buds. J Cell Biol 105:275a, 1987.
36. Heldin P, Laurent TC, Heldin C-H: Effect of growth factors on hyaluronan synthesis in cultured human fibroblasts. Biochem J 258:919–922, 1989.
37. Westergren-Thorsson G, Särnstrand B, Fransson L-Å, Malström A: TGF-β enhances the production of hyaluronan in human lung but not in skin fibroblasts. Exp Cell Res 186:192–195, 1990.
38. Tomida M, Koyama H, Ono T: Effects of adenosine 3′:5′-cyclic monophosphate and serum on synthesis of hyaluronic acid in confluent rat fibroblasts. Biochem J 162:539–543, 1977.
39. Knudson W, Biswas C, Toole BP: Stimulation of glycosaminoglycan production in murine tumors. J Cell Biochem 25:183–196, 1984.
40. Knudson W, Biswas C, Toole BP: Interactions between human tumor cells and fibroblasts stimulate hyaluronate synthesis. Proc Natl Acad Sci USA 81:6767–6771, 1984.
41. Tomida M, Koyama H, Ono T: A serum factor capable of stimulating hyaluronic acid synthesis in cultured rat fibroblasts. J Cell Physiol 91:323–328, 1976.
42. Knudson W, Toole BP: Properties of a membrane-bound tumor cell factor which stimulates hyaluronate synthesis in fibroblasts. J Cell Biol 101:339a, 1985.
43. Knudson W, Toole BP: Membrane association of the hyaluronate stimulatory factor from LX-1 human lung carcinoma cells. J Cell Biochem 38:165–177, 1988.
44. Biesecker JL: Cellular and humoral immunity after allogenic transplantation in the rat. I. Cellular and humoral immunity as measured by a ^{51}Cr cytoxicity assay after allogenic tumor and renal transplantation. Transplant 15:298–307, 1973.
45. Decker M, Chiu ES, Dollbaum C, et al.: Hyaluronic acid stimulating activity in sera from the bovine fetus and from breast cancer patients. Cancer Research 49:3499–3505, 1989.
46. Longaker MT, Chiu ES, Harrison MR, et al.: Studies in fetal wound healing. IV. Hyaluronic acid-stimulating activity distinguishes fetal wound fluid from adult wound fluid. Ann Surg 210:667–672, 1989.
47. Mulvihill SJ, Stone MM, Fonkalsrud EW, et al.: Trophic effect of amniotic fluid on fetal gastrointestinal development. J Surg Res 40:291–296, 1986.
48. Dahl LB, Hopwood JJ, Laurent UBG, et al.: The concentration of hyaluronate in amniotic fluid. Biochemical Medicine 30:280–283, 1983.
49. Longaker MT, Adzick NS, Hall JL, et al.: Studies in fetal wound healing: VII. Fetal wound healing may be modulated by hyaluronic acid stimulating activity in amniotic fluid. J Pediatr Surg 25:430–433, 1990.
50. LeBoeuf RD, Raja RH, Fuller GM, Weigel PH: Human fibrinogen specifically binds hyaluronic acid. J Biol Chem 261:12586–12592, 1986.
51. Weigel PH, Fuller GM, LeBoeuf RD: A model for the role of hyaluronic acid and fibrin in the early events during the inflammatory response and wound healing. J Theor Biol 119:219–234, 1986.
52. Weigel PH, Frost SJ, LeBoeuf RD, McGary CT: The specific interaction between fibrin (ogen) and hyaluronan: possible consequences in haemostasis, inflammation and wound healing. In: Tengblad L (ed), Hyaluronan, Ciba Symposium 145, Ciba Press, Paris, pp 262–275, 1989.
53. Leven RM, Schick PK, Budzynski AZ: Fibrinogen biosynthesis in the isolated guinea pig megakarocytes. Blood 65:501–504, 1985.
54. Belloc F, Hourdille P, Fialon P, et al.: Fibrinogen synthesis by megakarocyte rich human marrow cell concentrates. Thrombosis Res 38:341–351, 1985.
55. Handagama P, Shuman MA, Bainton DF: Incorporation of intravenously injected albumin, immunoglobulin G, and fibrinogen in guinea pig megakaryocyte granules. J Clin Invest 84:73–82, 1989.
56. Handagama P, Rappolee DA, Werb Z, Levin J, Bainton DF: Platelet α-granule fibrinogen, albumin, and immunoglobulin G are not synthesized by rat and mouse megakaryocytes. J Clin Invest 86:1364–1368, 1990.
57. Morse BS, Nussbaum M: The detection of hyaluronic acid in the serum and urine of a patient with nephroblastoma. Am J Med 42:996–1002, 1967.
58. Allerton SE, Beierle JW, Powars DR, et al.: Abnormal extracellular components in Wilms' tumor. Cancer Res 39:679–683, 1970.
59. Longaker MT, Adzick NS, Sadigh D, et al.: Hyaluronic acid stimulating activity in the pathophysiology of Wilms' tumors. J Natl Cancer Inst 82:135–139, 1990.

60. Smith TJ, Murata Y, Horowitz AL, Philipson L, Refetoff S: Regulation of glycosaminoglycan synthesis by thyroid hormone *in vitro*. J Clin Invest 70:1066–1073, 1982.
61. Smith TJ: Dexamethasone regulation of glycosaminoglycan synthesis in cultured human skin fibroblasts. Similar effects of glucocorticoid and thyroid hormones. J Clin Invest 74:2157–2163, 1984.
62. Lacy BE, Underhill CB: The hyaluronate receptor is associated with actin filaments. J Cell Biol 105:1395–1404, 1987.
63. Underhill CB: The interaction of hyaluronate with the cell surface: The hyaluronate receptor and the core protein. In: Evered D, Whelan J (eds), The Biology of Hyaluronan, Ciba Foundation Symposium #143, John Wiley & Sons, New York, pp 87–99, 1989.
64. Philipson LH, Westley J, Schwartz NB: Effect of hyaluronidase treatment of intact cells on hyaluronate synthetase activity. Biochemistry 24:7899–7906, 1985.
65. Larnier C, Kerneur C, Robert L, Moczar M: Effect of testicular hyaluronidase on hyaluronate synthesis by human skin fibroblasts in culture. Biochim Biophys Acta 1014:145–152, 1989.
66. Cossman J (eds): Molecular genetics and cancer diagnosis. New York, Elsevier Scientific Publishing, 1990.

CHAPTER **13**

Hyaluronan-Protein Interactions

D. Andrew R. Burd
John Siebert
Hari Garg

Following injury, the skin has a tremendous capacity to heal. When the injury involves disruption of the dermis, postnatal wounds heal with a macrophage-effected,[1] fibro-proliferative repair process that results in the laying down of a new collagen-rich dermal matrix over which epidermal continuity can be re-established. This process of repair and the subsequent reorganization of the dermal matrix results in scar formation. A scar can be identified morphologically by a lack of organization of cellular and matrix elements when compared to surrounding uninjured skin.

Fetal wounds heal without scarring.[2–10] The mechanism for scarless repair in the fetus is unclear; immunohistochemical staining[11] and biochemical studies[10,12] indicate that there is a deposition of a collagen repair matrix that is rapidly organized. In an early third-trimester fetal sheep, there is no observable scar tissue by two weeks after wounding. What is notable is that while macrophages are present in these fetal wounds, polymorphonuclear leukocytes (PML) are not. Healing after the mid-third trimester in fetal sheep is associated with scarring[11] and this time point coincides with the appearance of PMLs in the wound matrix.[1] It appears that earlier fetal wounds have an ability to undertake an autonomous, site-specific repair, while classically activated macrophage-effected repair is not site-specific and ends in scarring.

There is now evidence to suggest that postnatal wound healing can be modulated to result in a decrease in scarring. Hellstrom[13] reported enhanced wound healing in tympanic membrane perforations in a rat model following the topical application of tissue-extracted hyaluronan (HA). Membranes treated with HA appeared otomicroscopically normal (translucent) three months later in contrast to untreated membranes that showed extensive opacification. In a follow-up study it was reported that this effect was independent of molecular size or rheological properties of the HA but related to the concentration of the preparation.[14] But what is the mechanism for the proposed effect of HA in wound healing and scarring? The possibilities include:

1. macrophage-effected postnatal repair process is suppressed,
2. an intrinsic tissue repair process is augmented, or,
3. a combination of the two effects occurs.

Whatever the case, a mechanism can be proposed where HA has a definite role in harnessing and manipulating the natural reparative capacity of tissue fibroblasts. This raises the question whether HA alone has the capacity to control events of such complexity as wound healing and scar maturation. Our preliminary studies identified a heterogeneous group of HA-protein complexes in normal skin and post-burn scar.[15] This work stemmed from the finding of strange banding patterns in cyanogen bromide digests of fetal wound extracts. We looked at cyanogen bromide digests of various highly purified tissue extracts and found serendipitously that there appeared to be collagen and other proteins associated with highly purified hyaluronan extracted from human tissues. We turned to postnatal human tissues because our initial fetal animal model, the fetal rabbit, yielded too little tissue and allowed sampling only over a short gestational period (see Chapter 11). In addition, the rabbit placenta allows large macromolecules to pass freely, unlike the human placenta, which may influence the fetal wound healing environment.[16] In this chapter we describe our initial investigations of this association and propose a hypothesis concerning the role of HA and associated proteins in the wound healing process.

A previous report described the appearance of a banded, fibrillar structure associated with hyaluronic acid extracted from rooster comb and human umbilical cord.[17] Viscosity changes after treatment with collagenase suggested that this structure might be collagen; however, this finding was not confirmed by amino-acid analysis, because no hydroxyproline or hydroxylysine could be detected. We began by re-examining the association between collagen and HA.

PREPARATION OF HYALURONAN

Normal skin and scar tissue were obtained from postburn patients. The scar tissue was defined as normal or hypertrophic by clinical and histological examination.[18] HA was prepared by using the procedure described by Swann et al.[19,20]

In brief, the tissue was frozen and ground in a Wiley mill. The powder was extracted with 4 M guanidinium chloride (Gdm.C1) containing proteinase inhibitors. This technique extracted HA and proteoglycans (PGs). DEAE-cellulose ion exchange chromatography was then used to separate HA from the other PGs. The first uronic acid positive peak (Peak A, Fig. 13.1, Swann et al., 1985) was then further fractionated using a cesium chloride dissociation gradient following the method of Swann et al.[21] The HA fraction (Fraction B, Figure 1) was dialyzed

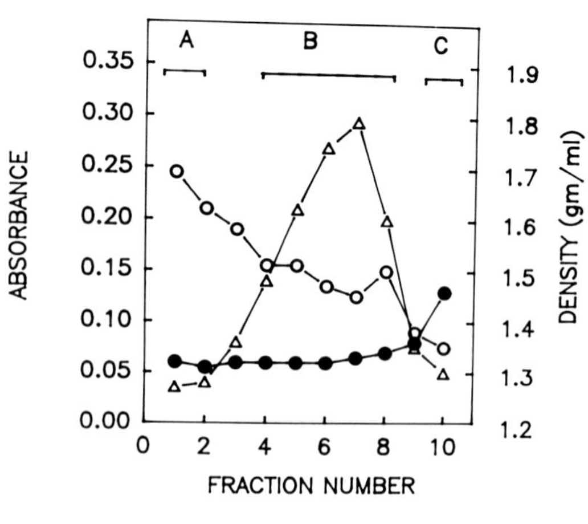

Figure 13.1 CsC1 density gradient fractionation of hypertrophic scar HA fraction after DEAE-cellulose chromatography. The distribution of uronic acid-containing constituents (△-△), the absorbance at 280 nm (·-·) and the density (o-o) following sedimentation. Fractions pooled as indicated.

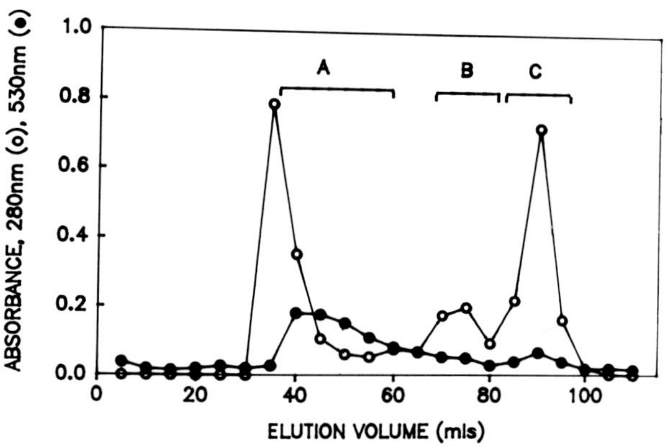

Figure 13.2 Sepharose CL-6B chromatography. Fractions pooled as indicated. A contains HA and protein, B and C are separate protein peaks.

against water, lyophilized, taken up in 3 M GdmCl and then further purified by running through a Sepharose CL-6B column under dissociative conditions. Fraction A in Fig. 13.2 was pooled and dialyzed against distilled water, then 1 M NaCl and finally distilled water again until salt-free. The dialyzed column fractions were lyophilized, and the proteins present were measured by their absorbency at 280 nm. The uronic acid content of the fractions was determined by the carbazole reaction.[22] The recovery of HA and protein eluted from the initial DEAE-cellulose column and those from the Sepharose CL-6B chromatography are given in Table 13.1. The HA fractions eluted from the Sepharose CL-6B column showed some absorption at 280 nm, indicating the presence of small amounts of protein. The fractions were pooled as shown in Figure 13.2 and the HA so obtained analyzed by cellulose acetate electrophoresis (Fig. 13.3). This HA fraction was found to electrophorese as a single band with a similar mobility to standard HA (lane 1), and disappeared after streptomyces hyaluronidase treatment (lane 4). Carbohydrate analysis of the HA fraction showed the following sugars associated with glycoproteins: N-acetylglucosamine, glucuronic acid, galactose, glucose, and

TABLE 13.1 Yield of HA and Protein in DEAE-Cellulose and Sepharose CL-6B Fractions

	DEAE cellulose fractions—yield (in mg) expressed as per gram dry tissue weight	
Tissue	HA (%)	Protein (%)
Normal skin	6.70 (6.95)	97 (93.5)
Normal scar	0.20 (0.30)	72 (99.7)
Hypertrophic scar	0.25 (0.25)	99 (99.8)
	Sepharose CL-6B fractions—yield (in mg) from pooled runs	
Tissue	**HA (Fraction A; Fig. 13.2) (%)**	**Protein (Fractions B, C; Fig. 13.2) (%)**
Normal skin	4.04 (74.6)	1.38 (25.4)
Normal scar	4.78 (62.1)	2.92 (37.9)
Hypertrophic scar	5.00 (83.2)	1.01 (16.8)

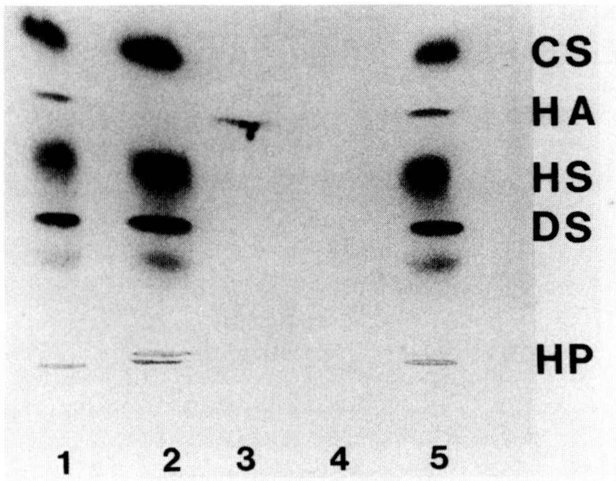

Figure 13.3 Cellulose acetate gel electrophoresis. Lane 1, standard; Lane 2, standard and HAdase; Lane 3, normal skin HA sample; Lane 4, normal skin HA sample and HAdase; lane 5, standard.

Standards: CS, chondroitin sulfate; HA, hyaluronan; HS, heparan sulfate; DS, dermatan sulfate; HP, heparin.

mannose. HA is composed of N-acetylglucosamine and glucuronic acid, whereas sugars associated with proteoglycans are iduronic acid and N-acetylgalactosamine (dermatan sulfate), glucuronic acid and N-acetylglucosamine (heparin), and glucuronic acid and N-acetylgalactosamine (chondroitin sulfate).

IDENTIFICATION OF COLLAGEN

Cyanogen Bromide (CNBr) Digestion

Tissue samples were suspended in nitrogen saturated 70% formic acid. Equal amounts of CNBr and sample were added, and the mixture was agitated in sealed tubes for 4 hr. at 37°C. The reaction was stopped by adding deionized water, freezing the mixture, and lyophilizing. The same sequence was then repeated.

Enzyme Digestion

Highly purified clostridial collagenase (Advance Biofactures Corp., NY) was mixed with the sample (2 units/5g) in 50 mM Tris HC1 pH 7.6, 100 mM NaC1 and 0.1 mM $CaC1_2$. The mixture was incubated for 30 min at 37°C and the reaction stopped by cooling to 40°C.

SDS-Polyacrylamide Gel Electrophoresis (SDS-PAGE)

CNBr digests with and without prior enzyme digestion were analyzed using SDS-PAGE on 12% polyacrylamide gels.[23] Samples were taken up in 0.625 M Tris pH 6.8, 2% SDS, 10% glycerol, 5% *b*-mercaptoethanol and 0.001% bromophenol blue, then heat denatured at 100°C for 3 min followed by electrophoresis in 12% SDS-polyacrylamide gels in a Tris-glycine buffer. Gels were fixed for 20 min in 50% methanol and 9% acetic acid, stained for 20 min in 0.25% Coomassie brilliant blue LR-250, and destained in 20% methanol and 7% acetic acid.

SDS-PAGE was performed by loading 500 ug samples of CNBr-digested HA fraction, with and without prior incubation, with collagenase. CNBr standards of human type I and III collagens were also run. Collagen peptides stained distinctly more reddish-purple than non-collagenous peptides, which appeared bluer. The banding pattern that appeared with the cyanogen bromide digestion of the HA samples demonstrated some reddish-purple bands, which corresponded to bands in the collagen standards. Samples treated with collagenase produced bands that varied depending on whether the enzymatic treatment preceded or followed CNBr digestion. When collagenase digestion preceded CNBr digestion, the appearance of CNBr collagen peptide bands was not altered, whereas when CNBr digestion occurred first, collagen peptide bands were absent on SDS-PAGE (Fig. 13.4).

Amino Acid Analysis

Samples were hydrolyzed in 6 N HC1 with phenol for 4 hr. at 110°C. Samples were then filtered and resuspended in citrate sample buffer (Bio-Rad, Richmond, CA). Amino acid analysis was performed using an automated Beckman 6300 amino acid analyzer using a citrate buffer system. Amino acid analysis was performed in the Protein Microsequencing Laboratory, Brigham & Women's Hospital, Boston. Amino acid analysis of the HA fractions after the initial purification and after the final purification with Sepharose CL-6B purification revealed hydroxyproline and hydroxylysine (Table 13.2). The percentage of collagen in the protein within the HA fraction was calculated on the basis that hydroxyproline constitutes approximately 10% of the collagen molecule.

Several factors must be considered when evaluating the evidence for collagen in the HA-protein complex: the purity of the HA preparation and whether or not unassociated protein contamination might come into play; whether HA is indeed complexed to collagen and not elastin or an associated microfibrillar protein; and whether the character of the association is chemical or physical.

In order to ensure the purity of the preparation, the HA fractions were isolated and chromatographed under denaturing conditions, with clear definition between

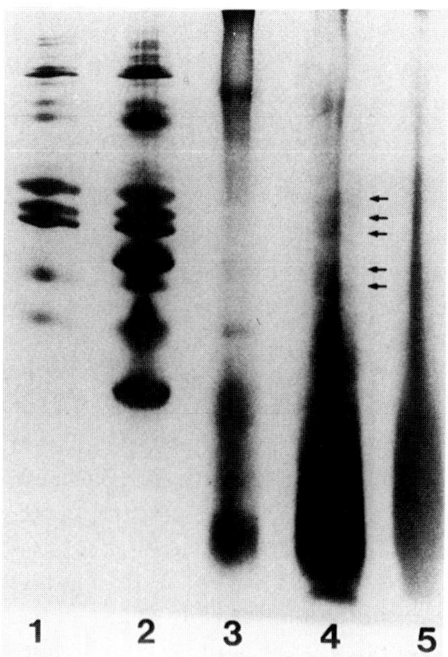

Figure 13.4 12% SDS-PAGE of CNBr-treated standard collagen and HA. Lane 1, CNBr peptides of human type I collagen; lane 2, CNBr peptides of human type III collagen; lane 3, 1 mg HA from normal skin; lane 4, 1 mg HA treated with CNBr (note the very faint bands [arrowed] that correspond with type III collagen peptides); lane 5, HA treated with CNBr, then collagenase (note absence of bands).

TABLE 13.2 Hydroxyproline and Hydroxylysine Residues/1000 Amino Acids

	After DEAE-cellulose	
	Hydroxyproline	Hydroxylysine
Normal skin	9	2
Normal scar	14	2
Hypertrophic scar	14	4

			Post Sepharose CL-6B		
	Hydroxyproline	Hydroxylysine	% Protein in HA Fraction	% Collagen in Protein	% Collagen in Protein
Normal skin	5	1	27.5	5	1.4
Normal scar	6	1	16.0	6	1.0
Hypertrophic scar	3	1	4.0	3	0.1

protein peaks as measured by absorbency at 280 nm. Although collagen contains a dearth of aromatic amino acids which absorb at 280 nm, 95% of the protein in the final extract was non-collagenous protein. Thus, the protein eluting with the HA peak in the final Sepharose chromatogram did not represent overlap contamination from other non-associated protein peaks. The convenient biochemical marker for collagen is hydroxyproline. Hydroxyproline is found abundantly in collagen, but it is also present in smaller quantities in other proteins, including elastin and micro-fibrillar protein.[24] Hydroxylysine, however, is not found in either elastin or microfibrillar protein.[25] The possibility that elastin and microfibrillar protein are associated with HA is not supported by either the CNBr digest peptide maps or the collagenase digests. The CNBr digestion maps produce bands that correspond with those of collagen standards and disappear with collagenase digestion, indicating that the hydroxyproline present is from collagen.

The evidence presented here supports a collagen-HA complex, but this does not necessitate covalent bonding; other chemical ionic and non-ionic interactions may be involved, as well as a purely steric interaction. Thus, repeated chromatographic purification of the HA would leave some protein "contamination." The resistance of the collagen within the HA-collagen complex from collagenase digestion is supportive of a functional association. In addition, collagen is by far the most abundant component of skin and scar tissue, yet it represents only 5% of the protein associated with the HA extracts. If the association represented random contamination, a much higher proportion of collagen would be expected. Whether the association between HA and collagen in vivo is of biological design may be relevant. Newly synthesized HA is released into the extracellular space, where collagen fibrillogenesis is taking place, and an HA-collagen complex might form at that time. This complex formation may be associated with the control of matrix deposition and the remodeling process.

The concept that an HA-collagen complex is involved in the organization of connective tissues is teleologically attractive when considering such phenomena as wound healing, growth, and development. These processes all involve matrix remodeling. Healing involves the deposition of new collagen and its subsequent remodeling. The poor quality of scar tissue is the result of the failure of the remodeling process to achieve as high a degree of connective tissue organization as seen in normal dermis. The absence of scarring in fetal skin wound healing suggests either more complete remodeling or more organized deposition of collagen.

Amino-acid analysis of highly purified HA, as well as of sugar components, indicates a major non-collagen protein element is present. What are these other proteins, and what are their significance? Conceivably, the HA-protein complex represents a transport stage, which allows proteins to gain access to specific regions without threat of enzymatic degradation or dilution in the extracellular space. Release of these proteins by hyaluronidase (HAdase) digestion of the associated HA would then allow them to fulfill their biological role. Collagen is a structural protein, and these initial fibrils might be serving as a framework to guide the subsequent construction of collagen fibers. Other protein elements might be peptide factors that influence cell movement and metabolism or the synthesis of new matrix materials by neighboring cells. While extremely speculative, this concept is open to investigation.

Commercially available HA produced by fermentation is almost free of protein "contamination." This HA can be compared with HA extracted from the tissues for its effect on healing. If the tissue-extracted HA produces an enhanced effect in the wound healing process compared to bacterially produced HA, then associated proteins may play a role in the modulation of wound healing and subsequent scarring.

PROTEIN COMPONENT'S BIOLOGICAL ACTIVITY

Highly purified HA extracted from human skin and scar along with several commercially available HA preparations from different sources including human umbilical cord extract (Sigma Grade 1), rooster comb extracts (Pharmacia and MedChem), and bacterial fermentation (Genzyme) were studied. These commercially available HA preparations were analyzed for protein content using an automated amino acid analyzer as described earlier.[26] The results (Table 13.3) show that all preparations did contain some protein. The laboratory prepared tissue-derived HA extracts contained the largest amount of protein. The amount of associated protein seemed to correlate directly with the relative degree of tissue organization present in the tissue source. The combination of both hydroxyproline and hydroxylysine residues is strongly supportive of the presence of collagen, although in small amounts. Nearly 95% of the protein is non-collagenous. The commercial preparations from rooster comb and the bacterial fermentation product did not contain hydroxyproline.

The initial experiment was designed to assess the biological heterogeneity of various HA preparations. The effects of HA-protein complexes on epidermal cell proliferation was first studied. The use of dermal explant cultures in serum free

TABLE 13.3 Protein Composition of HA Preparations

	Sigma	Genzyme	Pharmacia	Medchem	Epidermis	Dermis	Normal Scar
% protein in HA	0.17	0.06	0.15	0.15	1.83	4.63	1.58

medium removes extrinsic variables. Standardization of results can be achieved by comparing the zone of epithelialization around the hair follicle to the diameter of the hair follicle from which epithelialization is occurring. This index of epithelialization serves as a measurement of the propensity to increase epithelialization by each HA-protein complex. The heterogeneous nature of the HA preparations in stimulating re-epithelialization is evident in Figure 13.5. The superiority of the human HA, particularly from the epidermis and normal scar, is evident when compared to a pure HA preparation from bacterial fermentation.

Having determined that the HA preparations are indeed different biologically, attention was focused to find out whether these differences were due to the structure of different HAs or the content/structure of the protein component. The fibroblast proliferation assay was chosen because of its simplicity and reproducibility and also because ultimately cutaneous scarring follows dermal disruption, and the fibroblast is the predominant cell in the dermis. HA extracts from human

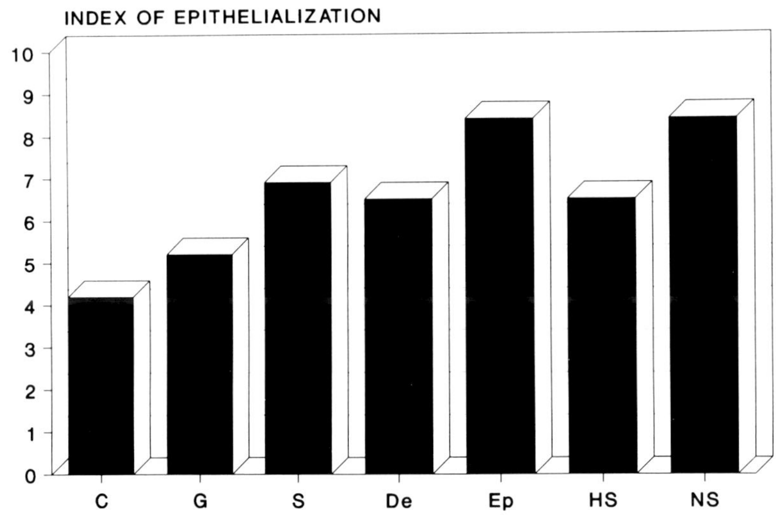

Figure 13.5 Effect of HA preparations on epidermal cell proliferation. Dermal sheets from the paravertebral areas of 5–6 months old pure bred Yorkshire pigs were harvested under aseptic conditions with a Pagett's dermatome at a setting of 0.5 mm after removing a 0.5 mm thick split-thickness graft containing the epidermis. Dermal strips were cut into 5 × 10 mm segments and transferred onto sterile dressing sponges in multiwell petri dishes to raise the explant to the air-liquid interface. Orientation of the dermis was maintained. Explants were maintained in 10% CO_2 environment with 95% humidity in serum free Dulbecco's Modification of Eagles Medium (DMEM) supplemented by 10 ng/ml hydrocortisone without antibiotics. 300 μg of HA extracts were suspended in sterile PBS and applied topically to the explants on Day 0. The medium was changed at four days and cultures were harvested after 4 and 8 days and fixed in 10% formalin. Re-epithelialized areas around the hair follicles were visualized by staining with 1% rhodamine solution for a few seconds and washing in formalin. Re-surfaced areas were photographed at a 10x magnification and their size determined using computerized morphometric analysis. The ratio of area of re-epithelialization to the cross sectional area of the hair follicle was determined to give an index of re-epithelialization. Statistical analysis was performed using analysis of variance in the CLINFO program. The ratios for the various experimental groups are depicted (C = control, DMEM and hydrocortisone; G = HA from bacterial fermentation; S = HA from rooster comb; De = Human HA from dermis; Ep = Human HA from epidermis; HS = Human HA from hypertrophic scar; NS = Human HA from normal scar). Duncan's multiple comparison demonstrated significant differences between NS and C, G and S at four days (data not shown) and between NS and Ep and C, G and S at eight days.

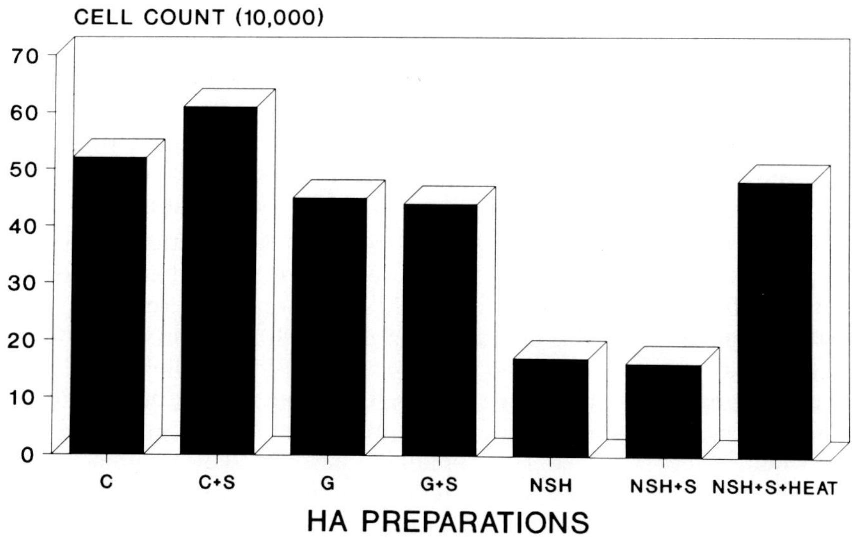

Figure 13.6 Fibroblast proliferation in monolayer culture. Normal human dermal fibroblast cultures were maintained in a humidified incubator at 37°C with 5% CO_2 and air. Medium for cell cultures consisted of DMEM supplemented with 10% fetal bovine serum and gentamicin 15 mg/mg. Experimental cultures were set up in 24 well culture dishes with 50,000 cells and 0.5 ml of medium per well. 200 μg/ml HA preparations were added at the time of plating. Cells were harvested at 48 hours using trypsin/EDTA solution 250 μg/well. Cell number was determined using a Coulter counter. Experiments were performed in triplicate and analyzed using Duncan's Multiple comparison test. (C = control [PBS]; G = HA from bacterial fermentation [Genzyme]; NSH = Human HA from normal scar; +S = predigestion with streptomyces hyaluronidase). This demonstrates significant inhibition of fibroblast proliferation when HA from NS is added. This effect is unaltered by predigestion with HAdase, but disappears when the associated protein is heat denatured or subjected to protease after HAdase predigestion.

postburn normal scar produced a significant inhibition of fibroblast proliferation (Fig. 13.6). Using selective enzyme digestion to degrade the HA (confirmed on cellulose acetate plate electrophoresis) we have found that this inhibitory effect persists. Treatment of the HA preparation by heating to 100°C for 5 min., to denature the proteins, eliminated the inhibition. Interestingly, if the HA-protein complex was subjected to a protease, inhibition of fibroblast proliferation persists. If the complex is treated with an HAdase the inhibition continues. However, if the HAdase treated HA-protein complex is then subjected to a protease the inhibition of fibroblast proliferation is lost. These results support the hypothesis that the associated proteins have biological activity and that HA protects the associated protein from enzymatic digestion. We should not be surprised by this as several glycosaminoglycans have been found to stabilize soluble protein growth factors. For example, both heparan sulfate and heparin have been found to increase the radius of diffusion and action of basic fibroblast growth factor.[27]

The effects of HA-protein complexes on an in vitro wound healing model developed in our laboratories were also studied.[28] A particular advantage of this model is that the control wound in fetal sheep skin does not heal. There is re-epithelialization and preservation of the gross morphology of the tissue, but the dermal cleft remains open at seven days (see Chapter 17). When the explant is treated daily with the HA produced by bacterial fermentation, which contains the least amount of associated protein, the healing is only slightly better than the control wound. Wounds treated topically with HA extracted from human normal scar demonstrate complete re-epithelialization by four days and the progressive reconstitution of the dermal matrix, so that by seven days only a small "dead space" exists in the upper dermis.

This experiment is relevant to the putative nature of the fetal tissue repair process. As tissue repair demonstrates more autonomy, what directs the fibroblasts in the repair process? It would appear that fetal wound healing in vitro is not a self-directed process in that the fibroblasts are present and viable in the control wounds, but healing of the dermal matrix does not occur. Similarly, the possibility of epidermal control of the dermal healing process can be excluded as the epidermis is viable, proliferates, and restores continuity, but again no dermal matrix repair occurs. DePalma and colleagues[29] have suggested that the HA enriched environment of fetal wounds creates a permissive environment for dermal repair. However, the application of HA alone does not result in dermal repair. It is only when tissue-extracted HA containing associated proteins is added that healing occurs. This suggests that in fetal wounds, as in postnatal wounds, extrinsic factors are important in initiating repair. The macrophage, the quarterback of postnatal wound healing, may also coordinate fetal wound healing via soluble protein products directing cellular interaction.[30]

THE HA-PROTEIN COMPLEXES OF FETAL TISSUES

Differences between fetal and postnatal wound repair are due to the different degrees of organization of collagen deposition in a dynamic extracellular matrix. This changing matrix has become a focus of our next series of studies. Many reports have demonstrated glycosaminoglycans (GAGs) playing a role in wound repair. HA, a non-sulfated GAG, has specific binding sites for fibrinogen.[31] Further, HA degradation products stimulate in vitro angiogenesis.[32,33] HA has also been shown to alter the phagocytic properties of monocytes and macrophages.[34,35] Finally, Toole[36] demonstrated HA to be an integral part in the dysmorphogenesis and regeneration of a severed newt limb.

The sulfated GAGs are characterized by sulfated side chains and various protein cores, and they temporally follow HA in the healing process. These GAGs have been shown to regulate collagen organization[37] and by binding to specific binding sites on collagen control its rate of degradation.[38]

The unique fetal ability to heal skin wounds without scarring and a transition to adult-like healing with scar formation midway through the last trimester may reflect changes in GAG content of fetal skin differentiating as a function of gestational age. We set out to identify the age-related changes in both quantity and quality of GAGs in fetal sheep skin. Fetal sheep allowed us to obtain specimens over a long gestational period (gestation = 145 days), in large sample sizes, and at an early fetal age. Chronological analysis of HA-protein complexes from a gestational age of 80 days to 145 days allows a unique window into fetal tissue repair.

Our results for uronic acid content (a measure of total glycosaminoglycan concentration) as a function of gestational age is shown in Figure 13.7. We observed the largest amount of uronic acid (528 ± 9 μg/gm tissue) in the youngest (80 day) specimen. The uronic acid content dropped in an age-related fashion to a low at 130 days (174 ± 11 μg/gm). From 135 days old to birth, the uronic acid content rose significantly from 189 to 337 μg/gm ($p<0.05$).

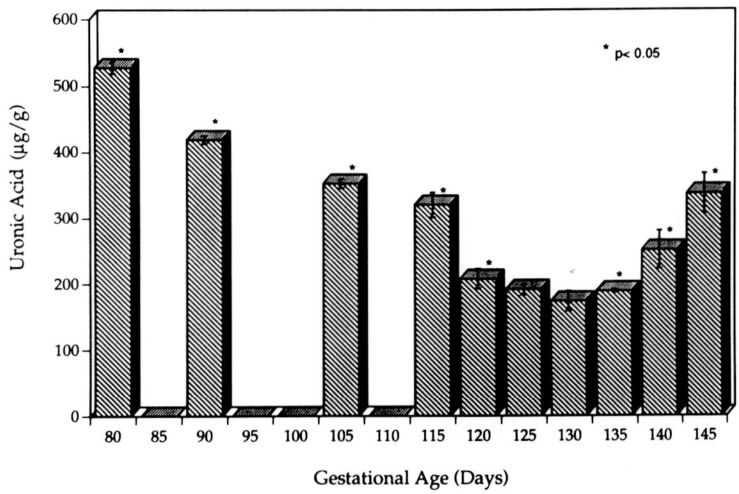

Figure 13.7 Uronic acid content in fetal sheep skin as a function of gestational age.

The total glycosaminoglycan content and relative percentage of each specific GAG were determined by densitometry and integration. The results are tabulated in Table 13.4. Heparin was present at all ages within a small range of concentrations. Dermatan sulfate (DS) and heparan sulfate (HS) became evident at 120 days gestation and increased in concentration with age. The appearance of both sulfated GAGs coincides with the appearance of scarring in fetal sheep.

The elevated levels of HA at 80 days gestation supports a study that demonstrates an HA stimulatory factor in fetal sheep serum, with its peak activity in 60 day fetal serum.[39] The decline of HA may also be associated with an increase in the concentration of hyaluronidase. Toole[36,40] has demonstrated that in morphogenesis, the decrease in HA levels are associated with a rise in hyaluronidase activity in the tissue. However, the increase in HA at the latter part of gestation cannot be explained by hyaluronidase activity unless it is also neutralized late in gestation.

TABLE 13.4 Percent of Total Glycosaminoglycans in Fetal Lamb Skin

Gestational Age (Days)	Hp	DS	HS	HA	CS
80	5.6%			94.4%	
90	3.7			96.3	
105	3.9			96.1	
110	4.1	1.0%		94.9	
115	4.0			96.0	
120	3.6	4.0	3.2%	89	
125	7.2	2.9		89	
130	2.6	6.4	3.7	87	
135	2.6	8.1	2.3	87.0	
140	4.3	14.9	5.5	74.6	0.7%
145	2.5	2.8	4.7	89.3	0.8

Hp = heparin; DS = Dermatan sulfate; HS = Heparan sulfate; HA = Hyaluronic acid; CS = Chondroitin Sulfate

Longaker and coworkers have shown the fetal lamb to heal with a disorganized scar after a gestational age of 120 days.[11] The appearance of sulfated GAGs (HS and DS) at 120 days gestation and their increase in concentration with age coincides with the timing of scarring in fetal skin. Toole has elegantly demonstrated the decline of HA and the appearance of sulfated GAGs to correlate with the onset of cytodifferentiation in developing tissues. Thus, the question arises, is scarless healing unique to the cellular differentiation of fetal skin at various gestational ages?

As we suspected, fetal skin-derived HA is complexed with various proteins. These proteins are stabilized during the extraction process. Following papain digestion of tissues the associated proteins are intact and identifiable. The percent protein in the extractable HA-protein complexes as a function of gestational age is shown in Figure 13.8. The protein component can be further identified by SDS-PAGE following HAdase degradation. When run against known molecular weight protein standards the molecular weight of the associated proteins for each gestational age can be determined (Table 13.5). Efforts are currently underway to further characterize the protein elements associated with scarless healing prior to 120 days gestational age in the fetal lamb. In addition, the role of sulfated glycosaminoglycans in wound healing needs further investigation. The onset of scarring in the fetal lamb corresponds to the accumulation of sulfated GAGs.

HA was first isolated by Meter and Palmer in 1934,[41] and has been shown to be a ubiquitous constituent of connective tissues. The chemical structure was established by enzymatic[42] and chemical[43] studies carried out on preparations obtained from human umbilical cord and consist of alternating 4-0 linked β-D-glucopyranosyluronic and 3-0-linked 2-acetamido-2-deoxy-β-D-glucopyranosyl residues. Because of its composition of hexosamine and uronic acid, and its method of biosynthesis, HA has been classified among the glycosaminoglycans such as dermatan sulfate, chondroitin sulfate, heparin sulfate, heparin, etc., although it is the only polymer of this class of compounds in which a linkage to a core protein backbone has not been demonstrated.[44] HA is also the only glycos-

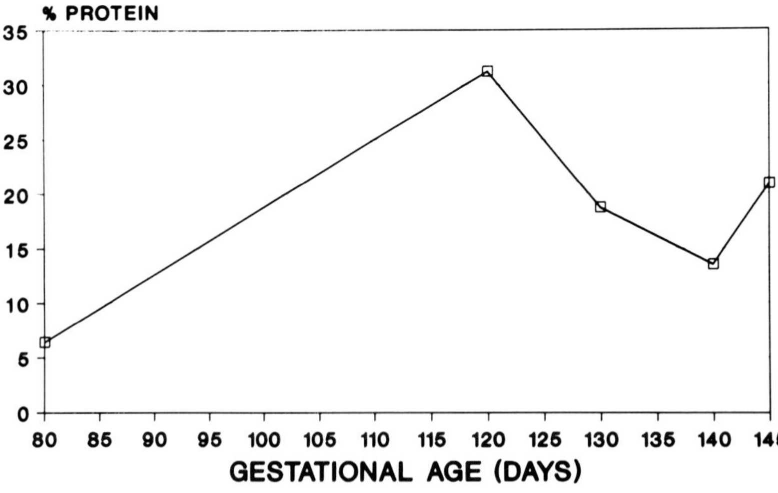

Figure 13.8 Percent protein component of HA-protein complexes derived from fetal sheep skin as a function of gestational age.

TABLE 13.5 Molecular Weights of Associated Proteins in HA-Protein Complex

Gestational Age (days)	Molecular Weight (kDa)		
80	35		61
120		42	61
130	35		61
140	35	42	
145		42	

aminoglycan to not have sulfated side groups in its molecular structure. The history of the structure determination of glycosaminoglycans, where new sugar components and new anomeric configurations have been found repeatedly, suggests that variations in the structure of HA are possible. Recently, N-deacetylated HA has been reported in old human skin.[45] Although a linear polysaccharide, its macromolecular structure is that of an expanded coil. This is susceptible to enzymatic degradation, resulting in the release of low-molecular weight oligosaccharides.

HA and its degradation products have been associated with a number of cell regulatory actions. Considerable attention has been directed toward the role of HA in growth and development,[46] and it would appear that the structural configuration of hyaluronic acid facilitates the movement of cells within the extracellular matrix.[47] In the early stages of repair, when HA levels are high, cell migration plays a prominent role in restoring cellular continuity.[48] Later, when HA concentrations fall and sulfated GAG concentrations are high, cell differentiation, collagen production, and tissue organization occur.[36,40] The high molecular weight HA seems to inhibit the formation of capillaries[49] while angiogenesis is induced by degradation products of HA.[33]

Weigel et al[50] have proposed a model for the role of HA in wound healing in which an HA-fibrin matrix forms that attracts inflammatory cells into the wound. This matrix is in turn modified by the cells entering the wound as they secrete hyaluronidase and plasminogen activator into the extracellular space to degrade hyaluronan and fibrin. The degradation products from both HA and fibrin are then seen as important regulatory molecules for controlling cellular functions involved in the inflammatory response and inducing new blood vessel formation in the healing wounds. The protein component of HA-protein complexes would fit into this model well. The breakdown of HA would allow the protein factors to fulfill their biological roles. They would be protected from breakdown by proteases present in early wounds in the HA-protein form.

Although Weigel's model for wound healing is attractive, the addition of soluble protein factors would better explain the degree of control that would be expected in such complex cell and matrix interactions as occur in wound healing and scar maturation. Our hypothesis also relates to the early events of the inflammatory response and wound healing. There is now increasing evidence to support the role of peptide factors in the control of acute phase healing[51–55] and it is very likely that such protein factors are involved in the longer term processes of remodeling the repair matrix.

The identification of the biological activity of various growth factors indicate that cells can respond to peptide messenger molecules in a profound and complex manner. It is almost certain that there are many more factors than have been presently identified and that these constitute the basis for intercellular communication and control. If this is the case, then it is possible that the behavior of the receptor cells will be determined by the combinations and quantities, and possible sequences, of the peptide factors to which they are exposed. The concept of being able to transport discrete collections of such factors for localized release would further enhance such a regulatory mechanism. The data presented in this chapter support such a hypothesis, but also raise many questions such as how the proteins become associated with the HA, which cells produce the factors, and do they provide the basis for a two-way communication? If so, what is the mechanism for targeting the HA-protein complex appropriately? While HA undoubtedly plays a major role in the growth, development, and repair of tissues, perhaps its obvious presence in these conditions has overshadowed the investigation of more critical determinants of tissue response.

REFERENCES

1. Knighton DR, Fiegel UD: The macrophage: Effector cell in wound repair. Prog Clin Biol Res 299:217–26, 1989.
2. Burrington JD: Wound healing in the fetal lamb. J Ped Surg 6:423–528, 1971.
3. Goss AN: Intrauterine healing of fetal rat oral mucosal, skin and cartilage wounds. J Oral Pathol 6:35–43, 1977.
4. Robinson BW, Goss AN: Intrauterine healing of fetal rat cheek wounds. Cleft Palate J 18:251–255, 1981.
5. Rowsell AR: The intra-uterine healing of foetal muscle wounds: Experimental study in the rat. Br J Plast Surg 37:635–642, 1984.
6. Adzick NS, Harrison MR, Glick PL, et al.: Comparison of fetal, newborn, and adult healing by histologic, enzyme-histochemical and hydroxyproline determination. J Ped Surg 20:315–319, 1985.
7. Hallock GG: In utero cleft lip repair in A/J mice. Plast Reconstr Surg 75:785–788, 1985.
8. Hallock GG, Rice DC, McClure HM: In utero lip repair in the rhesus monkey: An update. Plast Reconstr Surg 80:855–858, 1987.
9. Krummel TM, Nelson JM, Dieglemann RF, et al.: Fetal response to injury in the rabbit. J Pediatr Surg 22:640–644, 1987.
10. Siebert JW, Burd DAR, McCarthy JG, et al.: Fetal wound healing: A biochemical study of scarless healing. Plast Reconstr Surg 85:495–502, 1990.
11. Longaker MT, Whitby DJ, Adzick NS, et al.: Studies in fetal wound healing: VI. Second and early third trimester fetal wounds demonstrate rapid collagen deposition without scar formation. J Ped Surg 25:63–69, 1990.
12. Burd DAR, Longaker MT, Adzick NS, et al.: Fetal wound healing in a large animal model: The deposition of collagen is confirmed. Brit J Plast Surg 43:571–577, 1990.
13. Hellstrom S and Laurent C: Hyaluronan and healing of tympanic membrane perforations. An experimental study. Acta Otolaryngology Suppl 442:54–61, 1987.
14. Laurent C, Hellstrom S, Fellenius E: Hyaluronan improves the healing of experimental tympanic membrane perforations. Arch Otolaryngol Head Neck Surg 114:435–441, 1988.
15. Burd DAR, Siebert JW, Ehrlich HP, et al.: Human skin and postburn scar hyaluronan: Demonstration of the association with collagen and other proteins. Matrix 9:322–329, 1989.
16. Wild AE: Protein transmission across the placenta and foetal membranes. Sci Prog Oxf 54:351–364, 1966.
17. Swann DA, Caulfield JB, Ceselski A: Proteins associated with hyaluronic acid. Ann Rheum Dis 34 (Suppl.):98–100, 1975.
18. Linares HA, Kisher CW, Dobrikovsky M, et al.: The hypertrophic organization of the hypertrophic scar in humans. J Invest Dermatol 59:323–331, 1972.
19. Swann DA, Garg HG, Hendry CJ, Hermann H, et al.: Isolation and partial characterization of dermatan sulfate proteoglycans from human post-burn scar tissue. Collagen Rel Res 8:295–313, 1988.

20. Swann DA, Garg HG, Jung W, et al.: Studies on human scar tissue proteoglycans. J Invest Dermatol 84:527–531, 1985.
21. Swann DA, Powell S and Sotman S.: The heterogeneity of cartilage proteoglycans. J Biol Chem 254:945–954, 1979.
22. Bitter T and Muir HM.: A modified uronic acid carbazole reaction. Anal Biochem 4:330, 1962.
23. Laemmli, UK: Cleavage of structural proteins during the assembly of the head of the bacteriophage T4. Nature 227:680–685, 1970.
24. Adams, E and Frank, L: Metabolism of proline and hydroxyprolines. Ann Rev Biochem 49:1005–1061, 1980.
25. Ross R and Bornstein P: Elastic fibers in the body. Sci Amer 224 (June):44–52, 1971.
26. Garg HG, Siebert EP, Swann DA: Isolation and some structure analysis of a copolymeric chondroitin sulfate-dermatan sulfate proteoglycan from post-burn, human hypertrophic scar. Carbohydr Res 197:159–169, 1990.
27. Flaumenhaft R, Moscatelli D, Rifkin DB: Heparin and heparan sulfate increase the radius of diffusion and action of basic fibroblast growth factor. J Cell Biol 111:1651–1659, 1990.
28. Burd DAR, Longaker MT, Adzick NS, et al.: Fetal wound healing: An in vitro explant model. J Ped Surg 25:898–901, 1990.
29. DePalma RL, Krummel TM, Durham LA, et al.: Characterization and quantitation of wound matrix in the fetal rabbit. Matrix 9:224–231, 1989.
30. Longaker MT and Banda MJ: Inflammation and fetal wound healing. Presented at fetal wound healing symposia sponsored by Marion Laboratories, Nov. 1990, Dallas, Texas.
31. LeBoeuf RD, Raja RH, Fuller GM, Weigel PH: Human fibrinogen specifically binds hyaluronic acid. J Biol Chem 261:12586–12592, 1986.
32. Feinberg RN and Beebe DC: Hyaluronate in vasculogenesis. Science 220:1177, 1983.
33. West DC, Hampson IN, Arnold F, Kumar S: Angiogenesis induced by degradation products of hyaluronic acid. Science 228:1324–1326, 1985.
34. Ahlgren T and Jarstrand C: Hyaluronic acid enhances phagocytosis of human monocytes in vitro. J Clin Immun 43:246–249, 1984.
35. Forrester JV and Balazs EA: Inhibition of phagocytosis by high molecular weight hyaluronate. Immunology 40:435–445, 1980.
36. Toole BP and Trelstad RL: Hyaluronate production and removal during corneal development in the chick. Dev Biol 26:28–35, 1971.
37. Alexander SA and Donoff RB: The glycosaminoglycans of open wounds. J Surg Res 29:422–429, 1980.
38. Ruoslahti E: Structure and biology of proteoglycans. Ann Rev Cell Biol 4:229–255, 1988.
39. Longaker MT, Harrison MR, Crombleholme TM, et al.: Studies in fetal wound healing I: A factor in fetal serum that stimulates deposition of hyaluronic acid. J Ped Surg 24:789–792, 1989.
40. Toole BP: Hyaluronate turnover during chondrogenesis in the developing chick limb and axial skeleton. Dev Biol 29:321–329, 1972.
41. Meyer K, Palmer JW: The polysaccharide of vitreous humor. J Biol Chem 107:629–634, 1934.
42. Meyer K: Chemical structure of hyaluronic acid. Fed Proc 17:1075–1077, 1958.
43. Jeanloz RW: Chemistry of Mucopolysaccharide. Proc. 3rd Intl Congr Biochem pp.65–72, 1985.
44. Comper WW, Laurent TC: Physiological function of connective tissue polysaccharides. Physiol Rev 58:255–315, 1978.
45. Longas MO: Evidence for structural changes in dermatan sulfate and hyaluronic acid with aging. Carbohydr Res 159:127–136, 1987.
46. Toole BD, Goldberg RL, Chi-Rosso G, et al.: Hyaluronate cell reactions. In: Trelstad RL (ed): The Role of the Extracellular Matrix in Development. Alan R. Liss, Inc. New York, 43–66, 1984.
47. Docherty R, Forrester JV, Lackie JM, Gregory DW: Glycosaminoglycans facilitate the movement of fibroblasts through three dimensional collagen matrices. J Cell Sci 92:263–270, 1989.
48. Abetangelo G, Martelli M, Vecchia P: Healing of hyaluronic acid-enriched wounds: histological observations. J Surg Res 35:410–416, 1983.
49. Feinberg RN, Beebe DC: Hyaluronate in vasculogenesis. Science 220:1177–1179, 1983.
50. Weigel PH, Fuller GM, LeBoeuf RD: A model for the role of hyaluronic acid and fibrin in the early events during the inflammatory response and wound healing. J Theor Biol 119:219–234, 1986.
51. Nemeth GG, Bolander ME, Martin GR: Growth factors and their role in wound and fracture healing. Prog Clin Biol Res 266:1–17, 1988.
52. Davidson J, Buckley A, Woodward S, et al.: Mechanisms of accelerated wound repair using epidermal growth factor and basic fibroblast growth factor. Prog Clin Biol Res 266:63–75, 1988.

53. Sprugel KH, McPherson JM, Clowes AW, Ross R: The effects of different growth factors in subcutaneous wound chambers. Prog Clin Biol Res 266:77–91, 1988.
54. Pierce GF, Mustoe TA, Deuel TF: Transforming growth factor *B* induces increased directed cellular migration and tissue repair in rats. Prog Clin Biol Res 266:93–102, 1988.
55. Spencer EM, Skover G, Hunt TK: Somatomedins: Do they play a pivotal role in wound healing? Prog Clin Biol Res 266:103–116, 1988.

CHAPTER **14**

Glycosaminoglycan Processing During Tissue Repair: Degradation of Hyaluronic Acid

Charles N. Bertolami
Steven Berg
Earl G. Freymiller

HYALURONATE IN EMBRYOGENESIS

Glycosaminoglycan processing, properly understood, refers both to the synthesis and degradation of the long polyanionic polysaccharide chains that comprise the glycosaminoglycan class of molecules. This chapter discusses the much-neglected catabolic aspects of such processing, with a particular focus on hyaluronic acid,* the glycosaminoglycan thought to be most important in fetal repair processes.

Developmental biologists were the first to evince real interest in the role of glycosaminoglycans during embryonic development. After studying numerous different developmental systems,[1–5] a general pattern emerged in which predictable changes in glycosaminoglycan synthesis and breakdown were associated with specific changes in cellular proliferation, migration, differentiation, and synthesis. All of these processes were thought to be influenced by the effects of hyaluronic acid. In each developmental system studied, similar observations were made (summarized in Fig. 14.1).

From the standpoint of glycosaminoglycan metabolism, early embryogenesis was divided into two distinct periods. The first consisted of a morphogenetic phase characterized by high concentrations of hyaluronic acid. A subsequent phase of cytodifferentiation followed during which cells began to differentiate and to express a phenotype evidenced by synthesis and secretion of sulfated glycosaminoglycans and collagen. During the transition between morphogenetic and cytodifferentiative phases, an enzyme (hyaluronidase) specific for initiating hyaluronate catabolism became detectable in tissues. It acted on native hyaluronate as its preferential substrate and was associated with the removal of hyaluronic acid from developing tissues. At the same time, further hyaluronate synthesis ceased. The theory subsequently emerged that hyaluronic acid was important during early development as a means of promoting cellular growth, proliferation, and migration.[6] Furthermore, hyaluronidase was proposed as a signal for differentiation, functioning by promoting removal of hyaluronic acid from embryonic tissues. While the exact mechanisms for the putative effects of hyaluronate on cellular behavior were not known, they were presumed to arise purely as a consequence of the substance's known physical properties.

---

* Depending upon its chemical form, the terms hyaluronic acid, hyaluronate, and hyaluronan may be used. In this chapter, they are used essentially as synonyms.

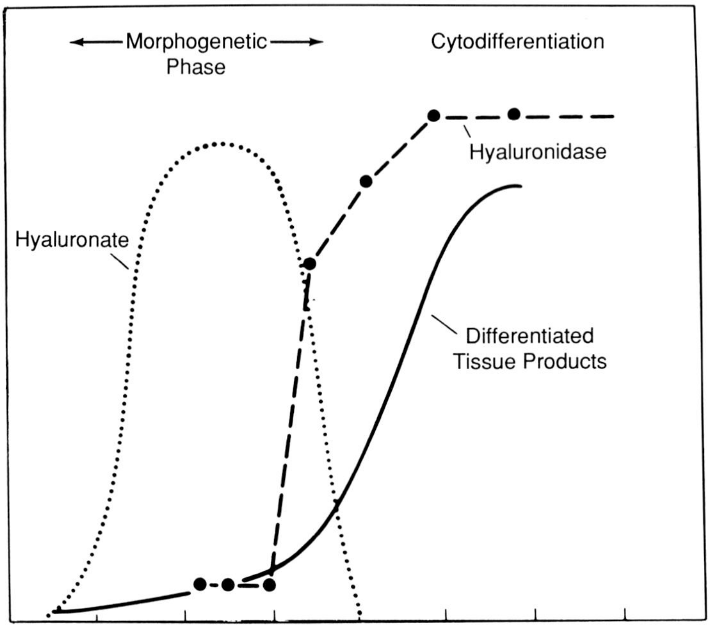

Figure 14.1 Generalized schematic of relationship between hyaluronate and hyaluronidase during embryonic development as conceptualized by Toole. Horizontal axis depicts relative time; vertical axis represents relative amount. The first, so-called morphogenetic, phase is characterized by high levels of hyaluronate which, presumably, favor cellular proliferation and migration. Near the end of the morphogenetic phase, hyaluronidase activity first becomes detectable and then rapidly increases. Existing hyaluronate is removed under the influence of hyaluronidase and additional hyaluronate synthesis ceases. Removal of hyaluronate is associated with the cessation of cell proliferation/migration and the onset of cytodifferentiation—evidenced by increased levels of characteristic differentiated cell products. (After Toole BP. Morphogenetic role of glycosaminoglycans [acid mucopolysaccharides] in brain and other tissues. In: *Neuronal Recognition* [SH Barondes, ed.], Plenum Press, New York, pp 275–329, 1976.)

HYALURONATE IN WOUND REPAIR

Conceptually, the existence of distinct and easily measurable events in embryogenesis corresponding to specific cellular behaviors leading to new tissue formation are of obvious interest to wound healing biologists. Since the nineteenth century, histologists had drawn analogies between embryonic development and wound healing. However, the analogy had a purely observational basis and was without substantiation at a biochemical level. Clearly, healing tissues show evidence of cellular proliferation, migration, differentiation, and synthesis, but whether the molecular mechanisms by which these events are regulated during healing resemble those of embryogenesis was unknown. The notion of examining the healing wound from a developmental perspective gained impetus because of the work on the role of hyaluronic acid, the other glycosaminoglycans, and the degradative enzyme hyaluronidase during embryogenesis. These components provided easily measurable criteria for making comparisons between repair and development.

Early investigators[7,8] attempted to measure the glycosaminoglycan content of healing wounds in experimental animals, but they were hampered by a lack of sufficiently sensitive and specific means for measuring glycosaminoglycans. More importantly, they were limited by the lack of a suitable developmental framework for understanding the importance of changes in glycosaminoglycan content. As methodology advanced and a clear understanding of the potential relevance of changes in glycosaminoglycan composition of reparative tissues emerged, the next step involved quantitating the content of glycosaminoglycan over time and measuring hyaluronidase activities to establish if the changes in hyaluronate observed for embryonic systems were also seen in healing tissues. Specifically, were large quantities of hyaluronate seen early in postnatal healing, and did they decline under the influence of a hitherto unrecognized wound hyaluronidase?

Figure 14.2 depicts the result of efforts to identify a wound hyaluronidase. The enzyme was present in wound granulation tissue and enzyme activity increased markedly during and after the second week of healing. Initially high levels of hyaluronic acid declined under the apparent influence of the enzyme, in much the same way as reported for developmental systems.[9–11] Efforts at purifying wound hyaluronidase were only partially successful (Fig. 14.3). Nevertheless, it was possible to increase the enzyme's specific activity sufficiently to allow characterization. Of special note was wound hyaluronidase's pH optimum (Fig. 14.4). The enzyme exhibited maximal activity at a low pH (in the vicinity of pH 4.5)

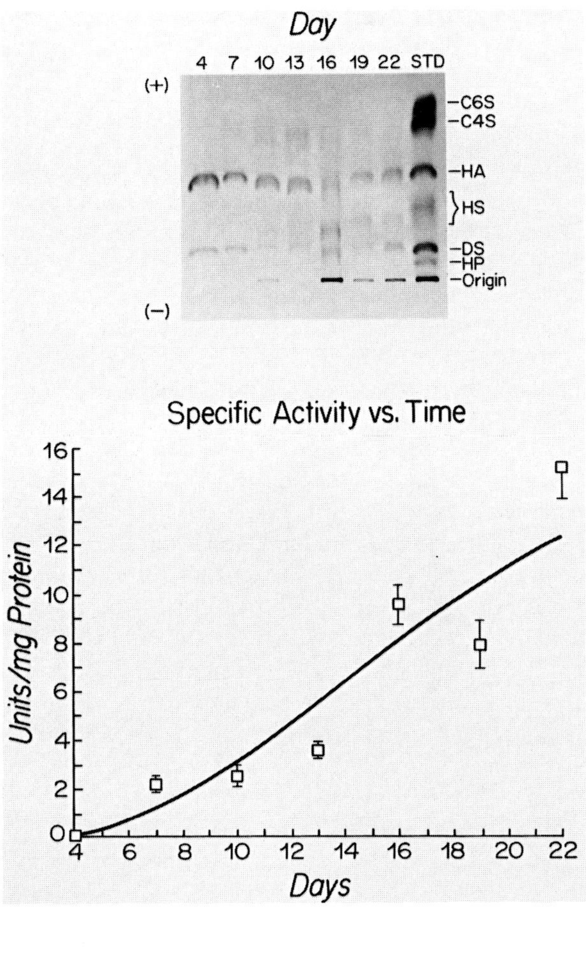

Figure 14.2 Upper panel shows a cellulose acetate electrophoretogram of the glycosaminoglycans (GAGs) in rabbit wound granulation tissue over a 22 day period. Authentic GAGs have been used as standards and are shown in the lane labelled STD. Relative migration positions are shown for chondroitin 6-sulfate (C6S), chondroitin 4-sulfate (C4S), hyaluronate (HA), heparan sulfate (HS), dermatan sulfate (DS), and heparin (HP). Alcian blue stain was used. Focusing on the hyaluronate migration position, it can be seen that staining of hyaluronate is greater for days 4, 7, 10 and 13 than for days 16, 19, or 22.

Correspondingly, the lower panel depicts hyaluronidase activities for the same tissues and postwound days. Hyaluronidase activity is minimal during days 4, 7, 10 and 13 but increases markedly for days 16, 19, and 22. Thus, wound hyaluronate is highest when hyaluronidase activity is absent or minimal. Hyaluronate levels decline when hyaluronidase activity increases. This general relationship is consistent with that described by Toole and co-workers in developmental systems and is even more evident when hyaluronate levels are quantified colorimetrically.[9,10]

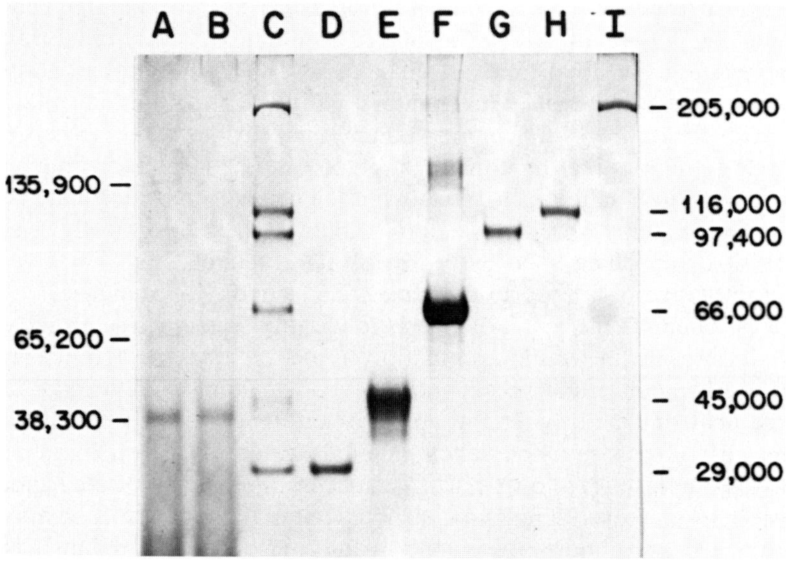

Figure 14.3 Sodium dodecyl sulfate (SDS)-polyacrylamide gel of partially purified rabbit mucosal wound granulation tissue hyaluronidase under reducing conditions. Lanes A and B show partially purified enzyme with fragments having molecular weights of 38.3, 65.2, and 135.9 Kd. Mixture of molecular weight markers is shown in lane C and individual markers are shown in lanes D-I. (After Bertolami and Ellis, J Dent Res 64:913–918, 1985.)

which resembled other hyaluronidases and, more significantly, showed a pH optimum typical for a lysosomal hydrolase.

In addition to a temporal change in hyaluronidase activity over the course of healing, a topographic change in enzyme distribution occurred as healing progressed. Hyaluronidase activity was highest near the wound's center. Correspondingly, the center of the wound showed the lowest levels of the enzyme's preferred substrate, hyaluronic acid. The periphery of the wound, particularly beneath migrating epithelium, showed threefold more hyaluronic acid than central wound regions and also revealed an absence of hyaluronidase for the longest period of time. The practical consequence of this observation is unknown, but

Figure 14.4 Typical pH-activity profile for mammalian wound hyaluronidase. Specific activity (expressed in relative absorbance units) is shown along the vertical axis, pH is shown along the horizontal axis. The preparation depicted here was derived from rabbit mucosal wound granulation tissue and exhibited a pH optimum of approximately 3.8. Cutaneous wound hyaluronidase shows maximal enzyme activity at a somewhat higher pH (approximately 4.5); however, in all cases, hyaluronidase's pH optimum is quite low (below 5.0) and is consistent with the view that it is a lysosomal hydrolase. (After Bertolami and Ellis, J Dent Res 64:913–918, 1985.)

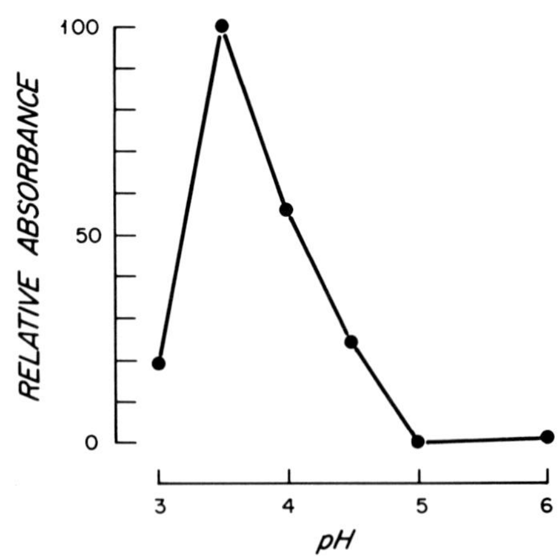

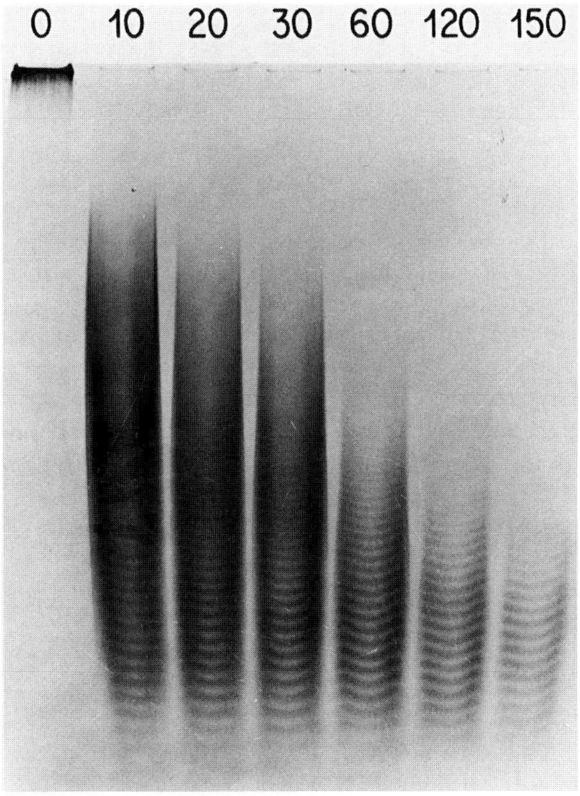

Figure 14.5 Sensitivity-enhanced polyacrylamide gel electrophoresis (SE-PAGE) of intact hyaluronate (time 0) and hyaluronate incubated with testicular hyaluronidase for progressively longer periods (10–150 minutes). Intact hyaluronate does not migrate into the gel, whereas, a ladder-like sequence of oligosaccharide cleavage products results from the endoglycosidic action of hyaluronidase. The difference in size between each band in the sequence is one disaccharide unit. Even at the shortest time interval (10 minutes), cleavage is evidenced at numerous sites within the hyaluronate chain. As incubation duration increases, there is a progressive downward shift in the average size of depolymerization product.

remains of interest in relation to the phenomenon of wound contraction. Wound contraction can be dramatic in healing cutaneous wounds and may be favored by a hyaluronate-enriched zone along the periphery—the area most affected by the contractile process.

The exact site of hyaluronidase action may be significant. In the work described thus far, wound hyaluronidase showed properties consistent with those of a lysosomal enzyme and, therefore, would represent an enzyme functioning exclusively intracellularly. Major differences in biological response can be inferred from the locus of hyaluronate depolymerization. For instance, as an endoglycosidic enzyme, hyaluronidase is not thought to lead to the complete breakdown of hyaluronate. Instead, it initiates the depolymerization process within the polysaccharide chain leading to variably-sized oligosaccharide cleavage products (Fig. 14.5) that possess biological activity in their own right. West[12] showed that partial degradation products of hyaluronate (4–25 disaccharides in length) are relatively potent angiogenic agents.

If hyaluronidase action occurs within the extracellular space, such oligosaccharides could be immediately available to influence cells, possibly leading to the expression of important biological behaviors. In contrast, if hyaluronidase functions exclusively within lysosomes, then biologically active breakdown products could not be formed from hyaluronic acid without some mechanism for limiting lysosomal digestion and for exteriorizing partial degradation products into the extracellular space. The exact site of hyaluronidase action and the nature and fate of resulting cleavage fragments have important biological significance not only in postnatal wound healing, but also in embryonic healing and embryonic development. Bernanke and Orkin[13–14] showed that hyaluronic acid is degraded exclusively intracellularly in the case of the chick cardiac cushion cell. However, a similar unequivocal observation has never been made in any mammalian system.

THE CELLULAR ORIGIN OF WOUND HYALURONIDASE

In identifying the origin of wound hyaluronidase, several candidate cells can be considered. Although inflammatory cell origin is logical in view of the known presence of such cells in healing wounds and the well-defined role of polymorphonuclear leukocytes and macrophages in lysis of bacteria and removal of necrotic debris, hyaluronidase activity is not present to a significant degree when the inflammatory infiltrate is the most intense. Hyaluronidase does not become evident until rather late in the healing sequence, that is, during or after the second week of repair when most of the inflammatory response has subsided. When hyaluronidase activities peak, the predominant cell type in the healing wound is the fibroblast. Fibroblasts could be appropriate candidate cells for detailed examination to determine whether they contain hyaluronidase activity, whether they secrete hyaluronidase, and whether they are actively involved in the catabolism of wound hyaluronate.

When fibroblasts derived from healing wounds are grown in culture (Fig. 14.6), there is a time-dependent increase in hyaluronidase activity during three weeks of culturing.[15] Interestingly, all hyaluronidase activity is confined to the cell layer; none appears in the medium, provided the cells are fed regularly. Hyaluronidase becomes detectable in culture medium only when fibroblasts begin to die. Thus, in experimental animals, hyaluronidase activity is present in wound granulation tissue fibroblasts, but hyaluronidase activity is confined entirely to the cell layer and there is no evidence of active secretion into the extracellular space.

The obvious implication from identifying hyaluronidase within fibroblasts—confined to the cellular fraction—is that the enzyme functions exclusively intracellularly (presumably within lysosomes). This finding poses the immediate problem of reconciling the presence of a macromolecular polymer in the extracellular space, with the exclusively intracellular location of the enzyme responsible for initiating depolymerization. For extracellular hyaluronate to be degraded by intracellular hyaluronidase, it is necessary for the hyaluronate molecule to be internalized by cells as a prerequisite for degradation. Inasmuch as liver endothelium has been shown to be the primary cell type responsible for degrading any hyaluronic acid that gains access to the systemic circulation (and does so by

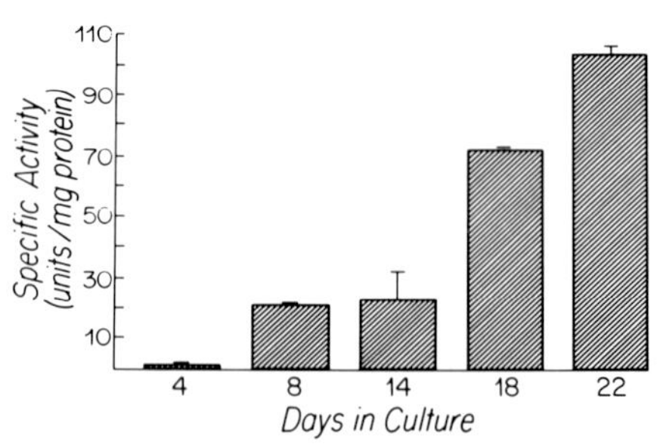

Figure 14.6 Hyaluronidase activity identified in the cellular fraction of normal dermal fibroblast cultures (in 10% serum, re-fed every third day) as a function of days in culture. Hyaluronidase activity increases progressively through day 22; free enzyme is not detectable in medium fractions as long as cells remain viable. (After Ruggiero et al., J Dent Res 66:1283–1287, 1987.)

binding and internalizing hyaluronate), a similar mechanism may be involved for fibroblastic degradation of hyaluronate locally.

Endothelial cells and other cells possess receptors for hyaluronic acid.[16–21] Hyaluronate is known to bind to cell surfaces by receptor-mediated mechanisms as a prelude to internalization and degradation in lysosomal vacuoles. While non-specific binding of hyaluronic acid to the cell surface almost certainly occurs,[22] investigators have favored the notion that binding of hyaluronate occurs by means of receptors, and that if internalization occurs at all, such receptors play a pivotal role in the internalization process. Some component of local degradation of hyaluronate by fibroblasts has been strongly advocated.[14,23,24] Assuming a similar mechanism as that shown for liver endothelium, fibroblasts in developing or remodeling tissues should exhibit cell surface, hyaluronate-specific receptors that are involved in internalizing hyaluronate for subsequent degradation.

HYALURONATE BINDING BY HUMAN DERMAL FIBROBLASTS

Recent work in our laboratory has shown that human dermal fibroblasts, when exposed to radio-labelled hyaluronate substrate, exhibit extensive binding between the substrate and the cell surface.[25] Binding is dose-dependent and it reaches a plateau at 25–50 μg/ml. This observation is consistent with receptor-mediated binding inasmuch as the process is readily saturable. Binding can be markedly enhanced by pretreatment of cells with testicular hyaluronidase. A resultant upward shift in the binding curve might be explained by the removal of hyaluronate already bound to the cell surface, thereby making additional receptors available to bind labelled substrate.

To gain insight into potential differences in binding between normal fibroblasts and those associated with various cutaneous fibrotic disorders, fibroblasts from normal skin, normal scar, hypertrophic scar, and keloid scar have been compared. The comparison is particularly relevant because hypertrophic and keloid scarring are typically characterized by accumulations of hyaluronic acid and other glycosaminoglycans.[26–28] Surprisingly, when hyaluronate binding is compared, all the fibroblasts behave similarly regardless of their tissue of origin. Thus, differences in the accumulation of hyaluronic acid in various fibrotic conditions are not immediately attributable to intrinsically different propensities for binding substrate prior to internalization and breakdown.

One of the more interesting observations is that pre-exposure of fibroblasts to non-radioactive hyaluronic acid does not significantly diminish subsequent binding of radio-labelled material. This would be unusual for standard binding studies in which the receptor sites would be occupied by unlabelled substrate and, hence, would no longer be available for binding when exposed to labeled substrate. Although several explanations are feasible, given the use of procedures in these studies favoring viability of the cells under no growth conditions, neither increases in cell number nor formation of new hyaluronic acid receptors provide a persuasive explanation. Evidence in other systems for hyaluronate receptor cycling[16] give context to our observations and suggest that hyaluronate bound to the external cell surface is internalized and degraded, thus making the receptors available again for binding.

Finally, the mere presence of receptors for hyaluronate on the fibroblastic surface may be purely coincidental to internalization of substrate by cells. The process by which hyaluronate substrate binds to cell surface receptors could be unrelated to the process by which substrate is internalized. Although the overwhelming weight of evidence in liver endothelial cells is that internalization is dependent on receptor binding, alternatives do exist. In particular, hyaluronate could be taken up by fibroblasts through a fluid phase endocytotic process. For cutaneous fibroblasts, there is no definitive evidence to prove that internalization occurs through a receptor versus a fluid phase process. Relatively simple experiments should eventually allow this distinction to be made.

INTERNALIZATION OF HYALURONATE BY HUMAN DERMAL FIBROBLASTS

Despite legitimate questions over the mechanism by which hyaluronate enters the cutaneous fibroblast, recent work in our laboratory leaves little doubt that high molecular weight hyaluronic acid is in fact internalized by fibroblasts, whatever the mechanism. When moderate amounts (35 μg/ml) of high molecular weight radio-labelled hyaluronic acid are added to fibroblasts derived from normal human skin, normal scar, hypertrophic scar, and keloid, radioactivity appears in the intracellular compartment. Of the internalized radioactivity, a distinction can be made between intact hyaluronic acid and hyaluronate-derived cleavage products by virtue of the capacity of cetylpyridinium chloride (CPC) to precipitate intact hyaluronate, leaving radioactive hyaluronate degradation products in solution.[29] Approximately half of the internalized radioactivity in fibroblasts is in the form of intact, high molecular weight (CPC-precipitable) hyaluronic acid. The remainder is hyaluronate-derived breakdown product. The intracellular CPC-precipitable radioactivity is unequivocally identified as hyaluronate by cellulose acetate electrophoresis, which shows that the material recovered from the interior of cells co-electrophoreses with an authentic hyaluronate standard. The existence of cleavage product indicates that hyaluronate is being degraded. Of the hyaluronate degradation products detected within cells, none is apparently salvaged and reused for synthesis of new glycosaminoglycan.

This observation supports a lysosomal site of hyaluronic depolymerization, since lysosomal breakdown would require hyaluronate to be exposed to the whole spectrum of other lysosomal exoglysidases leading to complete hyaluronate breakdown. If degradation occurred only to the level of monosaccharides, some of the resulting labelled monosaccharide might become available for salvage and reincorporation into other glycosaminoglycan.

Another interesting point is that the rate of cell growth is inversely related to the capacity of cells to internalize and degrade hyaluronic acid. Subconfluent, rapidly growing fibroblasts have little capacity for internalizing radioactivity. Conversely, cells in the plateau-phase of growth show a 3.5–4.2 fold increase in capacity for internalization (expressed on a per cell basis). This is of particular interest in view of recent research showing the reverse for glycosaminoglycan synthesis.[30] Growing, preconfluent cells exhibit approximately six-fold higher synthesis of glycosaminoglycan in comparison to confluent cells. Thus, when cells are actively growing, they are in a glycosaminoglycan synthetic phase. When quiescent, cells initiate internalization and degradation.

Finally, direct evidence of hyaluronidase activity in human fibroblasts has not yet been obtained. Although hyaluronidase has been identified in the fibroblasts of granulation tissue from experimental wounds in animals,[15] inability to demonstrate the enzyme in human dermal fibroblasts has sometimes been interpreted to mean that local degradation of hyaluronic acid does not occur. As a family of enzymes, the hyaluronidases are notably labile and susceptible to inactivation through minor changes in conditions.[31–32] Also, hyaluronidase may be found with an inhibitor that could co-purify with the enzyme when standard biochemical procedures are used for isolation and purification.[33]

The failure to find hyaluronidase in human dermal fibroblasts notwithstanding, recent data obtained in our laboratory shows that co-culturing human dermal fibroblasts with medium containing high molecular weight hyaluronic acid leads to formation of hyaluronate-derived oligosaccharides. Consistent with the previous observation that confluent, plateau-phase cells internalize hyaluronate to a much greater extent then do cells in log-phase growth, a far higher quantity of hyaluronate-derived depolymerization product is formed when hyaluronate is incubated with confluent cells. Whether fibroblasts participate in the breakdown of hyaluronic acid through lysosomal endoglycosidic hyaluronidase or by some other means, the net result is the same: fibroblast-mediated degradation of hyaluronic acid. Furthermore, since cleavage product can be identified in the medium, some mechanism must exist for returning partial degradation products to the extracellular space. The presence of low molecular weight (i.e., CPC-non-precipitable) cleavage products indicates that breakdown of hyaluronate takes place and that it occurs as a cell-mediated phenomenon. Sizing of CPC-non-precipitable products by gel filtration chromatography suggests that such products may be oligosaccharides. If confirmed, biological importance could be attached to such products particularly when they are returned to the extracellular space where they are believed to be angiogenic.[12]

COMPARING FIBROBLASTS FROM NORMAL AND ABNORMAL TISSUES

A surprising feature of this research has been that relatively little difference is observed in the hyaluronate processing capacity of fibroblasts derived from normal versus fibrotic tissues. Accumulation of hyaluronate (and other glycosaminoglycans) in tissue fibrosis and scarring could be explained either by increased production or by decreased degradation of glycosaminoglycan. No difference in binding, internalization or breakdown of hyaluronate was observed for fibroblasts derived from normal versus abnormal scarring. However, other differences were observed between the cell lines. Whereas normal skin and normal scar showed population doubling times of approximately 40 hours, hypertrophic scar and keloid showed much slower rates of growth (the population doubling time for hypertrophic scar was 70 hours). While there has been inconsistency in the literature over whether hypertrophic scars and keloids exhibit a higher, lower, or normal rate of growth in culture,[34–37] it is clear that a given result is highly dependent on the specific procedures of culture initiation and maintenance.

Under the conditions used in our work, fibroblasts from fibrotic cutaneous conditions grow more slowly than normal. This may be significant because growing fibroblasts do not internalize and degrade very much hyaluronic acid. If fibroblasts from abnormal tissues grow more slowly and for a longer period of time, their overall capacity for internalizing and degrading substrate could be diminished (since growing fibroblasts internalize less substrate). In addition, the total number of cells available for internalizing and degrading substrate at the plateau-phase of growth is lower, approximately half of normal. Thus, a smaller number of cells may actually be available for internalizing and degrading hyaluronate in cultures of abnormal tissues. Both slower growth and fewer fibroblasts could favor accumulation of substrate even though the capacity of any individual cell may be normal.

Another subtle, but potentially significant, difference between fibroblasts from normal and abnormal tissues concerns the amount and nature of breakdown product within the culture medium. In preliminary experiments, a significant increase in the amount of medium cleavage product was associated with fibroblasts from normal scar as compared to either normal skin or hypertrophic scar. Normal scar fibroblasts had a greater capacity to generate medium cleavage product than either normal skin or hypertrophic scar fibroblasts. In one sense then, the hypertrophic scar fibroblasts more closely resembled cells from normal skin than from normal scar. This observation reemphasizes the importance of distinguishing between normal scar and normal skin tissue. Normal scar has a moderately high capacity for remodeling. In animal studies referenced earlier, only the fibroblasts from remodeling wound granulation tissue contained hyaluronidase activity, whereas normal skin fibroblasts did not.[15]

While it is tempting to equate fibroblasts from normal scar and normal skin, it may be the lack of remodeling capacity of hypertrophic scar fibroblasts compared to that of normal scar (not normal skin) that leads to matrix accumulation. The possibility that normal skin fibroblasts do not exhibit much capacity for processing hyaluronate may be of little importance since normal skin is, by comparison, relatively static and is not ordinarily engaged in generating large quantities of matrix. Scar tissue, on the other hand, generates large amounts of matrix. Scars containing fibroblasts resembling those of normal skin may therefore be unable to appropriately process the amounts of matrix produced at the repair site. If these conclusions are confirmed, they would lead to the startling conclusion that the problem with hypertrophic scar fibroblasts is that they are normal, that is, too much like normal skin fibroblasts, whereas they preferably should closely resemble normal scar fibroblasts in their capacity for processing matrix.

CONCLUSION

Clearly, much of the work described in this chapter is of a speculative nature. The findings provide an explanation for matrix accumulation seen in abnormal scarring. Application of similar methods to study glycosaminoglycan processing in fibroblasts from scarless fetal wounds should contribute to the mosaic of understanding of both fetal and postnatal healing.

REFERENCES

1. Toole BP and Gross J: The extracellular matrix of the regenerating newt limb: Synthesis and removal of hyaluronate prior to differentiation. Dev Biol 25:57–77, 1971.
2. Toole BP and Trelstad RL: Hyaluronate production and removal during cornea development. Dev Biol 26:28, 1971.
3. Toole BP: Hyaluronate turnover during chondrogenesis in the developing chick limb bud and axial skeleton. Dev Biol 29:321, 1972.
4. Toole BP, Jackson G, Gross J: Hyaluronate in morphogenesis: Inhibition of chondrogenesis in vitro. Proc Natl Acad Sci 69:1384, 1972.
5. Polansky JR, Toole BP, Gross J: Brain hyaluronidase: Changes in activity during chick development. Science 183:862–864, 1974.

6. Toole BP: Morphogenetic role of glycosaminoglycans (acid mucopolysaccharides) in brain and other tissues. In Barondes SH (ed): Neuronal Recognition. Plenum Press, New York, 1976, pp 275–329.
7. Bentley JP: Rate of chondroitin sulfate formation in wound healing. Ann Surg 165:186, 1967.
8. Dunphy JE and Udupa KN: Chemical and histochemical sequences in normal healing wounds. N Engl J Med 253:847, 1955.
9. Bertolami CN and Donoff RB: Hyaluronidase activity during open wound healing in rabbits: A preliminary report. J Surg Res 25:256, 1978.
10. Bertolami CN and Donoff RB: Identification, characterization and purification of mammalian skin wound hyaluronidase. J Invest Derm 79:417, 1982.
11. Alexander SA and Donoff RB: Identification and localization of wound hyaluronidase. J Surg Res 27:163–167, 1979.
12. West DC, Hampson IN, Arnold F, Kumar S: Angiogenesis induced by degradation products of hyaluronic acid. Science 228:1324–1336, 1985.
13. Bernanke DH and Orkin RW: Hyaluronidase activity in embryonic chick heart muscle and cushion tissue cells. Dev Biol 106:351–359, 1984A.
14. Bernanke DH and Orkin RW: Hyaluronate binding and degradation by cultured embryonic chick cardiac cushion and myocardial cells. Dev Biol 106:360–367, 1984B.
15. Ruggiero SL, Bertolami CN, Bronson RE: Hyaluronidase activity of rabbit skin wound granulation tissue fibroblasts. J Dent Res 66:1283–1287, 1987.
16. McGary CY, Raja RH, Weigel PH: Endocytosis of hyaluronic acid by rat liver endothelial cells: Evidence for receptor cycling. Biochem J 257:875–884, 1989.
17. Smedsrod B, Pertoft H, Eriksson S, Fraser RE, Laurent TC: Studies in vitro on the uptake and degradation of sodium hyaluronate in rat liver endothelial cells. Biochem J 223:617–626, 1984.
18. Underhill CB: The interaction of hyaluronate with the cell surface: The hyaluronate receptor and the core protein. In: The Biology of Hyaluronan, Ciba Foundation Symposium 143, p 87–106, 1989.
19. Underhill CB and Toole BP: Receptors for hyaluronate on the surface of parent and virus-transformed cell lines: Binding and aggregation studies. Exp Cell Res 131:419–423, 1981.
20. Green SJ, Tarone G, Underhill CB: Distribution of hyaluronate and hyaluronate receptors in the adult lung. J Cell Sci 89:145–156, 1988.
21. Alho AM and Underhill CB: The hyaluronate receptor is preferentially expressed on proliferating epithelial cells. J Cell Biol 108:1557–1565, 1989.
22. Krumbiegel M and Arnold J: Microelectrophoresis studies of the binding of glycosaminoglycans to phosphatidylcholine liposomes. Chem Phys Lipids 54:1–7, 1990.
23. Orkin RW: Discussion of "Turnover and metabolism of hyaluronan" by Fraser JRE and Laurent TC. Symposium on the Biology of Hyaluronan. Ciba Foundation Symposium 143:53–58, 1989.
24. Orkin RW: Discussion of "Enzymatic pathways of hyaluronan metabolism" by Rodèn L, Campbell P, Fraser JRE, Laurent TC, Pertoft J, and Thompson JN. Symposium on the Biology of Hyaluronan. Ciba Foundation Symposium 143:76–85, 1989.
25. Berg S, Ellis DG, Bertolami CN: Affinity of dermal pericellular matrix for hyaluronic acid. J Dent Res 69:Abst 1976, 1990.
26. Savage K and Swann DA: A comparison of glycosaminoglycan synthesis by human fibroblasts from normal skin, normal scar, and hypertrophic scar. J Invest Derm 84:521–526, 1985.
27. Donoff RB, Swann DA, Schweidt SH: Glycosaminoglycans of normal and hypertrophic human scar tissue. Exp Molec Pathol 40:13–20, 1984.
28. Shetlar MR, Shetlar GL, Chien SF, Linares HA, Dobrkovsky M, Larson DL: The hypertrophic scar. Hexosamine containing components of burn scars. Proc Soc Exp Biol Med 139:544–547, 1972.
29. Huey G, Stair S, Stern R: Hyaluronic acid determinations: Optimizing parameters. Matrix 10:67–74, 1990.
30. Huey G, Moiin A, Stern R: Levels of [^{3}H]glucosamine incorporation into hyaluronic acid by fibroblasts is modulated by culture conditions. Matrix 10:75–83, 1990.
31. Orkin RW and Toole BP: Chick embryo fibroblasts produce two forms of hyaluronidase. J Cell Biol 85:248–256, 1980.
32. Joyce C, Jeyendran RS, Zaneveld LJD: Release, extraction, and stability of hyaluronidase associated with human spermatozoa: Comparisons with the rabbit. J Androl 6:152–161, 1985.
33. Shapiro SS, Bishop M, Kuenzig W, Tkaczevski V, Kamm JJ: Effect of ascorbic acid on hyaluronidase inhibitor. Nature 253:479–480, 1975.

34. Diegelmann RF, Cohen IK, McCoy BJ: Growth kinetics and collagen synthesis of normal skin, normal scar and keloid fibroblasts in vitro. J Cell Physiol 98:341, 1979.
35. Russell J and Witt WS: Cell size and growth characteristics of cultured fibroblasts isolated from normal and keloid tissue. Plast Reconstr Surg 57:207–212, 1976.
36. Babu M, Diegelmann R, Oliver N: Fibronectin is overproduced by keloid fibroblasts during abnormal wound healing. Mol Cell Biol 9:1642–1650, 1989.
37. Russell SB, Trupin JS, Myers JC, et al.: Differential glucocorticoid regulation of collagen mRNAs in human dermal fibroblasts. J Biol Chem 264:13730–13735, 1989.

CHAPTER **15**

Acute Inflammation in Fetal Wound Healing

Bruce A. Mast
Thomas M. Krummel

INTRODUCTION

Acute inflammation is a prominent homeostatic response in postnatal mammals that is initiated by tissue injury. Following hemostasis, the infiltration of polymorphonuclear leukocytes (PMNs) or neutrophils heralds the process of tissue repair. In contrast to adult animals, the response to tissue injury in the fetus is conspicuously devoid of acute inflammation. Indeed, the absence of neutrophils is perhaps the most consistent observation in fetal wounds. In both primarily closed linear wounds and excisional wounds in fetal sheep, Burrington noted the absence of neutrophils at wound sites.[1] Sopher made similar observations in monkey wounds[2] and Goss reported a lack of acute inflammation in incisional wounds in fetal rats.[3] Viljanto and associates,[4] Adzick and coworkers,[5] Krummel and colleagues[6] and Siebert et al.[7] similarly found no neutrophilic infiltration within various wound implants removed from fetal rabbits.

This chapter will review acute inflammation in fetal wound healing. An understanding of acute inflammation in the fetal repair process is predicated on an understanding of the mechanisms by which acute inflammation is established at the site of injury and the role neutrophils play in injured tissue. Therefore, important biologic mechanisms responsible for the acute inflammatory response will be presented, followed by a discussion of the role of acute inflammation in postnatal healing. Additionally, aspects of the developing fetal immune system that are pertinent to the function and activity of neutrophils will be covered. Finally, experiments that have specifically examined the role of acute inflammation in fetal wound healing will be examined.

MECHANISMS OF THE ACUTE INFLAMMATORY RESPONSE

Inflammation is a general response to a variety of tissue insults. Indeed, the initial description of inflammation—rubor, calor, dolor, tumor—represents the gross manifestations of this microcirculatory process. Inflammation can be divided into an acute phase and a chronic phase. The chronic phase represents an established inflammatory process with the potential for being sustained; it is characterized by mononuclear leukocytes, i.e., macrophages and lymphocytes. The acute phase of inflammation is generally transient, setting the stage for the infiltration of the cells of the chronic response. The neutrophil is the icon of acute inflammation.

The neutrophil is a circulating leukocyte derived from the bone marrow. Neutrophils are derived from pluripotent stem cells that undergo progressive differentiation, such that promyelocytes yield metamyelocytes that become myelocytes. These cells further differentiate into neutrophilic band cells that finally mature into segmented, polymorphonuclear leukocytes, also known as neutrophils.[8,9] Approximately two weeks are required for this process of maturation, representing the longest period in the neutrophil's life.[10] The response to an inflammatory stimulus involves increased production of neutrophils, as well as the mobilization of reserves of mature and immature cells in the marrow; an estimated 90% of the total neutrophil population is contained within the marrow.[11] Such mobilization results in a higher proportion of neutrophilic band cells in the peripheral blood, thus causing the classic "bandemia" associated with acute inflammatory processes.

Neutrophils contain two types of cytoplasmic granules. Azurophilic or primary granules first appear during the promyelocytic stage, while specific or secondary granules are formed subsequently, within myelocytes.[12] There are approximately three times as many specific granules as there are azurophilic granules in the mature neutrophil.[9] These granules contain biochemically active substances that are instrumental in neutrophil function (Table 15.1). Azurophilic granules contain myeloperoxidase, lysosomal (acid) hydrolases and neutral proteases. Specific granules have collagenase, lactoferrin, vitamin B-12 binding proteins, cytochrome b, histaminase, and receptors for formyl-methionyl-leucine-phenylalanine and laminin. Lysozyme is found in both azurophilic and specific granules.[9,12,13]

The establishment of acute inflammation at a site of tissue injury requires that blood-borne neutrophils exit the circulation and specifically infiltrate the site of injury. Various chemoattractants are responsible for the attraction of PMNs to the site of injury (Table 15.2). Substances related to bacterial invasion, such as N-formylated oligopeptides, are among the most important neutrophil chemoattractants. N-formylated peptides are derived from the amino terminal regions of newly synthesized bacterial proteins and are released from nonviable bacteria.[13,14] The synthetic peptide formyl-methionyl-leucine-phenylalanine (FMLP) provides the same chemotactic stimulus as soluble bacterial factors and has been used

TABLE 15.1 Contents of Neutrophil Granules

Azurophilic or Primary Granules:
Myeloperoxidase
Acid hydrolases
Neutral proteases
Lysozyme
Specific Granules:
Collagenase
Lactoferrin
Vitamin B-12 binding proteins
Cytochrome b
Histaminase
Receptors for FMLP and laminin
Lysozyme

TABLE 15.2 Neutrophil Chemoattractants

N-formylated peptides
C5a
Leukotriene B4
Platelet activating factor
Interleukin 8 (Neutrophil-activating factor)

extensively in research.[13,14,15] Therefore, the neutrophil response to FMLP demonstrates a nonspecific stimulus for chemotaxis in response to bacterial invasion. Another chemoattractant associated with bacterial invasion is C5a, a by-product of complement activation generated in the presence of bacteria.[16] Unlike FMLP and C5a, the chemoattractant leukotriene B4 is a product of neutrophil activation[12,17] and may act as a neutrophil-mediated means of maintaining the acute inflammatory response. Platelet activating factor (PAF) is another known chemoattractant for neutrophils. Neutrophil-activating peptide 1 or interleukin-8 has also been shown to be chemotactic for neutrophils in vivo.[18]

The response of PMNs to chemoattractants begins with margination of circulating neutrophils as these leukocytes adhere to the endothelium of postcapillary venules.[19] A complex of cell membrane bound glycoproteins known as the neutrophil adherence receptor or CD 18 is at least partly responsible for neutrophil-endothelial adhesion.[20,21] The importance of this receptor is demonstrated by the observation that a monoclonal antibody to CD 18 causes a dose-dependent inhibition of neutrophil migration in vivo.[20] Neutrophil adhesion to a variety of surfaces has been stimulated in vitro by FMLP and the chemotactic fragment of C5.[22] Therefore, neutrophil adherence is apparently potentiated by chemotactic substances, which is further evidenced by an observed up-regulation of the CD 18 receptor by neutrophils exposed to chemoattractants.[21]

Margination and adherence of neutrophils to the venular endothelium is followed by migration out of the vessels into the tissue by a process termed diapedesis. Increased vascular permeability may or may not be associated with this process.[23] The movement of the PMNs is along the concentration gradient of chemoattractants; a gradient as small as 1% has been reported to affect the orientation of neutrophils.[24] Locomotion occurs via the extension of pseudopodia and is thought to involve the contractile protein actin.[9]

Within the tissue, the activated neutrophil is a capable phagocyte, ingesting microorganisms and particulate matter from cellular debris. This process is facilitated by opsonins and mediated by neutrophil membrane receptors for the Fc portion of antibodies and the complement activation by-product C3b.[9] Once ingested, organisms are subjected to efficient cytotoxic processes. The oxygen-independent systems lethal to microbes are multiple and include degradation with lysozyme, neutral proteases and acid hydrolases and the toxic effects of basic proteins, lactoferrin, and phagosome acidification.[9]

The prominence of oxygen-dependent cytotoxic systems is exemplified by the early observation that increased oxygen consumption was noted in phagocytes when incubated with bacteria in vitro.[25] This phenomenon, known as the respiratory burst, is necessary to drive the multiple oxygen dependent reactions that generate substances that are cytotoxic. Superoxide anion formation is thought to be toxic due to its subsequent conversion to hydrogen peroxide, hydroxyl radicals, and singlet oxygen. The reaction catalyzed by myeloperoxidase yields the toxic substance hypochlorous acid.[9] The importance of these compounds is exemplified by the disease state known as chronic granulomatous disease of childhood. Neutrophils from patients with this condition are unable to produce hydrogen peroxide and have an increased incidence of infection by bacteria that are capable of neutralizing the hydrogen peroxide they produce (catalase-positive organisms).[15]

Upon entry of PMNs into the site of tissue injury, activation and degranulation occurs. The contents of specific granules are released first, while azurophilic degranulation is only moderate until neutrophils undergo intense phagocytosis and cell death. In addition to the cytotoxic effects on bacteria, factors released from neutrophil granules may modulate the inflammatory process. For instance, factors from specific granules have been noted to activate the complement cascade, generate C5a, and attract monocytes.[9,26] This may cause amplification of acute inflammation or the initiation of the chronic inflammatory response, thus providing a bridge to the next step in the repair process. Collagenase and elastase released from azurophilic granules may alter the extracellular matrix, thereby providing a possible facilitation of further cellular infiltration. A role in down-regulation of inflammation may also exist since a product of azurophilic granules, which degranulate later in the inflammatory process, has been observed to inactivate C5a and other chemoattractants.[9,26]

Neutrophilic infiltration into a site of tissue injury is a normal response in the processes of damage control and tissue repair. However, a balance exists between the protective function of PMNs and pathologic consequences. The multitude of substances released from or produced by neutrophils are not only toxic to microorganisms but are potentially damaging to host tissue. Neutrophils are thought to mediate vascular injury associated with endotoxemic and septic shock, ischemia-reperfusion injury and multiple organ failure.[21,27]

ACUTE INFLAMMATION IN THE FETUS

As a general concept, the immune system of the developing fetus can be considered immature. This is perhaps best exemplified by the fetus' inability to produce immunoglobulin G (IgG). The IgG present in fetal and newborn blood is maternally derived via the placenta. In regards to the acute inflammatory component of the immune system, a degree of underdevelopment is also apparent. Experimental fetal animals have been noted to be neutropenic compared to adults.[1,2,5] Additionally, neutrophilic chemotactic and phagocytic abilities may be reduced. As an extension of observations made in the newborn, the defect in phagocytosis appears to be related to suboptimal opsonization by plasma factors, rather than an inherent defect in neutrophils.[28]

Fetal and neonatal neutrophils also demonstrate an immaturity related to their various enzyme systems. Activation and superoxide production from neonatal and second trimester human fetal neutrophils is equivalent to that of adult PMNs,[29,30] although the ability to convert this free radical into the hydroxyl radical is deficient in neonatal neutrophils.[9] This apparent deficiency in hydroxyl radical formation may contribute to the diminished microbiocidal ability observed in fetal and neonatal neutrophils.[31] Infant neutrophils also exhibit decreased viability, thought to result from autooxidation due to a deficiency in enzymes such as catalase and glutathione peroxidase that protect PMNs from damage by the free radicals they generate.[32,33] Obviously, a decreased capacity of neutrophils to survive the cytotoxic substances that they liberate can affect their ability to provide bacterial defense.

Other factors exist that potentially affect the fetus' ability to mount an acute inflammatory response. The fetal complement system is underdeveloped; although some complement components are detectable in the human fetus as early as eight weeks of gestation, components are present in the fetal serum in lesser quantities than in adults.[34,35] Since by-products of complement activation are potent PMN chemoattractants, a relative deficiency of these substances may cause impaired chemotaxis. An additional factor that may contribute to a meager acute inflammatory response in the fetus is the sterile intrauterine environment. The absence of contaminating bacteria may contribute to inadequate chemotactic stimulation and activation of neutrophils.

Despite the immaturity of the various constituents of the acute inflammatory response, situations exist that demonstrate the capacity of the fetus to mount an appropriate neutrophilic response following provocation. In a study designed to investigate biliary atresia, noxious substances were injected into the biliary tree of fetal dogs. Three days following injection of sodium morrhuate, both a periportal acute inflammatory infiltrate and periportal necrosis were apparent.[36] Another example of acute inflammation in the fetus is the bowel wall of newborns with gastroschisis, a congenital defect in which there is intrauterine, extra-abdominal herniation of the intestine. Neutrophils are plentiful within the bowel wall of the herniated intestine. Neutrophil infiltration also is present in the intestine of infants with meconium peritonitis, another intrauterine abdominal disorder.

ACUTE INFLAMMATION IN POSTNATAL HEALING

The initial response to tissue injury in postnatal animals centers around hemostasis. Vasoconstriction, platelet aggregation and fibrin deposition occur in an attempt to control local hemorrhage. The deposition of fibrin creates an early wound matrix that is thought to provide a scaffold on which inflammatory cells can enter the wound site.[37,38] Neutrophil infiltration occurs as vasoconstriction is reversed by various stimuli that cause vasodilation such that acute inflammation is established at the site of injury in 12 to 24 hours.

Acute inflammation in postnatal wound healing acts primarily as a control for local bacterial contamination that occurs at the time of injury. As described above, the neutrophil is an efficient phagocyte with multiple means with which to destroy microorganisms. The primary immunologic role of the neutrophil in adult wound healing is exemplified by clinical observations as well as animal experiments. Clinically, it is well recognized that patients rendered neutropenic as a result of cytotoxic chemotherapy seldom have difficulties with wound healing as long as the wounds do not become infected. The most common wound complications in these patients are septic in nature and these infections, rather than the meager acute inflammatory response, can lead to secondary healing impairments.

Several laboratory studies have corroborated the clinical observation that wound healing can occur without a striking acute inflammatory response. Stein and Levenson studied the effect on wound healing in rats following the induction of neutropenia using anti-PMN antibodies.[39] Compared to controls, the neutropenic rats demonstrated an absence of PMNs at the wound site at 24 and 48 hours postwounding. After five days of healing, wounds from these rats had similar histologic appearances and breaking strengths compared to wounds of the control animals. Furthermore, sponges removed from wounds of neutropenic rats and from control wounds had the same hydroxyproline content, indicating a quantitatively similar deposition of collagen. Similarly, Simpson and Ross created severe neutropenia in guinea pigs using antineutrophil serum and histologically studied the healing of incisional wounds 10 days later.[40] No difference in the degree of connective tissue formation could be discerned in the wounds from the neutropenic animals compared to the controls. Another study in neutropenic guinea pigs demonstrated the importance of PMNs in the control of contaminating bacteria. Anderson et al. created open palate wounds in these animals and noted that deeper bacterial invasion had occurred in the wounds of the neutropenic guinea pigs compared to normal controls.[41]

As discussed above, substances produced by the activation of the complement system are important chemoattractants for neutrophils. Wahl and colleagues studied the role of complement in the development of acute inflammation during wound healing.[42] Guinea pigs were wounded following depletion of complement by administration of cobra venom factor. A 50% reduction in PMN infiltration was noted in the wounds of the complement depleted animals up to 48 hours following wounding. However, no differences in fibroblast proliferation, neovascularization, or connective tissue formation was observed in these animals compared to controls. Since acute inflammation was not eliminated in these complement depleted animals, it seems that other factors share responsibility for the elicitation of neutrophil infiltration into a wound site.

These studies demonstrate that the primary role of acute inflammation in postnatal wound healing is to control bacterial contamination. A reduction or elimination of PMNs at the wound site does not alter subsequent healing events such that fibroplasia and connective tissue deposition are not altered. Therefore, it appears that PMNs are not necessary for the completion of postnatal wound healing.

STUDIES OF ACUTE INFLAMMATION IN FETAL WOUND HEALING

The process of scarless fetal healing in virtually all species studied is associated with an absence of acute inflammation. In attempts to understand the significance of the lack of neutrophils in fetal wound healing several studies have been performed in which the fetal wound site has been manipulated and an acute inflammatory response has resulted. Some of these studies have attempted to specifically induce neutrophil infiltration into a fetal wound and others have noted acute inflammation as a secondary finding.

In an attempt to induce acute inflammation within a fetal wound, Krummel et al. treated fetal rabbit wounds with FMLP. The chemoattractant was introduced into fetal wound sites by the subcutaneous placement of PVA implants (Fig. 15.1) containing FMLP.[43] As expected, histologic examination of implants removed from normal untreated wounds demonstrated no neutrophils (Fig. 15.2). However, in distinct contrast, implants removed from FMLP-treated wounds after one day of healing demonstrated an acute inflammatory infiltrate (Fig. 15.3). At postwound day five, numerous fibroblasts were noted, as well as deposited collagen within implants removed from wounds treated with the chemoattractant (Fig. 15.4). This

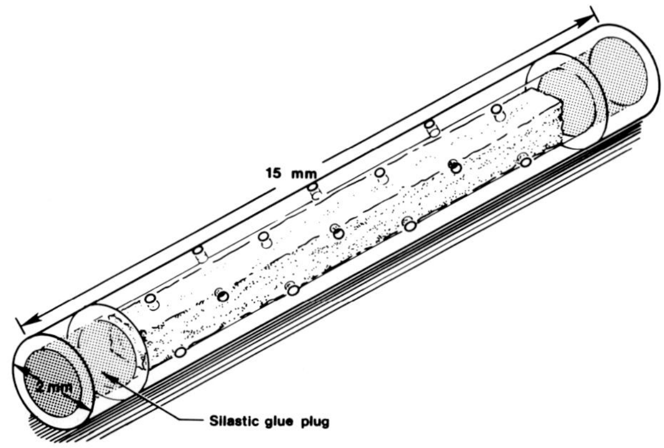

Figure 15.1 The PVA implant. This implant was initially designed for wound healing studies in humans and has been miniaturized for use in fetal studies. The implant contains a central polyvinyl alcohol sponge within a uniformly perforated silicone carrier. The entire implant is placed subcutaneously through a full thickness incision in the back of the fetus. Upon removal of the implant, the central sponge is withdrawn, thus providing easy, reliable and reproducible separation of wound tissue and surrounding normal tissue. The implant can also be used as a carrier to introduce substances into the fetal wound site. (Reprinted by permission of VCH Publishers, Inc., 220 East 23rd St., New York, NY., 10010 from: *Matrix,* Vol. 9, pp. 224–231, 1989, *Characterization and Quantitation of Wound Matrix in the Fetal Rabbit,* R. Lawrence DePalma, Thomas M. Krummel, Lucian A. Durham III, Barbara A. Michna, Brian L. Thomas, Jeffrey M. Nelson, Robert F. Diegelmann; figure 1, p. 226, a line drawing of a fetal implant).

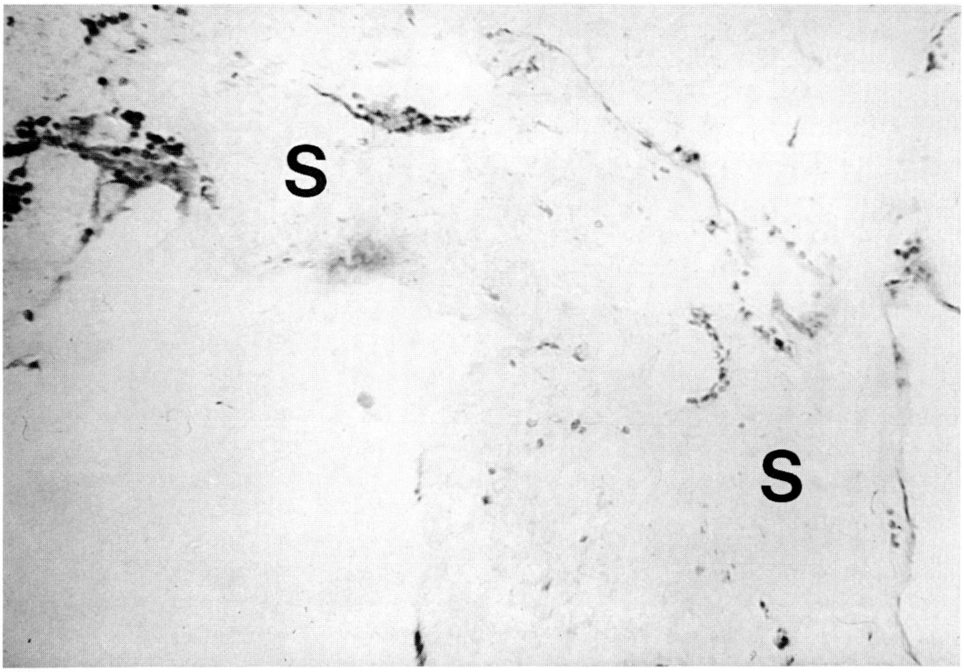

Figure 15.2 PVA implant removed from normal, untreated fetal rabbit wound after 5 days. There is an absence of infiltrating fibroblasts or collagen. Examination of implants removed after 24 hours showed no neutrophils. (Hematoxylin and eosin, magnification 64×; S is polyvinyl alcohol sponge).

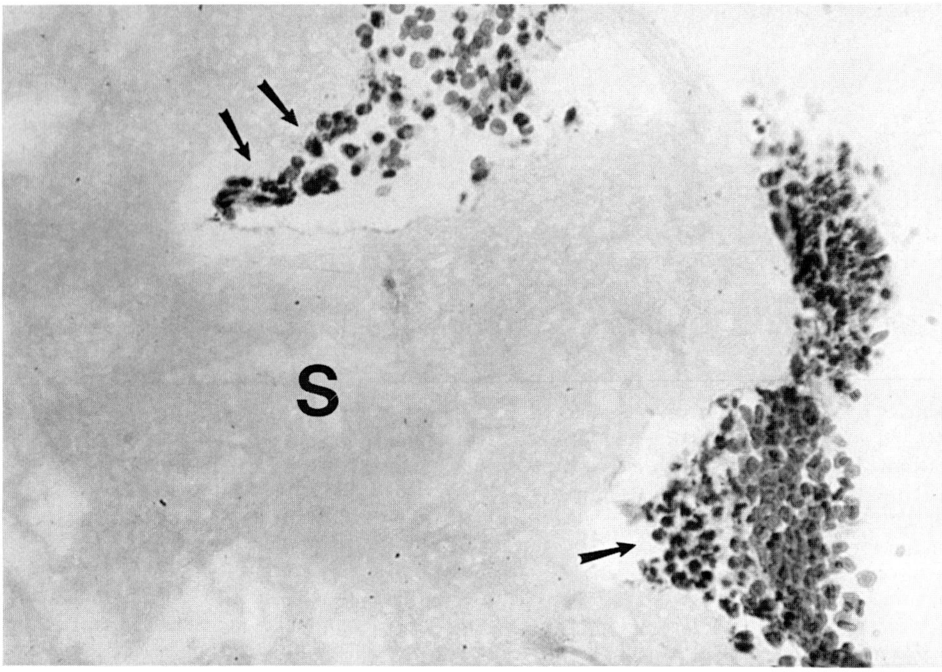

Figure 15.3 PVA implant removed after 24 hours from a fetal rabbit wound treated with 10ng of FMLP. An obvious infiltration of neutrophils (arrows) is present (Hematoxylin and eosin, magnification 100×; S is polyvinyl alcohol sponge).

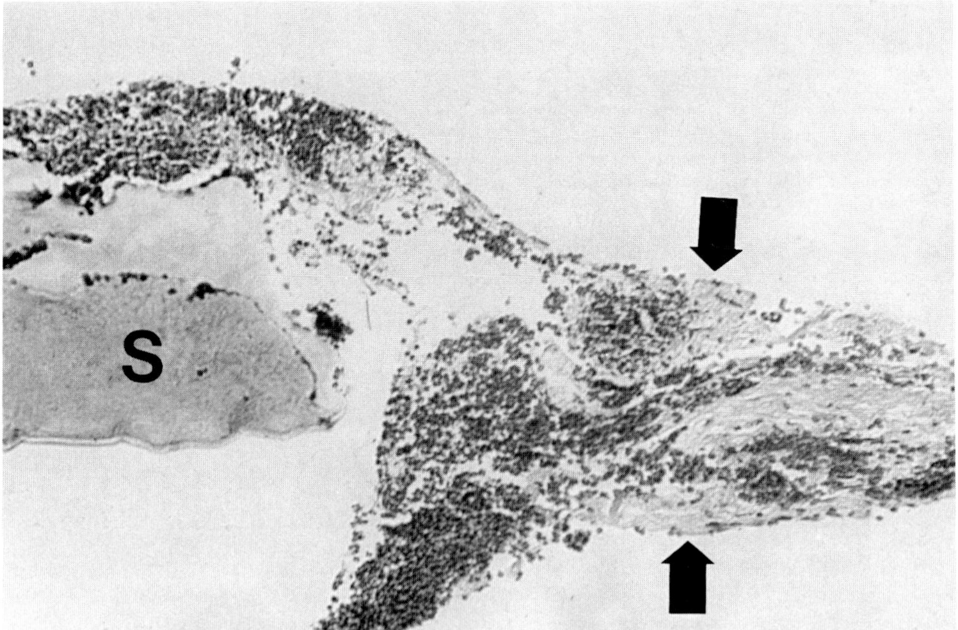

Figure 15.4 PVA implant removed after 5 days from a fetal rabbit wound treated with 50ng of FMLP. A prominent fibroblastic response (arrows) with many fibroblasts within a collagenous matrix is present surrounding the implant sponge. (Hematoxylin and eosin, magnification 40×; S is polyvinyl alcohol sponge).

was in marked contrast to the control PVA implants, which showed minimal fibroplasia and no infiltrating collagen. A moderate dose-dependent response was appreciated in that, compared to wounds treated with 10 ng of FMLP, wounds treated with 50 ng contained qualitatively more neutrophils early following injury and subsequently more fibroblasts and collagen. This study shows that fetal rabbit neutrophils can be attracted to the site of tissue injury by a known chemotactic agent. Furthermore, the establishment of acute inflammation within the fetal wound is associated with a change in the normal fetal healing response such that fibroplasia is more prominent.

A less artificial induction of acute inflammation in fetal wounds was attempted by Borchelt and colleagues by transferring the early adult wound environment into a fetal wound.[44] The rationale for this experiment was that the early adult wound environment contains factors that are responsible for the recruitment of neutrophils into the wound. PVA implants were removed from subdermal pockets on the backs of pregnant rabbits 6 to 24 hours following insertion (Fig. 15.5). The implants were then immediately inserted into fetuses of the same doe from which they were removed and then examined histologically five days later. Abundant neutrophilic infiltration was seen within the fetal implants, yet no fibroplasia or collagen deposition was noted (Fig. 15.6). Recruitment of fetal neutrophils in the wounds was inferred by the observation that the fetal wound implants contained significantly more PMNs than the adult implants (91.6 neutrophils per high power field for the fetal implants, versus 44.7 for the adult). Therefore, it appears that factors present within the early adult wound site are capable of initiating an acute inflammatory response in fetal wounds. However, unlike the provocation of acute

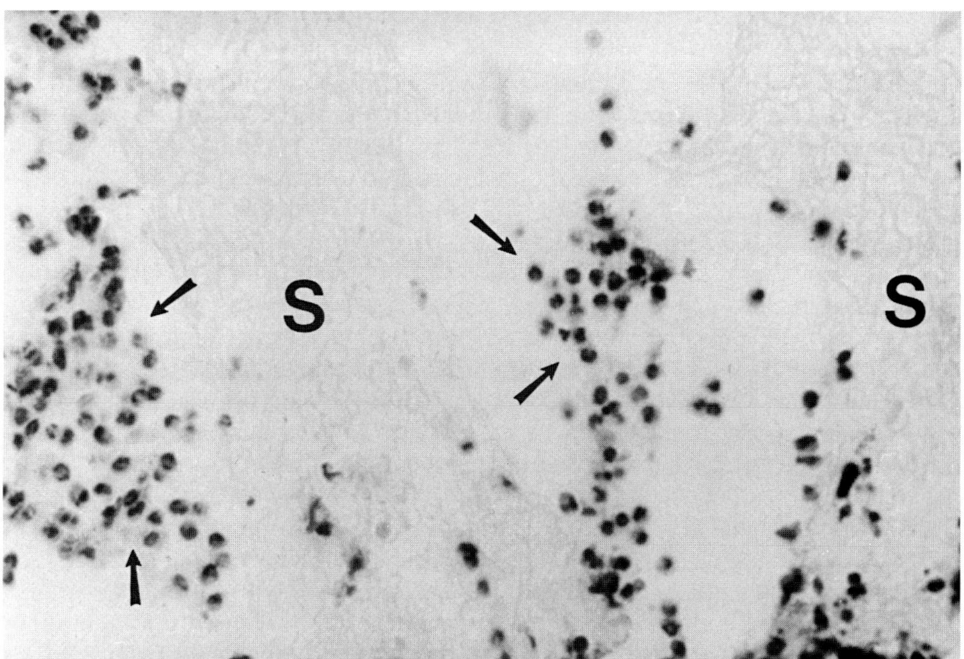

Figure 15.5 A prominent acute inflammatory response is seen in this PVA implant removed from an adult rabbit wound after 24 hours. Neutrophilic infiltration is denoted by the arrows. (Hematoxylin and eosin, magnification 100×; S is polyvinyl alcohol sponge).

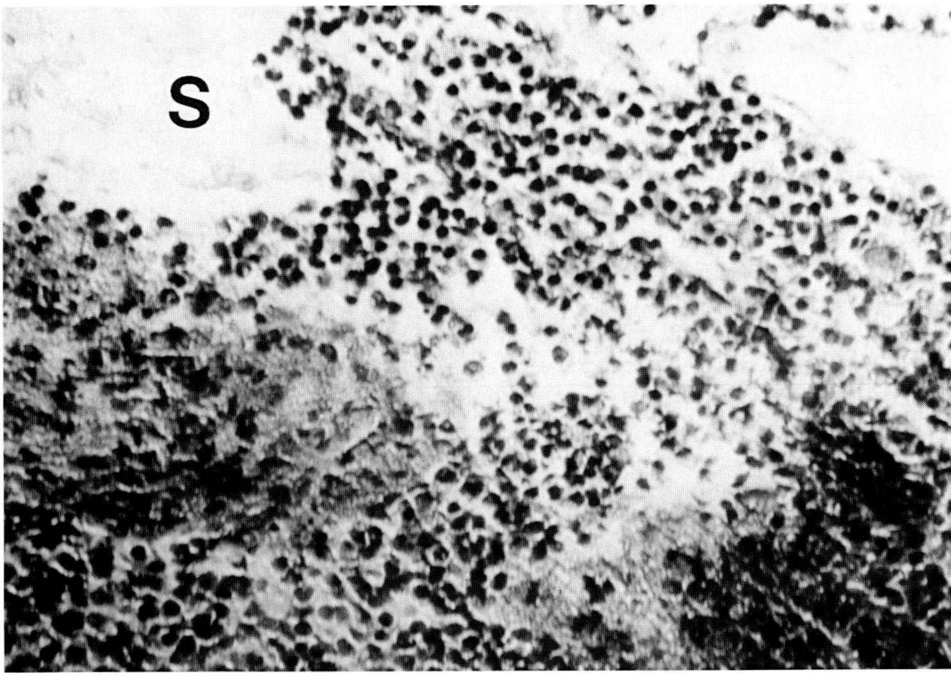

Figure 15.6 PVA implant removed from a fetal rabbit wound after 5 days. This implant was initially removed from an adult rabbit wound after 24 hours and then placed in the fetal wound site. An exuberant inflammatory response has resulted, consisting mostly of neutrophils. However, no fibroplasia or increased collagen deposition is noted compared to control wounds. (Hematoxylin and eosin, magnification 100×; S is PVA sponge).

inflammation by FMLP, neutrophils present in the wound following adult wound environment transfer, remain in the wound but do not lead to fibroplasia and collagen deposition.

Polypeptide growth factors are thought to be important mediators of granulation tissue formation during normal postnatal healing. Two such factors, transforming growth factor-β (TGF-β) and platelet derived growth factor (PDGF) have been studied extensively. Both of these factors are liberated from the alpha granules of platelets in the very early healing response and TGF-β is also secreted by macrophages. PDGF is an important mediator of postnatal healing in that it is a chemoattractant for vascular smooth muscle cells[45] and fibroblasts.[46] Similarly, TGF-β has been demonstrated to induce angiogenesis and fibrosis in vivo.[47]

The fetal response to these growth factors has also been studied by exogenously introducing TGF-β into fetal rabbit wound sites using the PVA implant.[48] After seven days of healing, the implants from TGF-β-treated wounds were encased in fibrous capsules and demonstrated abundant fibroplasia and collagen deposition. Additionally, implants removed only a few days following wounding contained neutrophils. In a similar experiment, Haynes et al. treated fetal rabbit wounds with PDGF and noted early acute inflammation and subsequent collagen deposition as well as neovascularization.[49] In both studies, implants from control, untreated wounds showed a fetal healing response characterized by a lack of acute inflammation, minimal fibroplasia, and no infiltrating collagen. Both these studies show that the fetal response to tissue injury can be converted into a healing response with typical postnatal features by the administration of growth factors important in postnatal healing. They also demonstrate that these growth factors are associated with the elicitation of acute inflammation at the fetal wound site. Since TGF-β and PDGF are not known to be chemoattractants for neutrophils, the results of this study suggest that neutrophils respond to these factors differently in fetuses compared to adults, or that the attraction of PMNs to the wound site is in response to a secondary factor that is initiated by these growth factors.

It is obvious from these studies that the absence of acute inflammation at a fetal wound site is not due to an intrinsic defect in the fetus' ability to mount an acute inflammatory response. The chemoattractive capacity of invading bacteria is thought to be simulated by the peptide FMLP. The elicitation of acute inflammation by FMLP within a fetal wound suggests that the sterile environment of the fetus fails to provide a bacterial stimulus for neutrophil recruitment, thus explaining the absence of this inflammatory response in fetal wounds. Furthermore, the observation that neutrophil infiltration occurs at the fetal wound site following placement of the early adult wound environment suggests that factors responsible for the elicitation of postnatal wound acute inflammation may be absent in the fetus. Such factors may include contaminating bacterial protein and adequate concentrations of complement activation by-products.

In normal postnatal wound healing, acute inflammation does not appear to be necessary for complete repair to occur; fibroplasia, collagen deposition and restoration of tissue integrity occur normally even when there is a muted acute inflammatory response. The establishment of neutrophil infiltration into fetal wounds by FMLP was associated with fibroblast infiltration and collagen deposition. When TGF-β and PDGF caused a fibrotic fetal healing response, it was similarly noted that neutrophils had accumulated within the wound. Therefore, an association between acute inflammation in a fetal wound and fibroplasia with increased collagen deposition appears to exist. The explanation for these observations is not clear. As discussed above, neutrophils secrete substances that modulate the immune response by further complement activation and monocyte recruitment. Perhaps the activated neutrophils within the fetal wound release such factors that affect subsequent healing events. Another explanation is that activated neutrophils may actually increase the degree of injury at the wound site by the generation of free radicals that are unable to act on ingested microorganisms in the sterile environment. The observed deficiency in the scavenger enzymes catalase and glutathione peroxidase in neonatal neutrophils suggests that a similar deficiency may exist in fetal neutrophils. The reduced activity of these enzymes may allow a longer duration of action of free radicals generated at the wound site and thus create more tissue damage. Such neutrophil-mediated injury is thought to be pathogenetically responsible for vascular damage in postnatal ischemia-reperfusion injury. This degree of injury in the fetal wound may be the nidus for causing supranormal fibroblast recruitment and collagen deposition.

Induction of acute inflammation at a fetal wound by means of transfer of an early adult wound into a fetal wound site was not associated with fibrosis. This apparent inconsistency may be explained in view of the second hypothesis offered above. Recruitment of acute inflammation into these wounds may be a manifestation of an immune response against maternal antigens or to bacterial protein contained within the implant. In this situation the activation of neutrophils would result in destruction of the foreign cells or clearance of foreign protein, rather than the unharnessed release of toxic substances that are free to injure the fetal tissue.

CONCLUSIONS AND FUTURE DIRECTIONS

One of the most consistent features of fetal wound healing, regardless of the species studied or the gestational age at which wounding occurred, is the absence of acute inflammation. The acute inflammatory response is a complicated process in which neutrophils leave the circulation and specifically infiltrate a site of tissue injury. The activated neutrophils provide a defensive role, engulfing and destroying invading microbes. Neutrophils also emit substances that may modulate the inflammatory response. The benefits of acute inflammation are not ubiquitous; neutrophils are also largely implicated in the pathogenesis of shock and associated ischemia/reperfusion injury. In normal postnatal healing, acute inflammation primarily provides a defensive role and does not appear to be necessary for the subsequent events involved in tissue repair.

Several studies presented in this chapter demonstrate that the fetus is capable of mounting an acute inflammatory response given various provocations. Therefore, neutropenia and neutrophil immaturity may not fully explain the lack of acute inflammation in fetal wounds. Furthermore, neutrophil accumulation within fetal wounds has been associated with increased fibroplasia and collagen deposition. Hypotheses are put forth that attempt to explain these observations and now the onus is on future investigators to determine the actual role fetal neutrophils may play in the repair of tissue injury. Further elucidation is required regarding the biology of the fetal neutrophils and the importance of the sterile environment as related to acute inflammation. It is becoming increasingly clear that the absence of acute inflammation in the fetal wound is not a superfluous observation. It is quite possible that the lack of neutrophils may be a vital feature that mechanistically distinguishes scarless fetal repair from fibrotic postnatal healing.

REFERENCES

1. Burrington JD: Wound healing in the fetal lamb. J Pediatr Surg 1971;6:523–528.
2. Sopher D: A study of wound healing in the foetal tissues of the cynomolgus monkey. Laboratory Animal Handbooks 1975;6:327–335.44.
3. Goss AN: Intra-uterine healing of fetal rat oral mucosal, skin and cartilage wounds. J Oral Pathol; 1977;6:35–43.
4. Viljanto J, Thomasson B, Pikkarainen J, et al.: Enzyme foetal connective tissue regeneration: A biochemical study in rabbits. Acta Chir Scand 1975;141:85–89.
5. Adzick NS, Harrison MR, Glick PL, et al.: Comparison of fetal, newborn and adult wound healing by histologic enzyme-histochemical and hydroxyproline determination. J Pediatr Surg 1985;20:315–319.
6. Krummel TM, Nelson JM, Diegelmann RF, et al.: Fetal response to injury in the rabbit. J Pediatr Surg 1987;20:315–319.
7. Siebert JW, Burd DAR, McCarthy JG, et al.: Fetal wound healing: A biochemical study of scarless healing. Plast Reconstr Surg 1990;85:495–502.
8. Riech PR: Hematology: Physiopathologic Basis for Clinical Practice. 2nd ed. Boston/Toronto: Little, Brown and Company, 1984:261–265.
9. Gallin JI: The neutrophil. In: Sampter M, Talmage DW, Frank MM, Austin KF, Claman HN, eds. Immunological Diseases. 4th ed. I. Boston/Toronto: Little, Brown and Company 1988:737–788.
10. Bainton DF, Ullyot JL, Farquhar MG: The development of neutrophilic polymorphonuclear leu-

kocytes in human bone marrow. Origin and content of azurophil and specific granules. J Exp Med 1971;134:907–934.
11. Boggs DR: Physiology of neutrophil proliferation, maturation and circulation. Clin Haematol 1975;4:535–551.
12. Baggiolini M, and Dewald B: The neutrophil. Int Archs Allergy Appl Immun 1985;76 (Suppl. 1):13–20.
13. Babior BM: Function of neutrophils and mononuclear phagocytes. In: Wyngaarden, JB, Smith, LH, eds. Cecil Textbook of Medicine. 17th ed. Philadelphia: WB Saunders, 1985:942–949.
14. Schiffmann E, Corcoran B, and Wahl S: N-formylmethionyl peptides as chemoattractants for leukocytes. Proc Natl Acad Sci USA 1975;72:1059–1062.
15. Robbins SL, Cotran RS, Kumar V: Pathologic Basis of Disease. 3rd ed. Philadelphia: WB Saunders 1984:48–52.
16. Craddock PR, Hammerschmidt P, White JG, et al.: Complement (C5a) induced granulocyte aggregation in vitro. J Clin Invest 1977;60:260–264.
17. Ford-Hutchinson AW, Bray M, Doig MV, et al.: Leukotriene B, a potent chemokinetic and aggregating substance released from polymorphonuclear leukocytes. Nature 1980;286:264–265.
18. Colditz IG, Zwahlen RD, Baggiolini M: Neutrophil accumulation and plasma leakage induced in vivo by neutrophil-activating peptide-1. J Leuko Biol 1990;48:129–137.
19. Smith RPC, Lackie JM, Wilkinson PC: The effects of chemotactic factors on the adhesiveness of rabbit neutrophil granulocytes. Exp Cell Res 1979;122:169–177.
20. Price TH, Beatty PG, Corpuz SR: In vivo inhibition of neutrophil function in the rabbit using monoclonal antibody to CD 18. Immunol 1987;139:4174–4177.
21. Welbourne R, Goldman G, Kobzik L, et al.: Neutrophil adherence receptors (CD 18) in ischemia. Dissociation between quantitative cell surface expression and diapedesis mediated by leukotriene B4. J Immunol 1990;145:1906–1911.
22. O'Flaherty JF, Kreutzer DL, Ward PA: The influence of chemotactic factors on neutrophil adhesiveness. Inflammation 1978;3:37–48.
23. Ryan GB, and Majno G: Inflammation. Kalamazoo: The Upjohn Company 1977:26.
24. Zigmond SH: The ability of polymorphonuclear leukocytes to orient in gradients of chemotactic factors. J Cell Biol 1977;75:606–616.
25. Baldridge CW, Gerard RW: The extra respiration of phagocytosis. Am J Physiol 1933;103:235–236.
26. Wright DG, Gallin JI: A functional differentiation of human neutrophil granules: Generation of C5a by a specific (secondary) granule product and inactivation of C5a by azurophil (primary) granule products. J Immunol 1977;119:1068–1076.
27. Vedder NB, Winn RK, Rice CL, et al.: Neutrophil-mediated vascular injury in shock and multiple organ failure. Perspectives in Shock Research: Metabolism, Immunology, Mediators, and Models. Alan R. Liss, 1989:181–191.
28. Koronos SB: The newborn: Perinatal pediatrics. In: Hughs, JG, Griffith, JF, eds. Synopsis of Pediatrics. 6th ed. St. Louis: CV Mosby, 1984:314.
29. Newburger PE: Superoxide generation by human fetal granulocytes. Pediatr Res 1982;16:373–376.
30. Shigeoka AO, Santos JI, Hill HR: Functional analysis of neutrophil granulocytes from healthy, infected, and stressed neonates. J Pediatr 1979;95:454–460.
31. Mills EL, Thompson T, Bjorkston B, et al.: The chemiluminescence response and bacteriocidal activity of polymorphonuclear neutrophils from newborns and their mothers. Pediatrics 1979; 63:429–434.
32. Strauss RG, Snyder EL: Neutrophils from human infants exhibit decreased viability. Pediatr Res 1981;15:794–797.
33. Strauss RG, Snyder EL, Wallace PD, et al.: Oxygen-detoxifying enzymes in neutrophils of infants and their mothers. J Lab Clin Med 1980;95:897–904.
34. Kohler, PF: Maturation of the human complement system. I. Onset, time and sites of fetal C1q, C4, C3 and C5 synthesis. J Clin Invest 1973;52:671–677.
35. Adinolfi, M: Human complement: Onset and site of synthesis during fetal life. Amer J Dis Child 1977;131:1015–1023.
36. Holder TM, Ashcroft KW: The effects of bile duct ligation and inflammation in the fetus. J Pediatr Surg 1967;2:35–40.
37. Schilling JA: Wound healing. Surg Clin North Amer 1976;56:859–874.
38. Weigel PH, Fuller GM, LeBoeuf RD: A model for the role of hyaluronic acid and fibrin in the

early events during the inflammatory response and wound healing. J Theor Biol 1986;119:219–234.
39. Stein JM, Levenson SM: Effect of the inflammatory reaction on subsequent wound healing. Surg Forum 1966;17:484–485.
40. Simpson DM, Ross R: The neutrophilic leukocyte in wound repair: A study with antineutrophil serum. J Clin Invest 197;51:2009–2023.
41. Andersen L, Attstrom R, Fejerskov O: Effect of experimental neutropenia on oral wound healing in guinea pigs. Scand J Dent Res 1978;86:237–247.
42. Wahl SM, Arend WP, Ross, R: The effect of complement depletion on wound healing. Amer J Pathol 1974;75:73–83.
43. Krummel TM, Thomas BL, Diegelmann RF, et al.: Chemoattraction of neutrophils into a fetal wound site results in fibrosis. Unpublished observations.
44. Borchelt BD, Krummel TM, Cawthorn JW, et al.: Transposition of an early adult wound to a fetal rabbit wound does not result in recruitment of fibroblasts. Surg Forum 1989;40:555–557.
45. Grotendorst GR, Chang T, Seppa HEJ, et al.: Platelet-derived growth factor is a chemoattractant for vascular smooth muscle cells. J Cell Physiol 1983;113:261–266.
46. Seppa HE, Grotendorst GR, Seppa SI, et al.: The platelet-derived growth factor is a chemoattractant for fibroblasts. J Cell Biol 1982;92:584–588.
47. Roberts AB, Sporn MR, Assoian RK, et al.: Transforming growth factor type β: Rapid induction of fibrosis and angiogenesis in vitro and stimulation of collagen formation in vitro. Proc Natl Acad Sci USA 1986;83:4167–4171.
48. Krummel TM, Michna BA, Thomas BL, et al.: Transforming growth factor-β induces fibrosis in a fetal wound model. J Pediatr Surg 1988;23:647–652.
49. Haynes JH, Johnson DE, Flood LC, et al.: Platelet-derived growth factor induces fibrosis at a fetal wound site. Surg Forum 1990;41:641–643.

CHAPTER **16**

Metabolic Aspects of Fetal Wound Repair

Mark N. Ahrendt
Michael T. Longaker
Michael D. Caldwell

The healing fetal wound has a unique environment that is influenced by the maternal circulation, placenta, fetal circulation, and amniotic fluid. To understand the metabolism of the fetal wound, it is necessary to review the effect of these different compartments on fetal metabolism.

FETAL CARBOHYDRATE METABOLISM

Fetal metabolism has been an intensively investigated area particularly in the ovine (sheep) model. Glucose is the major source of energy for the ovine fetus. Sheep are ruminants and have low plasma glucose concentrations. Ovine fetal plasma glucose concentrations average 20 mg/dl, well below maternal levels (50 mg/dl). In the basal state, fetal plasma glucose is derived from the mother via the placenta. This occurs by facilitated diffusion and is concentration gradient dependent.[1] Anand using [^{14}C]-labeled glucose has shown that fetal sheep lack gluconeogenesis.[2] In the basal state there is also no fetal hepatic glucose production from glycogenolysis. Fetal glycogenolysis can be stimulated by infusion of epinephrine[3] or supraphysiologic concentrations of glucagon.[4] The absence of basal and the presence of stimulated glycogenolysis is consistent with an immature developmental state. Thus glycogenolysis has an insignificant role in fetal glucose homeostasis.

The disposition of fetal plasma glucose is by either oxidation or tissue accretion. Approximately 50% of fetal glucose is oxidized for immediate energy use. This accounts for about 50% of basal fetal oxygen consumption.[5] Glucose disposal is regulated by several mechanisms. Plasma glucose concentration is the prominent regulatory mechanism.[2,6] Several glucoregulatory hormones also have effects on fetal glucose metabolism. Insulin can potentiate and enhance fetal glucose utilization.[7,8] As mentioned above, glucagon causes a glycemic response at supraphysiologic doses[4] and catecholamines are highly potent in inducing fetal glucose production.[3] These hormonal effects are secondary in importance to the primary control, glucose availability.

Fetal ovine blood is unique in that the fructose concentration is three to four times higher than glucose.[9] Glucose is converted in the placenta to sorbitol, then transported to the fetal liver where it is converted to fructose. There is insignificant umbilical uptake and there is a slow fetal turnover of fructose.[10] Therefore fructose has minimal importance as an energy substrate during fetal fasting, and its major role appears to be the regulation of the osmotic pressures in fetal sheep plasma.[11]

FETAL LACTATE METABOLISM

Lactate is a substantial metabolite in fetal sheep. The fetal plasma concentration of lactate is twice that of the maternal ewe. The lactate/pyruvate ratio is similar in mother and fetus. Fetal lactate comes from three sources: endogenous aerobic production from glucose (50%), non-glucose substrates (25%), and placental glycolysis (25%).[12] The actual disposition of fetal lactate is unclear. It is thought that the majority of the lactate is used in aerobic metabolism, via the citric acid cycle. Lactate oxidation may account for 15%–25% of the fetal sheep's oxygen consumption.[13] The sites of fetal lactate consumption are not well defined. The only fetal sites shown to consume lactate are the heart and portal venous drained viscera.[12] In contrast to adult sheep, lactate consumption has not been shown in the fetal liver or kidney. The low fetal hepatic phosphoenolpyruvate carboxykinase (PEPCK) activity should prevent gluconeogenesis.

FETAL AMINO ACID METABOLISM

In addition to glucose and lactate, amino acids contribute to the energy and tissue accretion needs of the fetal sheep. The umbilical uptake of nitrogen in the ovine fetus is 1.5 gm/kg/day. Approximately 40% of this is used for tissue accretion and the rest is used as a fuel.[9] Amino acids contribute approximately 25% of the fetal sheep's oxygen consumption.[14]

The concentration of most amino acids is higher in fetal circulation than in the maternal plasma. Several authors have suggested that this is related to active transport of amino acids from the ewe to the fetus.[15,16] Lemons et al. showed that neutral amino acids (glutamine, glycine, alanine, proline, threonine, valine, serine, leucine, tyrosine, asparagine, isoleucine) and basic amino acids (arginine, lysine) are actively transported by the placenta into fetal blood, while the acidic amino acids (glutamine, aspartate, and taurine) are not.[17] These data on the umbilical uptake of amino acids correlate well with the plasma concentrations of these amino acids. Interestingly, the ovine fetus delivers large amounts of glutamate to the placenta. This suggests that glutamate and aspartate are produced in the fetus. Raiha has shown that the urea cycle is less active in the immature fetus, thus the transfer of glutamate to the placenta may represent a major pathway of nitrogen excretion in early intrauterine life.[18]

Bell et al. have examined the ovine fetal uptake of amino acids.[19] Figure 16.1 shows the plasma amino acid concentrations in arterial blood of the mid- and late gestation fetus. Mid-gestational fetal blood has a higher glycine/serine ratio, lower concentration of valine, and higher concentrations of the acidic amino acids glutamate and aspartate as well as of lysine, ornithine, methionine, and histidine compared to late gestation fetal blood. These investigators found a similar pattern between mid- and late gestational uptake of most amino acids (Figure 16.2). The one exception was the relatively large placental uptake of fetal serine during mid-gestation. Again, this indicates production of serine in the fetus but the reason for this is unclear. It has been suggested that there is limited degradation of serine in pathways such as the transsulphuration pathway for cysteine.[19]

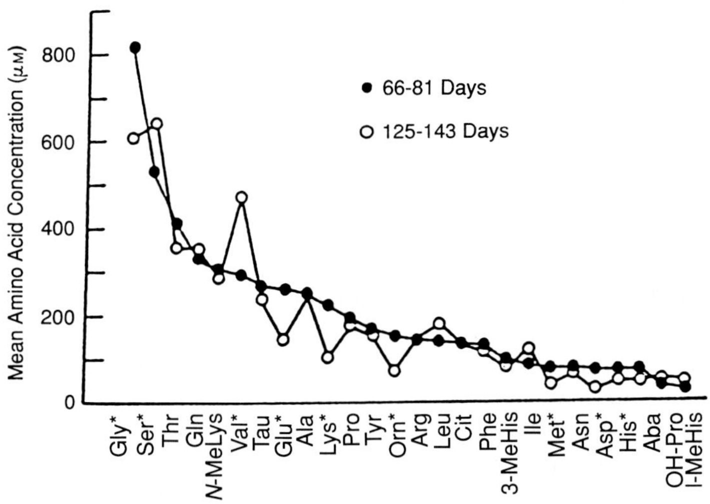

Figure 16.1 Mean amino acid concentrations in arterial blood of mid- and late-gestation fetuses. The mid-gestation values are plotted in order of decreasing concentrations. Amino acids with significantly different concentrations at the two gestational ages are marked by an asterisk. (From Bell AW, Kennaugh JM, Battaglia FC, Meschia G. Uptake of amino acids and ammonia at mid-gestation by the fetal lamb. QJ Exp Physiol 74:635–643, 1989.)

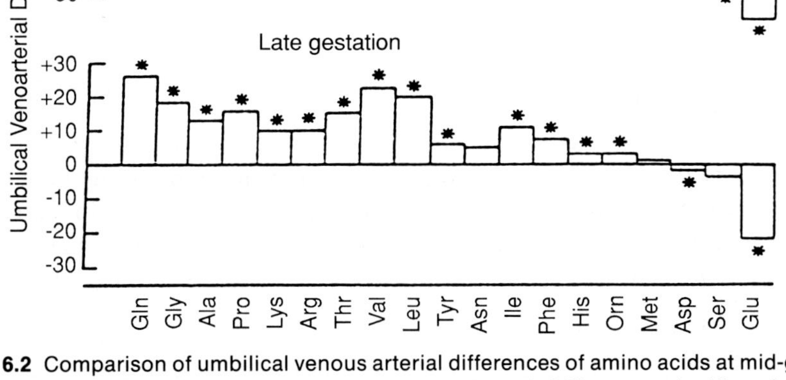

Figure 16.2 Comparison of umbilical venous arterial differences of amino acids at mid-gestation (age range 66–81 days) and late gestation (age range 125–143). Differences significantly different from zero are marked by an asterisk. (From Bell AW, Kennaugh JM, Battaglia FC, Meschia G. Uptake of amino acids and ammonia at mid-gestation by the fetal lamb. QJ Exp Physiol 74:635–643, 1989.)

FETAL FREE FATTY ACID METABOLISM

The source of fetal lipids is either from placental transfer of free fatty acids (FFA) or from endogenous production of nonessential fatty acids. There is an obligatory requirement for placental transfer of essential fatty acids. In the ovine fetus, there is a low umbilical uptake of long-chain FFA, β-hydroxybutyrate, and acetoacetate and there is no correlation with maternal levels in the fed and fasted states.[20,21] The above findings, in addition to the observed low plasma concentration of FFA and keto acids, suggests that these substrates would contribute negligibly to the caloric intake of the ovine fetus.

ADULT OVINE METABOLISM

The majority of the dietary carbohydrate in the adult sheep is fermented in the gut to acetic, propionic, and butyric acids. A small amount of the carbohydrate is absorbed from the gut. The majority of the plasma glucose is derived from hepatic gluconeogenesis. Substrates for this process are amino acids and propionic acid from the gut, glycerol from triglyceride breakdown, lactate from glycolysis (in muscle, erythrocytes, and brain), and amino acids from skeletal muscle protein turnover. Up to 50% of the glucose may be produced from propionic acid absorbed from the gastrointestinal tract.[22] In contrast to nonruminants, glucose is constantly released into the blood by the liver.[23] Interestingly, more glucose is released in the fed state than the fasted state. This occurs because in the fasted state there is less substrate for hepatic gluconeogenesis. Another factor in this setting is the low potential for glycogen storage.

Short-chain fatty acids account for 50%–80% of the digestible energy in sheep. The primary fatty acids used in energy production are acetic and butyric acids. These fatty acids are unable to be used for gluconeogenesis and are therefore used for oxidation and lipogenesis. This spares the ruminant's small supply of glucose for more important pathways.

OVINE PLACENTAL METABOLISM

The maternal metabolism does not always have a direct influence on fetal metabolism. Substances from the mother may take either of two pathways to the fetus. In the first pathway the placenta acts only to transport a substance from one vascular compartment to the other. In the second pathway the placenta will take up the substance and modify it prior to its release in the fetal circulation.

The placenta is one of the most complex mammalian tissues. It provides nutrients, gas exchange, and excretes wastes for the fetus. In addition, it is a complex endocrine organ that affects both fetus and mother. This review will focus on the metabolic processes of the placenta.

PLACENTAL CARBOHYDRATE METABOLISM

Glucose transported to the placenta can be transferred to the fetus by a facilitated diffusion system or can be taken up by the placenta for its own metabolism. Battaglia has found approximately two-thirds of the glucose is used by the placenta and the remainder is transported to the fetus.[24] The placenta also consumes 50% of the oxygen supplied to it.

Once in the placenta, glucose can enter a pathway toward glycogen synthesis or toward glucose oxidation. Both the glycolytic and hexose monophosphate shunt pathways for glucose have been described in the placenta.[25] The glycolytic pathway is the most significant route for placental glucose utilization. The lactate is produced under aerobic glycolysis. The lactate is transported to the fetus and may be an important substrate for the fetus.

Other important carbohydrates are glycogen and fructose. Glycogen is found in the placenta, but its function is unclear. It has been suggested that the placenta may store glucose in the form of glycogen for later release, but this has never been substantiated. The other important placental carbohydrate is fructose. As discussed above, fructose is found in high concentration in the ovine fetal plasma. The placenta is important in the first step in fructose production: the conversion of glucose to sorbitol (catalyzed by aldose reductase). The sorbitol is then converted to fructose in the fetal liver.[26]

PLACENTAL FREE FATTY ACID METABOLISM

Free fatty acid (FFA) transport across the placenta is variable from species to species. In sheep and rats there is very little transport of free fatty acids.[25] Rabbits have substantially more FFA transport across the placenta,[25] which appears to take place by an active transport system.

PLACENTAL AMINO ACID METABOLISM

The placenta obtains amino acids (AA) from the maternal plasma. Early in gestation AA are used primarily for protein synthesis related to rapid placental growth. Later in gestation, placental protein synthesis is related to production of hormones and fetal plasma proteins. Maternal plasma FAA are modified by the placenta and then transported to the fetus. This protein synthesis is under the hormonal control of estrogen and insulin.[25]

Characteristics of placental AA transport have been summarized by Szabo and Grimaldi.[25] These characteristics include: 1) active transport; 2) discrimination among different amino acids; 3) competitive inhibition for certain AA.

PLACENTAL HORMONES

The placenta produces a variety of hormones. One in particular, placental lactogen (PL), influences fetal metabolism. It is a growth hormone-like placental protein that has anabolic effects on fetal amino acid and glycogen metabolism and stimulates insulin and somatomedin production by fetal tissues.[27] The biological actions of PL in the fetus are mediated through PL receptors. These receptors have recently been identified in the fetal ovine liver.[28] Placental lactogen stimulates glycogen synthesis and inhibits the glycogenolytic effect of glucagon in fetal hepatocytes. Human PL increases the uptake of the amino acid, α-aminoisobutyric acid (AIB), by fetal fibroblasts and myoblasts.[29]

Placental lactogen influences the production of insulin-like growth factors in maternal and fetal tissue. Insulin-like growth factor I and II are polypeptides with substantial sequence identity to and biological properties of insulin. They are noncovalently bound to a specific carrier protein. This carrier protein: 1) abolishes the acute insulin-like actions typical of the free polypeptides; 2) restricts their permeability through capillaries; and 3) inhibits their access to membrane receptors.[3] The properties of the native (protein bound) IGF have not been determined because purification procedures dissociate the polypeptide from the carrier protein.

The biological effects of IGF I and II can be divided into rapid and chronic effects. The rapid effects are qualitatively indistinguishable from those of insulin and include stimulation of glucose uptake, oxidation in adipose cells and rat heart muscle, and increased glycogen and RNA synthesis in rat osteoblasts.[31] The chronic effects include increased DNA synthesis, increased cell multiplication, enhanced differentiation of cells from chick embryo ectoderm, and enhanced growth in mice.[32]

AMNIOTIC FLUID

Since fetal wounds are continuously bathed in amniotic fluid (AF), the amniotic fluid components could play an important role in the healing wound. There are several fetal compartments that contribute to the composition of amniotic fluid. The fetal urine contributes the greatest volume to AF and continuously modifies its composition throughout gestation.[32] The fetal lung, nasopharyngeal cavity, and buccal cavity also contribute lesser amounts to the composition of AF. The AF can also be modified by the amnion.

Several investigators have determined the components of AF and their concentrations. Wales and Murdoch examined the AF components at several time points during the first trimester of sheep (Table 16.1).[33] The components remain relatively stable during this time period. The glucose concentration in AF is less than both fetal and adult serum concentrations while the fructose is slightly less than in fetal serum. In comparison, the lactate concentration in AF is greater than the adult serum concentration but less than in fetal serum. The individual concentrations of amino acids in sheep AF have not been reported. The amino acids of bovine AF have been determined and may be similar to those in sheep (Table 16.2).[34] All AF amino acid concentrations are less than the fetal and adult serum concentrations.

Growth factors are another important component of AF. Various growth fac-

TABLE 16.1 Concentration of Several Organic Compounds in Ovine Amniotic Fluid

Component	Amniotic Fluid* Day 44 (mM)	Serum†# Fetal (mM)	Serum†# Adult (mM)
Fructose	3.28	4.01	0.06
Glucose	1.39	0.98	2.58
Lactic Acid	1.44	1.98	0.82

* Adapted from Wales RG, Murdoch RN. Changes in the composition of sheep fetal fluids during early pregnancy. *J Reprod Fert* 1973;33:197–205.

† Adapted from Meznarich HK, Hay WW, Sparks JW, et al. Fructose disposal and oxidation rates in the ovine fetus. *QJ Exp Physiol* 1987;72:617–625.

Adapted from Char VC and Creasy RK. Lactate and pyruvate as fetal metabolic substrates. *Pediat Res* 1976;10:231–234.

TABLE 16.2 Concentrations of Amino Acids in Amniotic Fluid of the Bovine Fetus (μM)

Isoleucine	21.8
Leucine	34.0
Lysine	39.3
Methionine	12.4
Phenylalanine	16.2
Threonine	34.0
Valine	69.6
Arginine	30.3
Cystathionine	14.3
Glutamine & Asparagine	162.7
Histidine	16.1
Tyrosine	11.5
Alanine	222.4
Aspartic Acid	3.5
Glycine	219.9
Glutamic Acid	73.3
Proline	38.8
Serine	38.8

Adapted from Baetz AL, Hubbert WT, Graham CK. Developmental changes of free amino acids in bovine fetal fluids with gestational age and the interrelationships between the amino acid concentrations in the fluid compartments. *J Reprod Fert* 1975;44:437–444.

tors, if present, could have a significant influence on fetal wound healing. Of the many growth factors identified thus far only two have been isolated from AF: epidermal growth factor (EGF)[35] and insulin-like growth factor (IGF).[36] As mentioned above, IGF has properties that could be very beneficial to the healing fetal wound. Presumably there are other growth factors in AF that require identification.

ADULT MAMMALIAN WOUND METABOLISM

One of the initial events in the process of wound healing is the development of the cellular infiltrate. This occurs in an orderly fashion with the consecutive cell populations producing factors that modify or promote the function of subsequent cell types. The first cell type to enter the wound environment is the polymorphonuclear leukocyte (PMN). PMNs reach a peak during days one to three after injury and are followed closely by a macrophage and lymphocytic infiltrate. These two cell lines produce many different factors that modify the wound environment. Several of these factors augment fibroblast proliferation and function. The metabolism of these cell lines influence the progression of the healing wound.

It has been clearly shown by several investigators that the marked increase in tissue deoxyribonucleic acid (DNA) content in response to wounding is directly related to the developing cellular infiltrate.[37,38] The accumulation of DNA can be prevented by blocking the cellular infiltrate.[37] Therefore the increasing DNA content is consistent with an infiltration of new cells rather than proliferation of the native cells at the site of injury.

The metabolism of the cellular infiltrate in wounded tissue has been characterized. Wounded tissue shows an increase in glucose uptake and lactate production as compared to non-wounded tissue. Several investigators have shown this to be due to aerobic glycolysis.[39–41] It has also been determined that wounded tissue has comparable oxygen consumption to non-wounded tissue.[42] Thus with the aerobic glycolysis of wounded tissue, glucose and pyruvate are oxidized by the tricarboxylic acid (TCA) cycle and the increased lactate production is presumably due to decreased activity of the NADH shuttles.[43]

Most amino acids accumulate within the wound fluid over time. The exceptions are cystine, tryptophan, arginine, and citrulline. It has been suggested that the increase in many AA in wound fluid (hydroxyproline, threonine, glutamine, proline, alanine, valine, isoleucine, histidine, leucine) is secondary to proteolysis.[44] The increase in taurine, glutamic, and aspartic acids could be explained by cell lysis, since these AA are the major intracellular AA pool of inflammatory cells. The disappearance of arginine and the accumulation of ornithine appear to be related to the release of arginase from macrophage lysis.[45]

CELL CYCLE EVENTS

It has been shown in wound fibroblasts that early wound fluid stimulates and later wound fluid inhibits cell proliferation.[46] This is consistent with Pardee's work showing that extracellular factors determine whether quiescent cells will begin to proliferate and whether a normal proliferating cell in G_1 will continue to cycle or become quiescent.[47] Therefore, G_0 and G_1 would logically represent the sphere of influence within the cell cycle for the extracellular factors found in wound fluid. The term G_0 is used to define the quiescent state while G_1 was originally defined as the temporal gap between the easily observed events of mitosis and DNA synthesis.

The G_1 state has been divided into subphases.[48] In sequence from G_0 to S, these subphases are referred to as competence, entry, progression, and assembly (Fig. 16.3). Competence has been produced in untransformed BALB/C 3T3 mouse fibroblasts by platelet-derived growth factor.[49] Competent cells will further progress toward S-phase under the influence of EGF, insulin, or plasma.[49] However, in the absence of essential amino acids, the cell cycle stops and does not enter the progression subphase.[41] The only growth factor thought to be required by the fibroblasts during the progression subphase is insulin-like growth factor (IGF-1).[50] Little is known about the extracellular requirements for the assembly

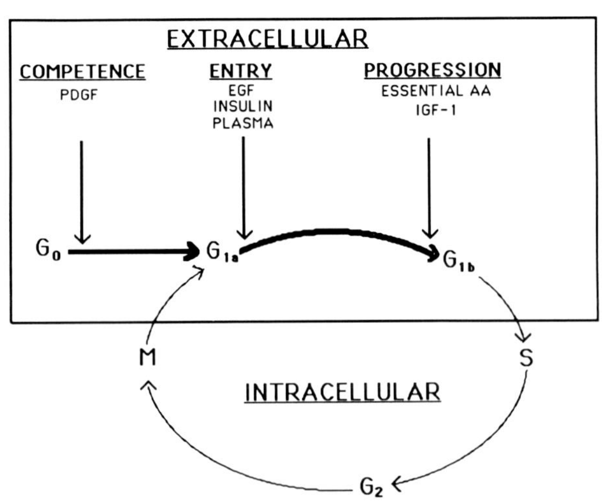

Figure 16.3 Cell cycle as adapted from Pardee. (From Pardee AB. G_1 events and regulation of cell proliferation. Science 246:603–608, 1989.)

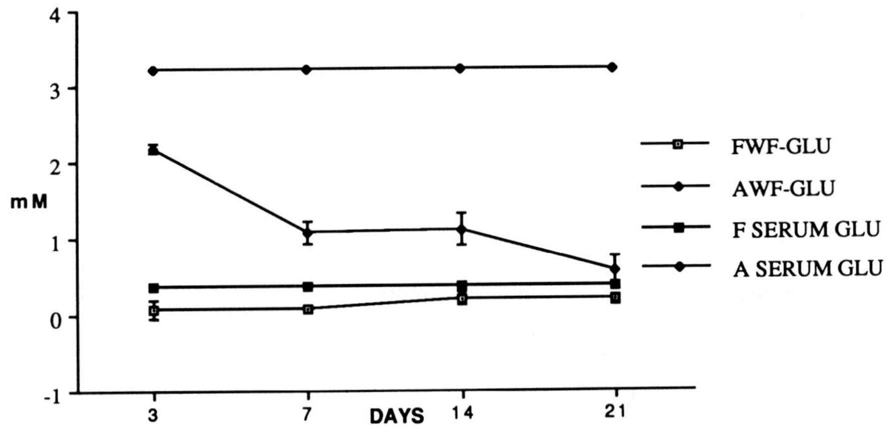

Figure 16.4 Glucose concentration of fetal (FWF) and adult (AWF) wound fluid in sheep.

subphase. Therefore, there are many factors, known and unknown, that are required by proliferating cells.

FETAL WOUND METABOLISM

Fetal wound metabolism is a new field. All of the work has been accomplished within the last year using the fetal sheep model.[51] Briefly, Hunt-Schilling wound chambers are implanted in the fetus of a 100 day gestation (early third trimester) pregnant ewe. Wound fluid was aspirated on days three, seven, 14, and 21 postimplantation. Fetal and maternal serum were also obtained at the same time points.

Fetal wound fluid (FWF) and adult wound fluid (AWF) glucose concentrations are compared in Figure 16.4. The AWF glucose gradually decreased over the three weeks of the study. The AWF glucose is less than the serum glucose. The FWF glucose remains constant over the same time period. As would be expected, the FWF and fetal serum glucose are less than in the adult. In the adult wound,

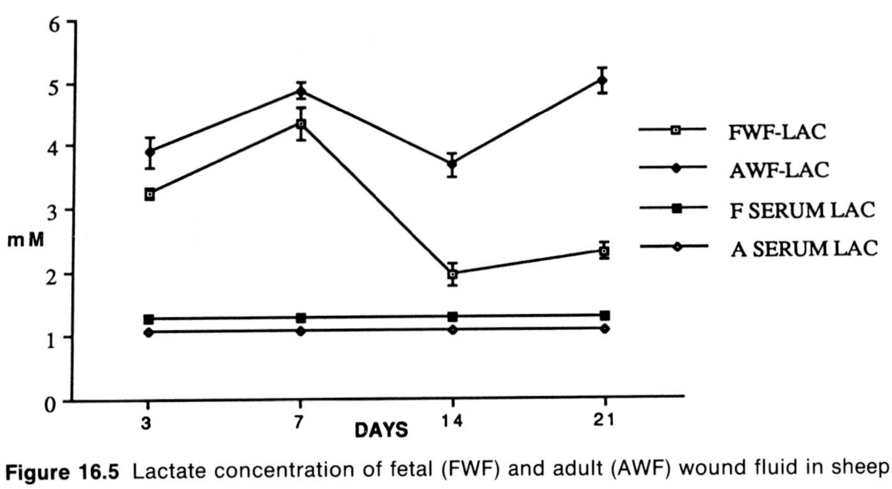

Figure 16.5 Lactate concentration of fetal (FWF) and adult (AWF) wound fluid in sheep.

the finding of decreasing glucose concentration is consistent with that seen in other adult mammalian wounds. As noted above, this is thought to be secondary to increased glucose uptake by inflammatory cells. In the fetal wound the glucose remains relatively constant. One might speculate that the glucose uptake may not be as large in fetal wounds as in adult wounds due to the absence of an acute inflammatory infiltrate in fetal wounds.

The ovine fetus uses lactate as one of its major substrates, therefore the lactate concentration in the wound was also of interest (Fig. 16.5). As compared to the serum lactate concentration, the FWF lactate concentration is two times higher. The AWF lactate is four times higher than the adult serum lactate level. In the AWF, the lactate concentration remains constant over this time period. In the FWF there is a decrease in the wound fluid lactate after the first seven days. This may indicate that the fetal wound preferentially uses lactate instead of glucose. It may also be possible that less lactate is being delivered to the wound environment.

Amino acid (AA) concentrations in fetal and adult wounds were also determined at days three, seven, 14, and 21. In fetal wounds the majority of AA decreased in concentration over time. This is distinctly different from other mammalian models and may be a characteristic of ruminant metabolism. Those AA which decrease include: arginine, lysine, histidine, ornithine, phenylalanine, tyrosine,

TABLE 16.3 Wound Fluid as a "Growth Medium"

Amino Acid	Eagle (1962)* (μM)	Fetal Wound Fluid Day (μM) 3	7	14	21
"Essential" AA					
Isoleucine	400	156	79	68	63
Leucine	400	286	163	155	152
Lysine	400	160	115	115	98
Methionine	100	133	63	72	92
Phenylalanine	200	111	76	72	75
Threonine	400	183	105	251	287
Tryptophan	50	46	53	69	62
Valine	400	475	307	266	246
(Arginine)	600	79	86	73	46
(Cystine)	100	22	16	20	18
(Glutamine)	2000	600	341	346	458
(Histidine)	200	57	69	74	85
(Tyrosine)	200	110	88	78	74
"Non-Essential" AA					
Alanine	100	302	241	235	271
Asparagine	100	57	46	43	59
Aspartic Acid	100	41	39	38	47
Glycine	100	782	436	454	987
Glutamic Acid	100	128	130	63	95
Proline	100	251	184	179	302
Serine	100	683	480	655	1124
Glucose	5500	63	85	200	187
Lactate	1000	3230	4330	1940	2290

* From Eagle H, Piez KA. Amino acid pools, protein synthesis and protein turnover in human cell cultures. In Holde JT (ed.) "Amino Acid Pools," Amsterdam: Elsevier, pp 694–707.

leucine, valine, isoleucine, methionine, and glutamine. The AA which increase are: tryptophan, taurine, serine, hydroxyproline, glycine, and threonine. The group of AA which are unchanged include: cysteine, proline, alanine, citrulline, aspartate, and asparagine.

The results of the adult wound fluid amino acid pattern are similar to that of the fetal wound fluid. The majority of AA decreased over time. Those AA that decrease include: arginine, lysine, histidine, ornithine, tyrosine, leucine, valine, isoleucine, alanine, aspartate, glutamate, and asparagine. The AA that increase are: tryptophan, hydroxyproline, and citrulline. The group of AA that are unchanged: cysteine, taurine, proline, methionine, glutamine, phenylalanine, serine, and threonine.

As discussed in the cell cycle section, extracellular factors found within wound fluid can affect cell proliferation. Eagle's work in 1962 showed that the extracellular amino acid concentration is a crucial determinant of the rate of cell proliferation.[52] Listed in Table 16.3 are Eagle's minimum substrate concentrations necessary for optimal mammalian cell proliferation in culture. Listed next to these recommended values are the concentrations of various substrates found within fetal wound fluid. The amino acids listed in parentheses under "essential" amino acids are those which Eagle found to be necessary for cell proliferation, although these amino acids are not felt to be essential to the entire mammalian organism. Eagle's work was done in nonruminants but several investigators have used Eagle's medium to successfully grow fetal ovine cell cultures.[53,54] Examination of the table reveals that almost all amino acids fail to reach the minimum concentrations required by cells to proliferate. How this may influence cell proliferation in the healing wound is unclear, but it is tempting to speculate that factors must be present within the ovine wound fluid which will increase amino acid uptake and thereby allow an appropriate intracellular amino acid concentration for cell replication. These data raise many questions about fetal wound metabolism and only further work will help elucidate the answers.

REFERENCES

1. Simmons MA, Battaglia FC, Meschia G: Placenta transfer of glucose. J Dev Physiol 1:227–243, 1979.
2. Anand RS, Sperling MA, Ganguli S, et al.: Bidirectional placental transfer of glucose and its turnover in fetal and maternal sheep. Pediatr Res 13:783–787, 1979.
3. Sperling MA, Ganguli S, Leslie N: Fetal-perinatal catecholamine secretion: Role in perinatal glucose homeostasis. Am J Physiol 247:E69–E74, 1984.
4. Deveskar SU, Ganguli S, Styer D, et al.: Glucose dynamics in sheep: Evidence for glucagon resistance in the fetus. Am J Physiol 246:E256–E265, 1984.
5. Hay WH Jr, Myers SA, Sparks JW, et al.: Glucose and lactate oxidation rates in the fetal lamb. Proc Soc Exp Biol Med 173:553–563, 1983.
6. Hay WH Jr, Sparks JW, Wilkening RB, et al.: Fetal glucose uptake and utilization as a function of maternal glucose concentration. Am J Physiol 246:E237–E242, 1984.
7. Hay WH Jr, Meznarich HK: The effect of hyperinsulinemia on glucose utilization and oxidation and on oxygen consumption in the fetal lamb. QJ Exp Physiol 71:689–698, 1986.
8. Carson BS, Philipps AF, Simmons MA, et al.: Effects of a sustained insulin infusion upon glucose uptake and oxygenation of the ovine fetus. Pediatr Res 14:147–152, 1980.
9. Battaglia FC, Meschia G: Principal substrates of fetal metabolism. Physiol Rev 58:499–527, 1978.
10. Tsoulos NG, Colwell JR, Battaglia FC, et al.: Comparison of glucose, fructose and oxygen uptakes by fetuses of fed and starved ewes. Ann J Physiol 221:234–237, 1971.
11. Faber JJ, Thornburg KL: Transfer of nutrients and wastes. In Placental Physiology. Raven Press, New York, 1983, p 153.

12. Sparks JW, Hay WW Jr, Bonds D, et al.: Simultaneous measurements of lactate turnover rate and umbilical lactate uptake in the fetal lamb. J Clin Invest 70:179–192, 1982.
13. Burd LI, Jones MD Jr, Simmons MA, et al.: Placental production and foetal utilisation of lactate and pyruvate. Nature (London) 254:710–711, 1975.
14. Lemons JA, Schreiner RL: Amino acid metabolism in the ovine fetus. Am J Physiol 244:E459–466, 1983.
15. Dancis J, Money WL, Springer D: Transport of amino acids by placenta. Am J Obstet Gynecol 101:820–829, 1968.
16. Feldman BH, Christensen HN: Placental transport of model amino acids. Proc Soc Exptl Biol Med 109:700–702, 1962.
17. Lemmons JA, Adcock EW, Jones MD Jr, et al.: Umbilical uptake of amino acids in the unstressed fetal lamb. J Clin Invest 58:1428–1434, 1976.
18. Raiha NCR, Kekomaki M: Developmental aspects of amino acid metabolism in the human. In Ghadimi H (ed): Total Parenteral Nutrition. John Wiley & Sons, Inc., New York, 1986, p 208.
19. Bell AW, Kennaugh JM, Battaglia FC, Meschia G: Uptake of amino acids and ammonia at mid-gestation by the fetal lamb. Quert J Exp Physiol 74:635–643, 1989.
20. James E, Meschia G, Battaglia FC: A-V differences of free fatty acids and glycerol in the ovine umbilical circulation. Proc Soc Exptl Biol Med 138:823–826, 1971.
21. Morriss FH Jr, Boyd RDH, Makowski EL, et al.: Umbilical V-A differences of acetoacetate and betahydroxybutyrate in fed and starved ewes. Proc Soc Exptl Biol Med 145:879–883, 1974.
22. Leng RA, Steele JW, Luick JR: Contribution of propionate to glucose synthesis in sheep. Biochem J 103:785, 1967.
23. Barker JM: The metabolism of carbohydrate and volatile fatty acids in the marsupial, Setonix Brachyurus. Quert J Exptl Physiol 46:54, 1961.
24. Battaglia FC: Placental transport and utilization of amino acids and carbohydrates. Federation Proc 45:2508–2512, 1986.
25. Szabo AJ, Grimaldi RD: The metabolism of the placenta. Adv Metab Discord 4:185–228, 1970.
26. Hers HG: Sorbitol in seminal vesicles and in foetal blood of the sheep. Biochem J 66:30, 1957.
27. Freemark M, Comer M, Mularoni T, et al.: Nutritional regulation of the placental lactogen receptor in fetal liver: Implications for fetal metabolism and growth. Endocrinology 125:1504–1512, 1989.
28. Freemark M, Handwerger S: The glycogenic effects of placental lactogen and growth hormone in ovine fetal liver are mediated through binding to specific fetal oPL receptors. Endocrinology 118:613, 1986.
29. Hill DJ, Crace CJ, Strain AJ, Milner RDG: Regulation of amino acid uptake and deoxyribonucleic acid synthesis in isolated human fetal fibroblasts and myoblasts: Effect of human placental lactogen, somatomedin-c, multiplication-stimulating activity and insulin. J Clin Endocrin Metab 62:753–760, 1986.
30. Zapf J, Schoenle E, Jagars G, et al.: Inhibition of the action of non-suppressible insulin-like activity on isolated rat fat cells by binding to its carrier protein. J Clin Invest 63:1077–1084, 1979.
31. Zapf J, Schmid CH, Froesch ER: Biological and immunological properties of insulin-like growth factors I and II. Clinics in Endo and Metab 13:3–30, 1984.
32. Mellor DJ, Slater JS: Some aspects of the physiology of sheep foetal fluids. Br Vet J 130:238–247, 1974.
33. Wales RG, Murdoch RN: Changes in the composition of sheep fetal fluids during early pregnancy. J Reprod Fert 33:197–205, 1973.
34. Baetz AL, Hubbert WT, Graham CK: Developmental changes of free amino acids in bovine fetal fluids with gestational age and the interrelationships between the amino acid concentration in the fluid compartments. J Reprod Fert 44:437–444, 1975.
35. Scott SM, Buenaflor GG, Orth DN: Immunoreactive human epidermal growth factor concentrations in amniotic fluid, umbilical artery and vein serum, and placenta in full-term and preterm infants. Biol Neonate 56:246–251, 1989.
36. Merimee TJ, Grant M, Tyson JE: Insulin-like growth factors in amniotic fluid. J Clin Endocrinol Metab 59:752–755, 1984.
37. Ross R: The fibroblast and wound repair. Biol Rev 43:51–96, 1968.
38. Falcone PA, Caldwell MD: Wound metabolism. Clin Plast Surg 17:443–456, 1990.
39. Caldwell MD, Shearer J, Morris A: Evidence for aerobic glycolysis in lambda-carrageenan wounded skeletal muscle. J Surg Res 37:63–68, 1984.
40. Hunt TK, Twomey P, Zederfeldt B: Respiratory gas tensions and pH in healing wounds. Amer J Surg 114:302–307, 1967.
41. Silver I: Tissue pO_2 changes in acute inflammation. Adv Exp Med Biol 94:769–774, 1977.

42. Caldwell MD: Carbohydrate and energy metabolism in healing wounds. In Barbul A, Pines E, Caldwell M, et al (eds): Growth Factors and Other Aspects of Wound Healing: Biological and Clinical Implications. Alan R. Liss, Inc., New York, 1988, pp 183–213.
43. Lehninger AL: Biochemistry. Worth Publishers, New York, 1975.
44. Caldwell MD, Mastrofrancesco B, Shearer J, Bereiter D: The temporal changes in amino acid concentration within wound fluid—A putative rationale. Prog Clin Biol Res 365:205–222, 1990.
45. Alvina JE, Caldwell MD, Henery WL, Mills CD: Regulation of macrophage functions by L-arginine. J Trauma 29:842–846, 1989.
46. Mills CD, Pricolo VE, Albina JE, Caldwell MD: Concomitant macrophage and fibroblast/lymphocyte inhibition by wound fluid: The "arginine-deficiency of inflammation" is a partial explanation. Prog Clin Biol Res 365:193–204, 1990.
47. Pardee AB: G_1 events and regulation of cell proliferation. Science 246:603–608, 1989.
48. Temin HM: Stimulation by serum of multiplication of stationary chicken cells. J Cell Physiol 78:161, 1971.
49. Cross F, Weintraub H, Roberts J: Simple and complex cell cycles. Ann Rev Cell Biol 5:341, 1989.
50. Leof EB, et al.: Epidermal growth factor (EGF) is required only during the traverse of early G_1 in PDGF stimulated density-arrested BALB/C 3T3 cells. Exp Cell Res 147:202, 1983.
51. Longaker MT, Chiu ES, Harrison MR, et al.: Studies in fetal wound healing. IV. Hyaluronic acid-stimulating activity distinguishes fetal wound fluid from adult wound fluid. Ann Surg 210:667–672, 1989.
52. Eagle H, Piez KA: Amino acid pools, protein synthesis, and protein turnover in human cell cultures. In Holde JT (ed): Amino Acid Pools; Amsterdam, Elsevier, 1987, pp 694–707.
53. Godkin JD, Bazer FW, Roberts RM: Protein production by cultures established from day 14–16 sheep and pig conceptuses. J Reprod Fert 74:377–382, 1985.
54. Godkin JD, Bazer FW, Moffatt J, et al.: Purification and properties of a major, low molecular weight protein released by the trophoblast of sheep blastocysts at day 13–21. J Reprod Fert 65:141–150.

CHAPTER 17

In Vitro Fetal Wound Healing Models

D. Andrew R. Burd
Michael T. Longaker
N. Scott Adzick

Postnatal wound healing is a complex, macrophage-effected, fibroproliferative repair which results in scarring. Fetal and postnatal healing appear to differ both in rate and result; fetal repair is more rapid and is associated with a lack of scarring.[1–5] The mechanisms underlying these differences are unknown.

In vitro wound healing models eliminate systemic circulatory factors and permit elucidation of the effect of local factors on wound healing. Considering the central role played by circulating cells which have become incorporated into the wound, it is not surprising that wound healing does not occur in explants of postnatal skin. In contrast, fetal wounds appear to have more autonomy. If we hypothesize that local tissue fibroblasts are the architects and engineers of embryonic dermal development, then the process of regeneration following wounding in the fetus might be stimulated by giving the appropriate signal or signals to these fibroblasts. A fundamental question concerns the origin of the signal: macrophage, fibroblast, or epidermal cell? Perhaps it is not a cellular response at all but rather a signal from the extracellular matrix by peptide regulatory factors or an enzymatically manipulated mechanism. Whatever the case, the development of in vitro fetal wound healing models to study the effect of local factors on this process becomes a very attractive prospect.

The possibilities for studying fetal wound healing in vitro extend from looking at the behavior of cells to studying the entire fetus. Examples include laboratory created "tissues" using fetal cells and collagen such as the fibroblast populated collagen lattice (see Chapter 9) as well as the embryonic mouse and chick models (see Chapter 18). In this chapter, we will describe two in vitro fetal wound healing models: 1) a confluent fibroblast monolayer that is "wounded" with a scratch, and 2) a full-thickness fetal sheep skin explant model.

EXPERIMENTAL BACKGROUND

Research into maintaining fetuses or fetal tissue in laboratory conditions is not a recent phenomenon. Over 20 years ago, workers were reporting the maintenance of isolated fetuses in conditions which permitted certain physiological studies.[6] These cultures, however, did not result in growth or differentiation of the fetus.

Kistler and colleagues have studied fetal rat wound healing responses both in the normal intrauterine environment and in whole-limb organ culture at 19 days gestation.[7] Re-epithelialization and dermal regeneration of fetal rat skin wounds occurred in both groups. A subsequent study determined the serum factor requirements for in vitro closure of fetal skin wounds in limb buds at 13 days gestation.[8] While re-epithelialization did not occur in the absence of serum, addition of either fetal calf serum or Ultroser G (a serum substitute) resulted in wound closure within one day. Cyclohexamide, an inhibitor of protein synthesis, reversibly inhibited wound healing. Using dialysis, ultrafiltration and HPLC fractionation of Ultroser G, it was shown that high molecular weight factors (greater than 25,000 d) were required for epidermal wound closure.

A further report from this group examined the ontogenic transition of wound healing patterns in fetal rat skin.[9] Full-thickness defects were made in fetal rats of either 16 or 18 days gestation. These defects were then excised en bloc and cultured in a submerged system using pins mounted on a teflon ring to stretch the skin. The wounds from the 16 day gestation fetuses, maintained in a culture medium of buffered Dulbecco's Modified minimal essential media (DMEM), antibiotics, serum and aprotinin, closed in three days. The wounds from the 18 day gestation fetuses remained open in vitro. In contrast, wounds in 16 day fetuses in vivo appeared to close by co-optation of the surrounding skin, whereas wounds in 18 day fetuses demonstrated a "postnatal" type of healing with invasion of inflammatory cells and re-epithelialization.

THE FIBROBLAST SCRATCH MODEL

Wound healing in the adult is a dynamic process involving both cellular migration and repair. Fibroblasts migrate into the wound and form a connective tissue matrix. Directed migration has been observed in fibroblasts and is thought to be one of the controlling mechanisms of wound repair.[10–12] Fibroblast migration and the trophic factors involved are critical aspects of wound healing. Previous work has demonstrated that adult serum contains chemoattractants for fibroblasts in vitro.[10]

Several in vitro techniques have been used for analyzing cell migration into an artificially created acellular area on a confluent monolayer of cells.[11,13,14] Using a modification of the technique developed by Todaro et al.,[13] we studied the effect of fetal versus adult serum on the movement of fibroblasts. By employing in vitro models, it may be possible to identify and resolve some of the individual components that participate in the dynamic process of in vivo wound repair.[13]

We developed an in vitro model of wound healing, using scratches made in a confluent monolayer of human neonatal foreskin fibroblasts (Fig. 17.1).[15] The effects of either 120 day gestation fetal calf serum (FCS) or postnatal calf serum on the migration of fibroblasts were compared. Scratches were made on confluent fibroblasts grown on coverslips, creating a trough 10–12 cell diameters in width.

Differences between fetal and postnatal calf serum-incubated fibroblasts grown on coverslips were observed within 15 minutes of exposure. Cells in fetal serum began to change both shape and orientation and to move into the trough created by the scratch. The fibroblasts incubated in fetal calf serum completely filled in the trough within 16 hours while those incubated in calf serum did not do so even after 24 hours. We estimate that, at any point, there was a 50% lag time in the migration of the fibroblasts in the presence of postnatal calf serum (Fig. 17.2). This difference in migration and filling was not a function of mitogenesis; the mitogenicity of the two sera were comparable. The results suggest that fibroblast

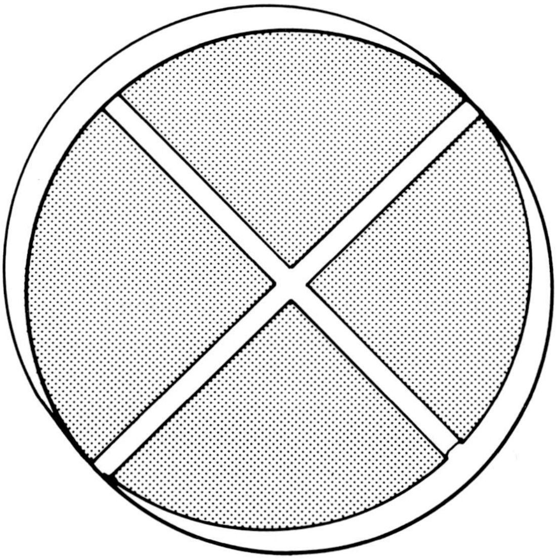

Figure 17.1 Confluent monolayer of human neonatal dermal fibroblasts were "scratched" diagonally in two directions, creating an "X" pattern. This "wound" trough was approximately ten to twelve cell widths in diameter. Serial phase photomicroscopy documented the temporal progression of wound closure.

migration in vitro is accelerated by the fetal serum. A similar mechanism may occur in vivo and may underlie the ability of the fetal wound to heal more rapidly.

The purpose of the scratch model experiment was to determine if fetal serum contained unique components that stimulated the process of wound healing in a fetal-like manner, i.e., that some of the unique properties of fetal wound healing could be attributed to the properties of fetal serum rather than being intrinsic to the fetal cells themselves. In our previous studies, a hyaluronic acid (HA) stimulating factor was detected, which enhanced HA deposition in cultured human fibroblasts.[16,17] In this study, we demonstrated that fetal calf serum also enhanced migration of fibroblasts. We postulate that the cell migration factor of serum and the HA stimulating factor are perhaps identical or related substances, but this will require direct evidence.

The 120 day FCS was selected because of our previous work showing that serum at this gestational age has peak HA-stimulating activity.[16] We have also shown previously that preconfluent fibroblasts synthesize large quantities of HA. This synthesis was sensitive to contact inhibition, which caused HA deposition

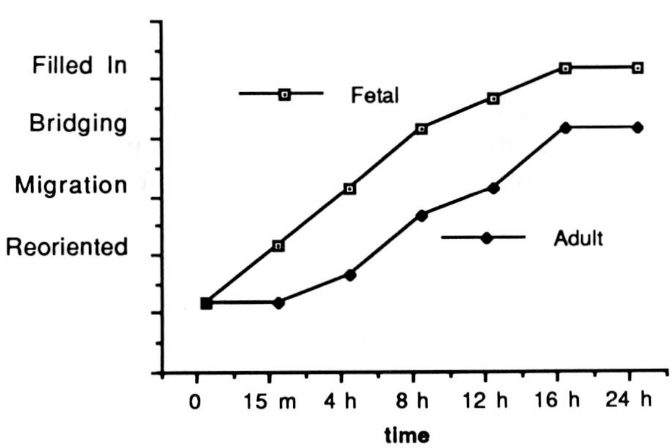

Figure 17.2 Schematic representation of the progression of fibroblast migration to eventually fill in the scratch wound. We estimated a 50% lag time in the migration of neonatal fibroblasts bathed in postnatal (*adult*) calf serum compared to *fetal* calf serum.

to shut down when cells reach confluence. We hypothesize that formation of the scratch separated fibroblasts and reversed the contact inhibition for the fibroblasts adjacent to the scratch, allowing them to synthesize HA once again. Under the influence of greater levels of HA stimulating factor in the 120-day FCS, the ability of fibroblasts to synthesize HA was enhanced further and an environment conducive to cell motility and migration was created.[18–20] On the other hand, postnatal calf serum contains very little HA-stimulating activity, resulting in far less HA production by fibroblasts.[16,17]

Fibroblasts incubated in the "fetal" environment filled in the scratch more quickly than those in the "adult" environment. We suggest that a similar mechanism may underlie the ability of the in vivo fetal wound to heal more rapidly, and that a component of the unique properties of fetal wound healing may be attributed to components of fetal serum.

This in vitro wound healing model has limitations. There is a lack of a dermal-epidermal component, and angiogenesis is entirely absent. We are now attempting to use fetal and adult dermal-epidermal combinations to explore further mechanisms of accelerated fetal wound healing. By mixing fetal and adult dermis and epidermis, we expect to identify additional signals that modulate the rate and quality of fetal wound healing, and focus on events that allow for healing without scar formation.

THE FETAL SHEEP SKIN EXPLANT MODEL

The concept of using wounded explant cultures of fetal skin stemmed from the work of Dr. Sigrid Regaur, who was able to maintain multiple adult skin explants in culture and then treat them with a wide range of topically applied growth factors. By placing the explants on gauze in the culture dishes she was able to keep the surface of the explant above the level of the culture medium and yet maintain adequate nutritional exchange within the entire explant to maintain viability.[21]

Using this basic physical concept and fetal skin, we developed an in vitro fetal wound model that fulfilled certain criteria: a) was in viable tissue but isolated from the circulation, b) retained morphological integrity, and c) allowed us to evaluate dermal and epidermal healing separately. After preliminary studies with fetal rabbit and adult pig skin which demonstrated no re-epithelialization, we successfully achieved a suitable model using fetal sheep skin.[22]

The initial problem was to determine an optimum culture medium for the composite tissue. The major cell types within the skin are keratinocytes in the epidermis and fibroblasts in the dermis. In monolayer culture these cells have different requirements for optimum growth. Initial experiments were performed using the complete medium for either pure fibroblast or pure epidermal cell culture. Medium for fibroblast cell cultures consists of DMEM (Gibco, Grand Island, NY) with 10% fetal bovine serum (FBS) and gentamicin 15 μg/ml. Medium for secondary keratinocyte cultures consists of DMEM with 20% FBS, hydrocortisone and epidermal growth factor (EGF).[23] Full-thickness fetal sheep skin was initially maintained in Roswell Park Memorial Institute-1640 (RPMI-1640; Gibco, Grand Island, NY). Our current medium is an empiric combination of the three media. Epidermal growth factor (EGF) which extends the life of monolayer cultured keratinocytes, was not included; insulin was added to facilitate transportation of the enriched RPMI-1640 used in preference to DMEM (Table 17.1).

TABLE 17.1 Enriched Culture Medium for Fetal Sheep Skin Explants

RPMI-1640
10% fetal calf serum
Hydrocortisone (0.4 μg/ml)
Insulin (5 μg/ml)
Bicarbonate (5 mg/ml)
L-glutamine (2 Mm)
Gentamicin (15 μg/ml)

Full-thickness skin was harvested from 100 day gestation (term = 145 days) fetal sheep immediately postmortem. This gestational age was selected because previous work has demonstrated scarless incisional skin healing at this stage of development. The skin was collected and transported at 4°C in serum free RPMI 1640 with 10,000 U/ml penicillin, 10 μg/ml streptomycin and 25 μg/ml amphotericin B. Within 24 hours, the fetal skin was rinsed extensively in sterile, phosphate buffered saline, carefully defatted, and cut into strips 10 mm × 40 mm. A linear, partial thickness incision was made along the middle of the long axis of the skin using a guarded blade to produce a reproducible wound. Each rectangle of tissue was cut into eight pieces 10 mm × 5 mm to provide two control wounds and six experimental wounds (Fig. 17.3). The two end pieces were immediately pinned on cardboard and fixed in 10% formalin to serve as controls for the depth of incision. The remaining six strips were transferred to sterile gauze dressing sponges in 24 well petri dishes to raise the explant surface to the air-liquid interface. The orientation of the skin was maintained with the epidermis superficial. The explants were kept in a 10% CO_2, 90% air environment with 95% humidity at 37°C. Five hundred μl of medium were added and 450 μl replaced on alternate days. Explants were harvested at two, four, and seven days and were frozen for cryosectioning or fixed in 10% formalin.

The most obvious difference in effect between the fibroblast culture medium and the keratinocyte culture medium was the reduction in sub-epidermal liquefaction. Hydrocortisone is necessary for the preservation of normal keratinocyte morphology in secondary culture. In the explant culture, hydrocortisone suppresses collagenase production which is crucial since focal collagenase activity at the dermal-epidermal junction results in tissue separation (Fig. 17.4).

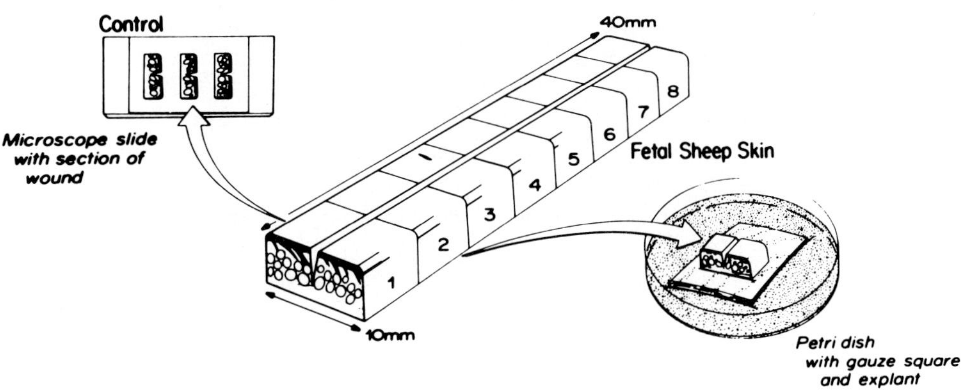

Figure 17.3 A schematic representation of the explant model showing the method of creating the wound. *Reprinted with permission.*[22]

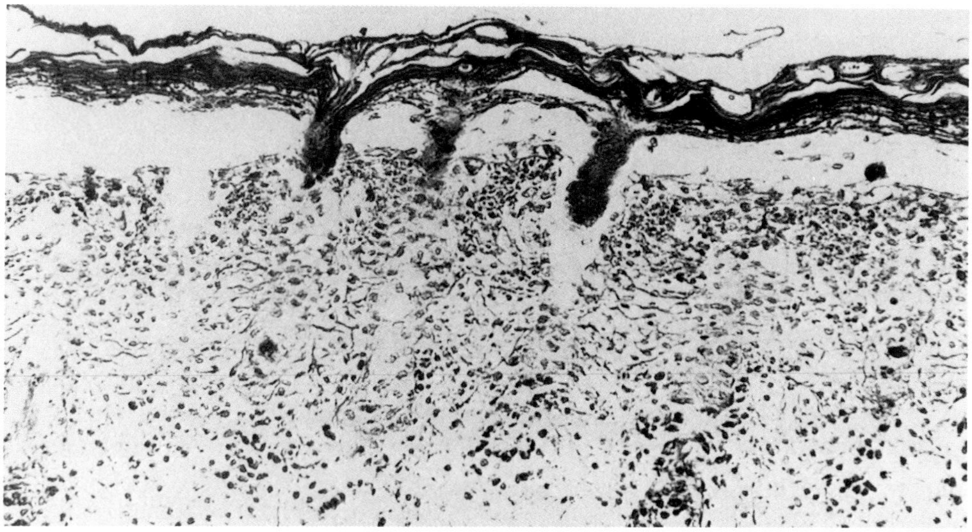

Figure 17.4 An example of separation of epidermis from dermis due to subepidermal liquefaction. The specimen was adult pig skin grown in DMEM. (Magnification ×100)

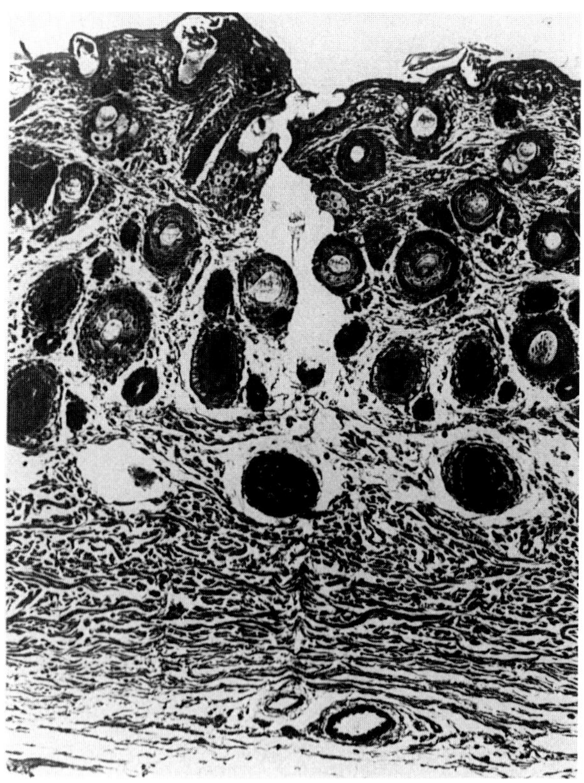

Figure 17.5 Control wound in fetal sheep skin. Note the thickened papillary dermis containing multiple hair shafts. (Magnification ×150)

The response of fetal sheep skin was different. The control wound at time zero is shown in Fig. 17.5. An epidermal layer 3–4 cells thick overlies a wide papillary dermis invested with multiple hair follicles. An incision has been made through the epidermis and the papillary dermis. Four days later the epidermis has closed the wound but the cleft through the papillary dermis remains open (Fig. 17.6). At seven days postwounding the epidermis is showing aberrant differentiation of keratosis and is much thicker (6–8 cells) overlying the dermal cleft (Fig. 17.7). A convenient marker for the wound is the overlying focal hyperkeratosis. Although the dermal wound appears smaller, it does reach down to the reticular dermis as in the control wound at time zero. The general morphology of the tissue on either side of the wound has been preserved throughout the seven days in culture.

This study demonstrates that it is possible to achieve conditions in culture which maintain fetal tissue viability and gross morphology. When fetal sheep skin is incised, the epidermis responds and epidermal continuity is re-established. However, dermal repair is not apparent. This observation suggests that in this model neither intrinsic fibroblast activity nor epidermal cell derived factors are sufficient to trigger the rapid dermal repair response seen in vivo. Extrinsic factors appear to be necessary. These could be produced in vivo by the macrophages which "police" the tissues[24] or be present in the circulation.[25]

We are continuing to modify the model and are aiming toward an objective assessment of the tissue response to manipulation. Various possibilities are being

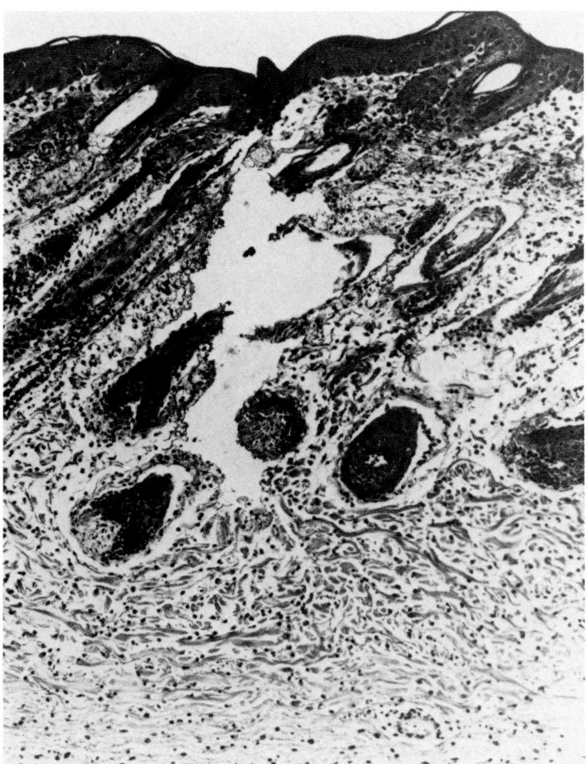

Figure 17.6 At four days postwounding, the epidermal layer has healed in culture. The dermal cleft remains open. (Magnification ×150)

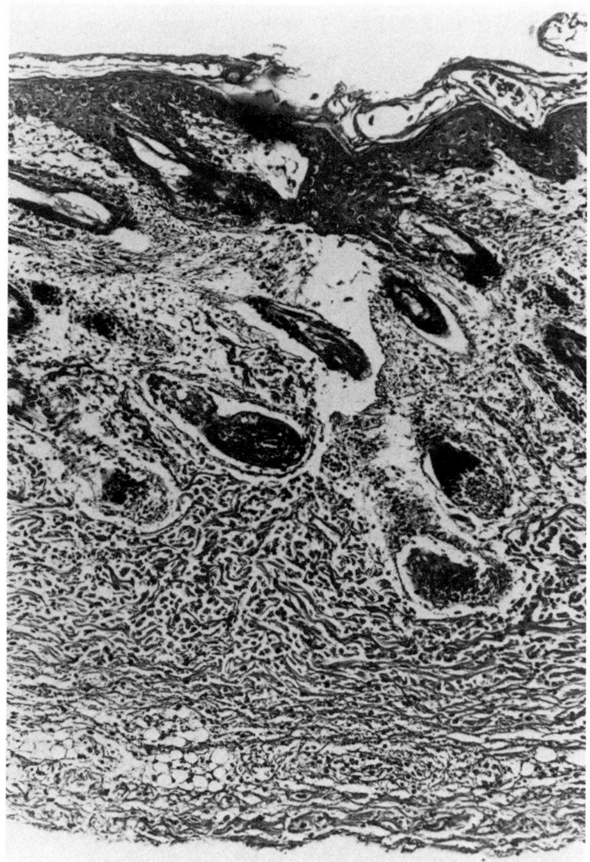

Figure 17.7 By seven days the epidermis is considerably thickened at the site of repair. There is an obvious dermal cleft. This begins immediately deep to the epidermis and reaches the reticular dermis. The dermal defect is smaller than at four days suggesting limited repair at the deeper level. (Magnification ×150)

studied. Trichrome staining for collagen and polarized optics to study birefringence patterns can demonstrate matrix organization. Computerized morphometric analysis can quantify the wound "dead space." Immunohistochemical studies using a wide range of antibodies to collagens,[26] other glycoproteins and proteoglycans are possible. Complementary DNA probes to procollagen alpha chains for type I, III, VI and IV are now available and can be used for in situ hybridization.[27] Finally it will be possible to subject control and wounded skin to biochemical and biomechanical analysis.

This model will permit manipulation of fetal sheep skin wound healing in a controlled fashion. One active area of interest involves the extracellular matrix of fetal wounds known to be rich in HA (see Chapter 12). We are currently evaluating the effect of amniotic fluid, HA-stimulating activity found in fetal serum and wound fluid, as well as either commercially available HA or HA-protein complexes derived from human scar tissue using this model. Preliminary studies demonstrate that when the explant wound is treated topically with HA extracted from human normal scar, then progressive reconstitution of the dermal matrix occurs. By seven days, only a small "dead space" exists in the dermis (see Chapter 13).

This in vitro wound healing model does have limitations. Our technique offers a normal epidermal-dermal architecture, but angiogenesis and inflammation are absent. Despite these limitations, the in vitro fetal skin explant wound healing model may allow us to elucidate some of the individual components that participate in the phenomenal process of scarless fetal skin repair.

REFERENCES

1. Rowsell AR: The intra-uterine healing of foetal muscle wounds: Experimental study in the rat. Br J Plast Surg 37:635–642, 1984.
2. Hallock GG, Rice DC, McClure HM: In utero lip repair in the rhesus monkey: An update. Plast Reconstr Surg 80:855–858, 1987.
3. Krummel TM, Nelson JM, Dieglemann RF, et al.: Fetal response to injury in the rabbit. J Pediatr Surg 22:640–644, 1987.
4. Adzick NS, Harrison MR, Glick PL, et al.: Comparison of fetal, newborn, and adult wound healing by histologic, enzyme-histochemical, and hydroxyproline determinations. J Pediatr Surg 20:315–319, 1985.
5. Siebert JW, Burd DAR, McCarthy J, et al.: Fetal wound healing. A biochemical study of scarless healing. Plast Reconstr Surg 85:495–502, 1990.
6. Alexander DP, Britton HG, Cohen NM, Nixon DA: In Wolstenholme GEW and O'Conner M (eds): Foetal Autonomy. Churchill, London, 1969, p 95.
7. Kistler A, Utsugi R, Ihara S: Wound healing in fetal limb organ culture. Ann Plast Surg 21:303–309, 1988.
8. Kistler A, Ihara S: Requirements of serum factors for wound closure of embryonic skin in vitro. Ann Plast Surg 23:479–487, 1989.
9. Ihara S, Motobayashi Y, Nagao E, et al.: Ontogenic transition of wound healing pattern in rat skin occurring at the fetal stage. Development 110:671–680, 1990.
10. Orredson SU, Knighton DR, Scheuenstuhl H, et al.: A quantitative in vitro study of fibroblast and endothelial cell migration in response to serum and wound fluid. J Surg Res 35:249–258, 1983.
11. Postlethwaite AE, Snyderman R, Kang AH: Generation of a fibroblast chemotactic factor in serum by activation of complement. J Clin Invest 64:1379–1385, 1979.
12. Stewart RJ, Duley JA, Allardyce RA: The migration of fibroblasts into an in vitro wound. Br J Exp Pathol 60:582–588, 1979.
13. Todaro GJ, Lazar GK, Green H: The initiation of cell division in a contact-inhibited mammalian cell line. J Cell Comp Physiol 66:325–333, 1965.
14. Sholley MM, Gimbrone MA, Cotran RS: Cellular migration and replication in endothelial regeneration: A study using irradiated endothelial cultures. Lab Invest 36:8–25, 1977.
15. Longaker MT, Harrison MR, Langer JC, et al.: Studies in fetal wound healing: II. A fetal environment accelerates fibroblast migration in vitro. J Pediatr Surg 24:793–798, 1989.
16. Decker M, Chiu ES, Moiin A, et al.: A hyaluronic acid-stimulating factor in fetal bovine serum. Cancer Res 49:3499–3504, 1989.
17. Longaker MT, Harrison MR, Crombleholme TM, et al.: Studies in fetal wound healing: I. A factor in fetal serum that stimulates deposition of hyaluronic acid. J Pediatr Surg 24:789–792, 1989.
18. Turley BP, Torrance J: Localization of hyaluronate-binding protein on motile and non-motile fibroblasts. Exp Cell Res 161:17–28, 1984.
19. Kujawa MJ, Tepperman K: Culturing chick muscle cells on glycosaminoglycan substrate: Attachment and differentiation. Dev Biol 99:277–286, 1983.
20. Toole BP: Glycosaminoglycans in morphogenesis. In Hay ED (ed): Cell Biology of the Extracellular Matrix. New York, Plenum Press, 1981, pp 259–294.
21. Regaur S and Compton CC: Cultured keratinocyte sheets enhance spontaneous re-epithelialization in a dermal explant model of partial thickness wounds. J Invest Derm 1991 (in press).
22. Burd DAR, Longaker MT, Adzick NS, et al.: Fetal wound healing: An in vitro explant model. J Pediatr Surg 25:898–901, 1990.
23. Rheinwald JG: Serial cultivation of normal human epidermal kerotinocytes. Methods in Cell Biol 21A:229–254, 1980.

24. Rappolee DA, Mark D, Banda MJ, et al.: Wound macrophage express TGF-α and other growth factors in vivo: Analysis by MRNA phenotyping. Science 241:708–712, 1988.
25. Longaker MT, Harrison MR, Crombleholme TM, et al.: Studies in fetal wound healing: I. A factor in fetal serum that stimulates deposition of hyaluronic acid. J Pediatr Surg 24:789–792, 1989.
26. Longaker MT, Whitby DJ, Adzick NS, et al.: Studies in fetal wound healing: VI. Second and early third trimester fetal wounds demonstrate rapid collagen deposition without scar formation. J Pediatr Surg 25:63–69, 1989.
27. Olsen DR, Peltonen J, Jaakola S, et al.: Collagen gene expression by cultured human skin fibroblasts. Abundant steady state levels of type VI procollagen messenger RNAs. J Clin Invest 83:791–795, 1989.

CHAPTER **18**

The Mechanics of Embryonic Skin Wound Healing: Limb-Bud Lesions in Mouse and Chick Embryos

Paul Martin
Julian Lewis

The mechanisms involved in embryonic wound healing interest us for three reasons. First, they offer us, as developmental biologists, insight into the machinery of cell proliferation and migration that the embryo has at its disposal for the purposes of normal morphogenesis. Secondly, embryonic wound healing may serve as a simplified model for adult wound healing: the embryonic tissues are simpler, and their healing is not complicated by an inflammatory response or hidden by a scab. Finally, fetal wound healing is now of direct clinical relevance as surgeons begin to operate in utero to correct deformities such as diaphragmatic hernia. Although there have been several previous studies of embryonic wound healing in amphibians,[1–7] birds,[2,8–15] and mammals,[16] the underlying mechanisms remain largely unknown.

We have chosen to work in two systems—the chick embryo at four days of incubation and the mouse embryo at 11.5 days of gestation; both are at the early limb bud stage.[17] The chick embryo has for many years been the classic system for 'cut and paste' embryologists because of the ease with which operations can be performed in ovo, while the mouse embryo, when removed from the uterus and grown in a small volume of medium in a roller culture bottle, offers special opportunities to manipulate the conditions biochemically. We have used the chick to study the basic ground rules and mechanics of embryonic wound healing: its timecourse, the relative contributions of mesenchymal contraction and epidermal movement, and the way in which the epidermis at the edge of the wound moves forward. In the mouse system we have begun to test the capacity of growth factors to enhance healing and the capacity of other molecules to affect healing by interfering with the binding of the cells to extracellular matrix.

A STANDARD SQUARE LESION ON THE CHICK LIMB BUD HEALS WITHIN 24 HOURS

At stage 23 (4 days of incubation), when we make our standard lesion on the chick wing bud, its skin has a very simple structure: the epidermis consists of just two layers—a cuboidal basal layer and a squamous outer layer known as the periderm—while the dermis is represented by a homogeneous mesenchyme that is not visibly different from the mesenchyme deeper in the limb bud, except that it has no blood vessels running through it.[18,19] For our standard lesion we make cuts with a sharpened tungsten needle to delineate a square measuring 0.5 mm × 0.5 mm (Fig. 18.1A). The square of skin is then dissected away to a depth of approximately 100 μm. This dissection inevitably damages some blood vessels in the cutaneous vascular plexus which sits 100 μm beneath the limb surface.[18–20]

At 0 hours (within 5 minutes of wounding), scanning electron microscopy reveals that the epidermis around the wound has a ragged edge of damaged cells, while the exposed mesenchymal cells have numerous blebs on their apical surfaces (Fig. 18.1B). One hour later after lesioning the wound edges have become neat and regular (though with some variation in the shapes of the epidermal cells) and the exposed mesenchymal cells have flattened down to form a pavement of cells that superficially resemble a squamous epithelium (although by transmission electron microscopy it clearly is not a true epithelium and lacks a basal lamina). The exposed mesenchymal cells retain their epithelioid phenotype (Fig. 18.1C) until the epidermis closes over them. After 12 hours of healing, wounds are usually about 75% closed (25% of the originally exposed area is still exposed). The appearance of the wound front—the moving free edge of epidermis around the lesion—at this stage is typical of most of the period of active healing. It is surprisingly different from what one would expect on the basis of descriptions of epidermal healing and migration in other systems.[5,6,21–26]

Around most of the wound front, the epidermal cells appear tightly adherent to one another, forming an epithelial surface with a free edge that is clean and straight or smoothly curved as seen by scanning electron microscopy (Figure 1D); in a few places, the cells are individually rounded up as though less tightly coherent (Fig. 18.1C). But in either case, whether we look by scanning EM (which reveals surface details) or by transmission EM (which lets us see the basal epidermal layer) or by light microscopy, we find scarcely any sign of lamellipodia at the epidermal wound front, in either the basal or the peridermal layer (Fig. 18.1C,D). In cross section, the wound front generally has a rounded or only bluntly angular profile rather than the flattened cellular protrusions one might expect at a leading edge that was actively crawling forward over the exposed mesenchyme.

Nonetheless, 24 hours after wounding, most of the lesions that had been healing without hindrance (without drying out or excess blood debris) have completely closed. At the focal point of closure we usually see a pimple, which at high magnification is clearly a pile-up of cells reflecting an overrun of the epidermal closure mechanism (Fig. 18.1E). Beneath the pimple the wound mesenchyme is less dense than elsewhere and has yet to attain the cell spacing present in the rest of the limb (Figure 18.1F). It seems unlikely, therefore, that the final closing-in of the epidermis is driven by contraction of the mesenchyme beneath.

The above description is necessarily based on a series of separate embryos fixed at different times after wounding. However, there is some unavoidable variability between individual wounds and so, to get a more accurate picture of the timecourse of healing, we followed the process in living embryos in ovo, observing the wound margins of single lesions and recording their positions with camera lucida drawings made at zero, one, two, three, six, 12, 18, and 24 hrs postwounding (Fig. 18.2). By measurement from these drawings, we find that the embryonic wound front moves in at approximately 12 μm per hour with no observable initial lag phase, until closure occurs usually at some time between 18 and 24 hours after wounding.

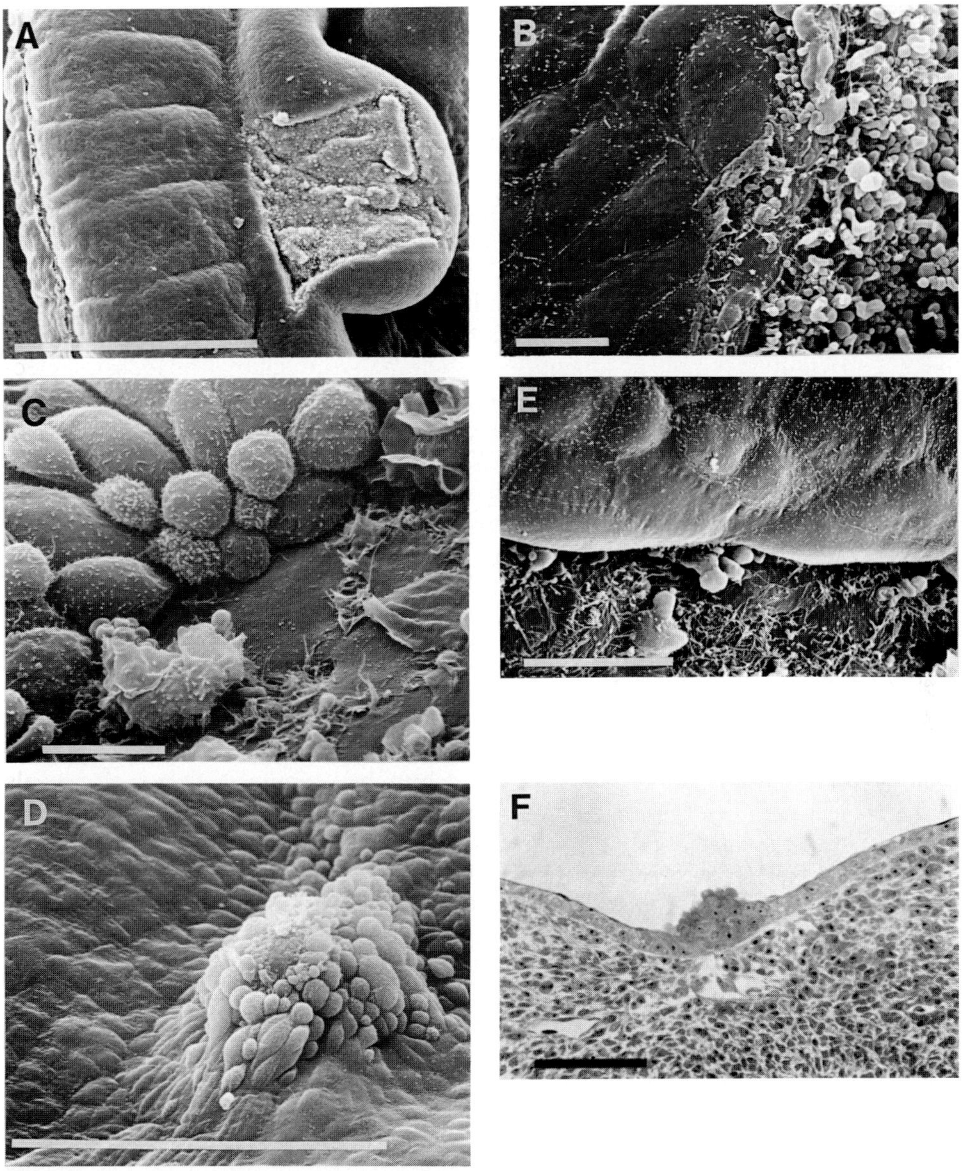

Figure 18.1 Normal healing of a wound made by cutting away a square patch of skin from the dorsum of the 4-day chick embryo wing bud. **A.** Overview of the 0-hour wound, i.e., immediately after the operation; the wing bud is to the right, the trunk of the embryo to the left. (Scanning EM; scale bar = 1mm.) **B.** Detail of 0-hour wound edge; epidermis is to the left, exposed mesenchyme to the right. (Scanning EM; scale bar = 10 μm.) **C.** Detail of 12-hour wound edge; epidermis to the upper left, flattened epithelioid surface of the exposed mesenchyme to the lower right. Note that in this picture the epidermal cells at the wound front are rounded, but more often, as in D, they appear tightly coherent, forming a smoother epithelial surface. (Scanning EM; scale bar = 10 μm.) **D.** Detail of another sample of 12-hour wound edge; epidermis above, exposed mesenchyme below. Note the smooth edge of the epidermis and the absence of lamellipodia. (Scanning EM; scale bar = 10 μm.) **E.** Epidermal pimple at the focal point of wound closure, 24 hours after wounding. (Scanning EM; scale bar = 100 μm.) **F.** Section through such a pimple, showing the pile-up of epidermal cells overlying mesenchyme that is less dense than elsewhere. (Toluidine blue stain; scale bar = 100 μm.)

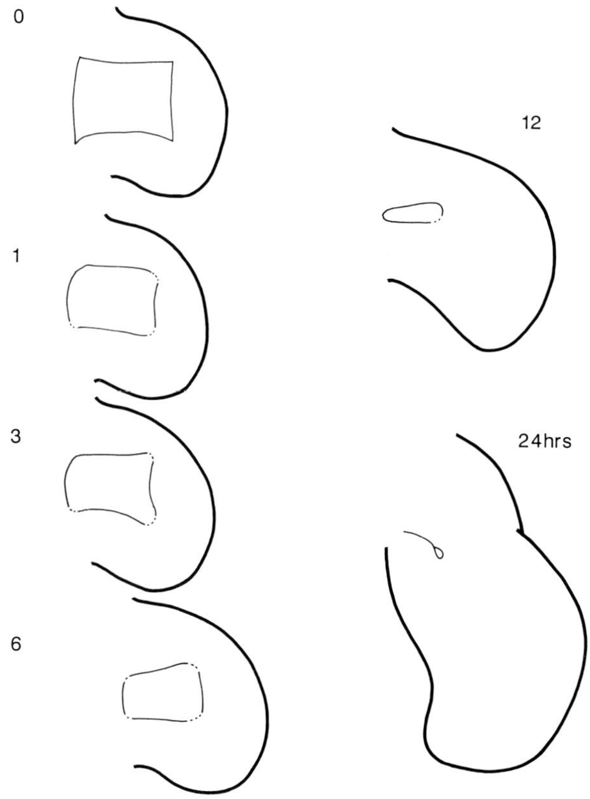

Figure 18.2 Camera-lucida drawings of a living specimen, showing the time course of healing of a standard square wound (as in Figure 18.1A) on the dorsum of a chick wing bud. The wound front is difficult to see clearly at its corners (dotted lines) in the living specimen; scanning EM of fixed specimens reveals that the corners are generally rounded.

EMBRYONIC HEALING INVOLVES ACTIVE EPIDERMAL MOVEMENT TO COVER THE EXPOSED MESENCHYME

Adult wound closure involves active movements of both connective tissue and epidermis.[27] The exposed connective tissue of the wound—the granulation tissue—contracts to tug the wound edges together,[28–30] and the epidermis migrates to cover over the exposed connective tissue.[26] We wanted to know whether these two types of movement are occurring during embryonic wound healing. For this, we marked the edges of the patch of exposed mesenchyme with the lipophilic cell marker DiI at the time of wounding, allowed 18 hours of healing to take place, and then observed the change in area of the patch of mesenchyme outlined with DiI and the relation of the epidermal wound front to the marked mesenchymal patch. We do find a modest decrease in the area of the marked mesenchyme (though more control experiments are needed to establish what this signifies). The observation we wish to stress, however, is that there is very clearly an active closure movement of the epidermis: over the 18 hour period, in all cases examined, the wound epidermis had swept in over the marked patch of mesenchyme, and in some cases had covered it completely (see Fig. 18.3 in color section).

Lesions to the Chick Limb Bud Caused by UV Light Do Not Heal

As described above, surgical lesions to the embryonic chick limb bud heal rapidly. However, we find that if we kill a patch of limb skin with short-wave (254 nm) UV light, the resulting lesion does not heal.[20,31] Rather, the lesion remains open and expands in size (at least until 10 days after wounding, which is as late as we have looked) (Fig. 18.4). By scanning EM and in light microscope sections, the irradiated cells can be seen to be dying within six hours after irradiation, and by about 24 hours the debris has largely disappeared, leaving a cleanly denuded patch, with no further obvious sign of dying cells. Around this patch the non-healing UV wound front consists of a rim of apparently healthy epidermal cells, similar to that seen around a healing surgical lesion (Fig. 18.4C).

The rate of proliferation of these cells, as judged by tritiated-thymidine autoradiography, seems normal.[32] Why then does the UV lesion not heal? One difference from a surgical lesion is that the irradiation procedure does not cause direct damage to blood vessels and so there is no bleeding. We wondered whether

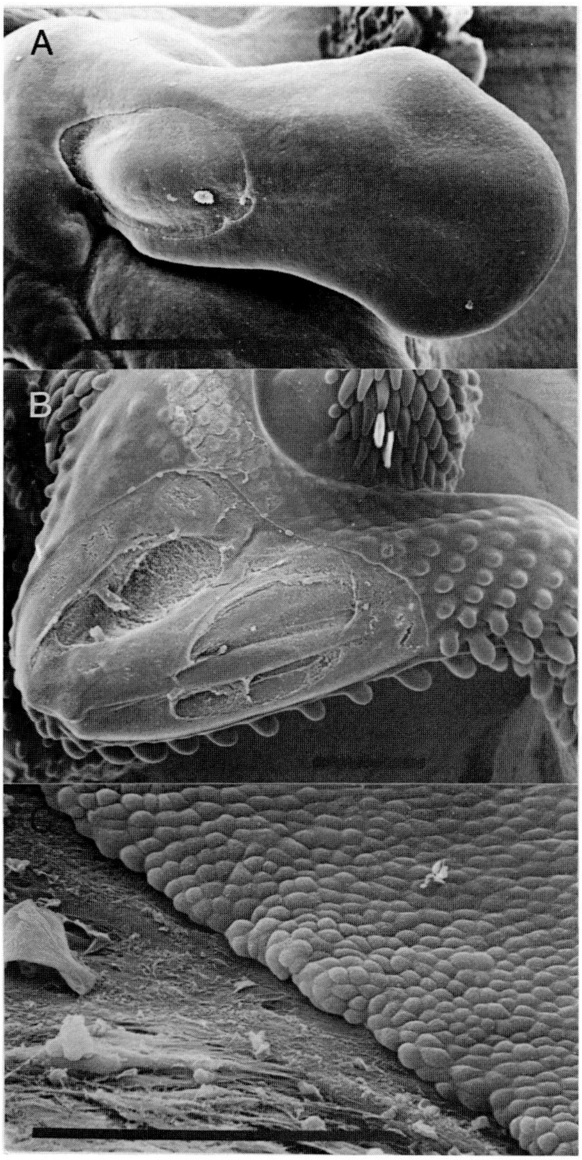

Figure 18.4 A lesion created by UV-irradiating a circular patch on the dorsum of the chick wing bud fails to heal. **A.** 48 hours after irradiation. The irradiated patch of limb surface is cleanly denuded of epidermis. (Scale bar = 1 mm.) **B.** 6 days after irradiation. The denuded patch has enlarged in parallel with the growth of the limb; there is no sign of healing. (Scale bar = 1 mm.) **C.** Detail from B, showing the non-healing epidermal wound front; epidermis is at upper right, exposed mesenchyme at lower left. (Scale bar = 100 μm.)

this absence of bleeding might be the explanation: the epidermal wound front might require a bloodborne trigger to initiate forward movement. This first guess at why UV wounds do not heal turned out to be easy to disprove. We simply scratched with a tungsten needle at the exposed mesenchymal surface of lesions 48 hours after UV irradiation, causing extensive bleeding; we were unable to trigger healing. We still have only tentative speculations as to the reason why healing fails in these UV specimens, but we remain interested in them as a possible model for non-healing ulcers in adult life, where again there are puzzling variations in the ability of the epidermis to heal.[33]

Islands of Embryonic Epidermis Tend to Shrink: A Pursestring Mechanism may Drive Movement of an Epidermal Free Edge

Since UV lesions do not heal, they provide ideal test beds on which to grow patches of normal embryonic skin. We grafted a small (250 μm × 250 μm) square patch of embryonic skin (epidermis and underlying mesenchyme) dissected from the dorsum of a stage 23 limb bud to the denuded mesenchymal surface of a 48-hour old UV lesion (Fig. 18.5). The graft was of quail origin so that donor and host (chick) tissues could be histologically distinguished. (Feulgen-stained quail cells show a prominent mass of heterochromatin associated with the nucleolus.) The host limb with graft was fixed after 12 or 24 hours and processed for resin

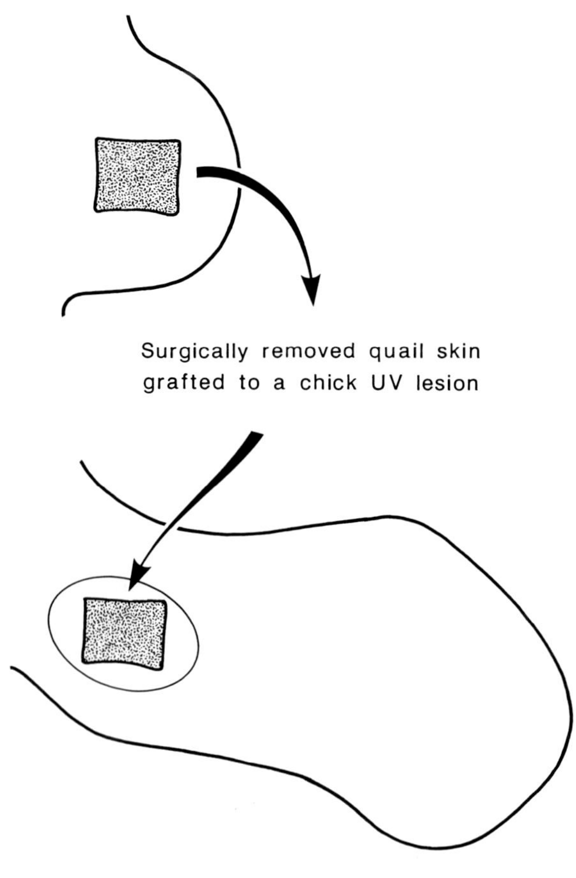

Figure 18.5 An island of normal quail skin is grafted into the middle of a patch of chick wing bud surface that has been denuded of epidermis by UV irradiation 48 hours beforehand.

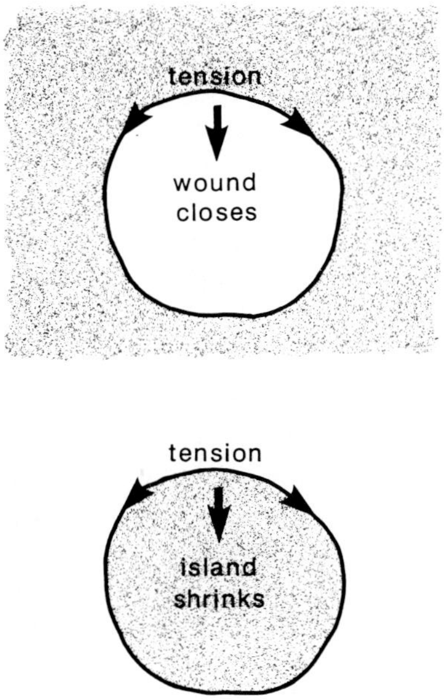

Figure 18.7 The pursestring mechanism: circumferential tension at the free epidermal edge will cause a wound to close and an island to shrink.

histology. Transverse sections through the graft region revealed that the quail epidermis had not only failed to spread out over the exposed chick mesenchyme but had actually shrunk back relative to its own underlying quail mesenchyme (see Fig. 18.6 in color section). Although we have only a small number of specimens, this observation that epidermal islands tend to shrink clashes with the conventional expectation for an epithelium with migratory tendencies, as did our earlier observation that the epidermal cells at a closing wound front do not send out lamellipodia. It occurred to us that both phenomena might be explained by the same unconventional mechanism for epidermal movement, operating at any free embryonic epidermal edge. The driving force could be a circumferential tension generated in the free margin of the epidermis, acting like a pursestring. Contraction of this pursestring would cause an epidermal island to shrink and a hole in the epidermis—a wound—to close (Fig. 18.7).

The Pursestring Corresponds to a Cable of Actin

If there is such a pursestring tension, the obvious guess would be that it would be generated by a structure containing actin. We therefore examined the actin distribution around the margins of wounds in embryos fixed at various times after wounding. We stained for filamentous actin using fluorescently tagged phalloidin[34,35] and viewed our specimens as wholemounts with a confocal laser scanning microscope, which lets us see a series of thin optical sections parallel to the wound surface. An optical section in the plane of the most superficial layer of cells at the wound margin reveals the peridermal cells clearly outlined by their cortical actin; but there is no actin specialization that makes peridermal cells at the wound margin appear different from those further back from the wound (Fig. 18.8a). A few micrometers deeper we move into the basal epidermal layer. Here we find a clear and dramatic cable of actin that appears to run continuously around most of the wound margin[36] (Fig. 18.8b). It is confined to the single row of basal

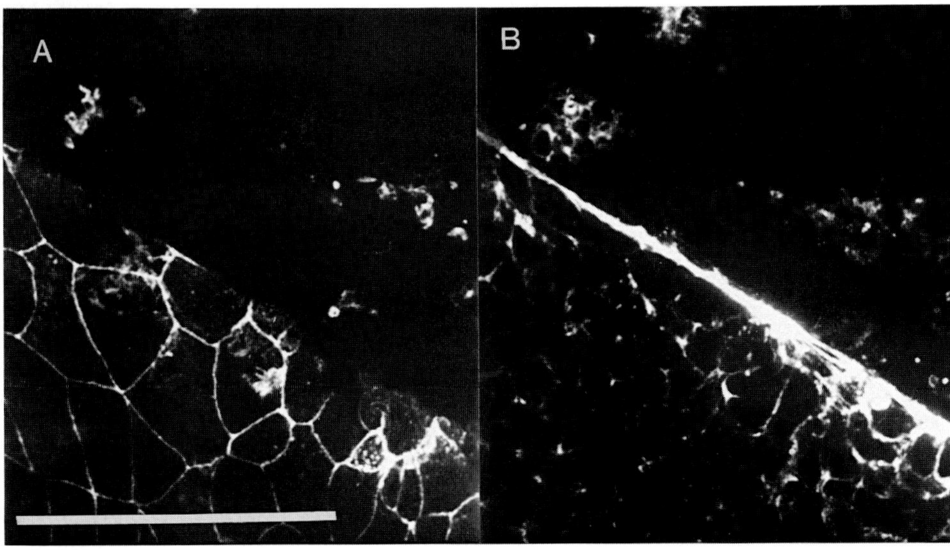

Figure 18.8 The epidermal wound front on the dorsum of a chick wing bud after 12 hours of healing, as seen in optical section by confocal scanning laser microscopy. The tissue has been stained with rhodamine-labelled phalloidin, which binds to filamentous actin, and the sections are parallel to the plane of the epidermis; epidermis is at lower left, exposed mesenchyme (largely below the plane of section) is at upper right. **A.** Superficial section, in the plane of the periderm, whose broad flat cells are outlined by their cortical actin. **B.** Section about 4 μm deeper, in the plane of the basal epidermal cells, showing the actin cable at the wound front. (Scale bar = 50 μm.)

cells at the wound front. The appearance of continuity from cell to cell presumably reflects the alignment of actin filament bundles in adjacent cells through anchorage at cadherin-mediated cell-cell junctions. The actin cable is occasionally interrupted by short stretches of disorderly actin with disorder also in the arrangement of the cells. These sites generally correspond to kinks in the wound front and might reflect epidermal attachment to the mesenchymal substratum. Around the whole margin of a wound there might typically be three or four such sites of interruption of the cable, although sometimes we see none at all.

The actin cable appears within the first hour of wounding and remains until the wound is closed. It varies a little in thickness and density from wound to wound and in different regions of the same wound, but its width is always less than that of a single basal cell; its average thickness seems to remain roughly constant throughout the course of healing. To gauge more accurately the time-course of establishment of the actin cable, we have begun looking at a much simpler type of lesion—a single slash wound running along the proximodistal axis of the limb.[37] It takes only seconds to make this cut as opposed to the 5–10 minutes required to dissect a square of skin from the limb bud. Our slash lesion data indicate that the actin cable begins forming along the wound margin within minutes of wounding, suggesting that the cable is constructed by reorganizing preexisting actin filaments and/or by converting some of the pool of monomeric actin into filamentous actin.[38,39] The formation of the cable is too rapid to be the result of transcriptional or even translational upregulation of cellular actin levels. In this respect, and in its maintenance of a roughly constant thickness by disassembly as it shortens, it resembles the contractile ring of actin filaments that brings about egg-cell cleavage, as described by Schroeder.[40] It is important to note, however, that in our system wound closure cannot be merely a matter of shortening of intracellular actin bundles, but must also involve changes of cell-cell contacts, since the number of cable-containing cells at the wound front steadily decreases during closure (if it did not, the cells there would have to become enormously elongated radially—a phenomenon that we do not see).

Although we do not as yet have any direct proof that the actin cable is generating the driving force for wound closure in our system, this seems much the most likely hypothesis. Moreover, several other studies of embryonic wound healing, in the chick,[2,9] in the rat[16] and in Xenopus,[2,4] show scanning EM pictures similar to ours; and although these accounts do not explicitly interpret the phenomena in terms of a pursestring mechanism, there is evidence that epidermal wound closure in these systems does depend on calcium-dependent forces generated by actin.[1,3,4] From a theoretical point of view, the formation of an actin cable of the type we see should come as no surprise in the light of what is known from the studies of Kolega[41] and others on the effects of tension on the organization of actin filaments inside cells in a taut epithelial sheet. At the wound edge, by making a cut, we have relaxed the component of epithelial tension at right angles to the edge, while the component parallel to the edge remains; this will tend to make the actin filaments align parallel to the edge, while suppressing motile activity at right angles to the edge. If, as is probable, the exposed mesenchyme is a poor substratum for the epidermal cells to adhere to, it will be doubly difficult for them to extend lamellipodia over it, leaving a pursestring mechanism as almost the only possible means of wound closure.

THE MOUSE EMBRYO IN CULTURE PROVIDES A SENSITIVE ASSAY FOR EMBRYONIC WOUND HEALING FACTORS

The chick embryo in ovo is ideal for studying many aspects of embryonic wound healing because it is so convenient for surgical manipulation. However, it is not good for biochemical experiments because of the vast volume of yolk and albumin which act as a sink for any exogenously added factor. Furthermore, mammalian embryonic wound healing holds greater interest from a clinical point of view. For these reasons we have begun to study wound healing in mouse embryos cultured in vitro.

We dissect the embryos from the uterus into Tyrode's saline at 11.5 days of gestation, when the hindlimb bud is about as long as it is broad. It has previously been shown that rat embryos at limb-bud stages can be cultured and will develop normally for up to two days.[42] The decidua is removed and the yolk sac carefully cut close to where it abuts the placenta, avoiding cutting any major yolk sac blood vessels. The embryos are then gently pulled out of their yolk sacs and the amniotic membranes are torn, exposing the embryo to the external medium without killing it; the heart continues to beat (Fig. 18.9). From a pair of litters, 10–15 embryos of very similar developmental stage and size can be collected. For biochemical experiments, where the rate of healing is the principal assay, we need to be able to make accurately standardized lesions. In place of the square wound on the dorsum of the limb bud that we have used in our chick studies, we have resorted to the more extreme but much more reproducible lesion resulting from simple amputation of the early hindlimb bud at its base. As with the chick wounds, the

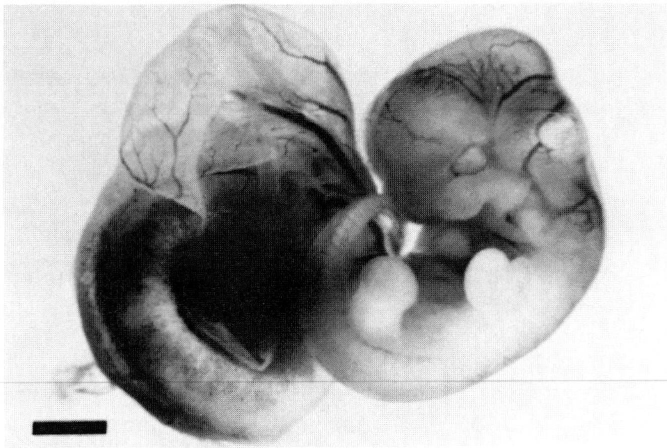

Figure 18.9 A mouse embryo at 11.5 days of gestation, ready for culture in vitro. The embryo proper is at the right, the placenta at the left. (Scale bar = 1 mm.)

mouse limb amputations are performed with sharpened tungsten needles. The lesions normally stop bleeding within a minute and the embryos are then transferred to roller culture bottles with 4 ml of a 1:3 mix of rat serum with Tyrode's saline and an atmosphere of 95% oxygen (regassed after 12 hours), in which they are rolled at 30 revolutions per minute at 37°C. Embryos cultured in this way develop normally, at the same rate as their peers in utero, for at least a day and sometimes for up to two days.

We find that the hindlimb stump lesions (Fig. 18.10) have all closed by 24 hours of culture, at which time most show an overrun pimple at the focal point of closure, like the chick lesions described above. At 6 hours of culture the mouse wounds are about 50% closed—that is, 50% of the originally exposed area has now become covered with epidermis. At 12 hours they are 75% closed; this value is variable by only ±6% (SD, n = 7). At both of these timepoints we see actin cables in the basal epidermal layer of the wound margin, just as in healing chick wounds, suggesting that the mechanisms driving epidermal forward movement are similar for our two systems. We have chosen 12 hours of healing as a convenient endpoint by which to judge the capacity of exogenously added factors to enhance or inhibit wound healing.

THE EMBRYONIC EPIDERMIS HEALS NORMALLY OVER A WOUND EVEN IN THE PRESENCE OF AN INHIBITOR OF CELL-MATRIX ATTACHMENT

According to many previous accounts,[26,43] epidermis heals over a wound by lamellipodial crawling, and this mode of locomotion requires adhesion of the epidermal cells to extracellular matrix components such as fibronectin.[44] Such adhesion depends on integrins in the membrane, and in several systems it has been found that the RGD or, more efficiently, the GRGDS peptide can inhibit adhesion and locomotion by competing with extracellular matrix molecules such as laminin and fibronectin for their RGD binding sites on integrins.[45] On the other hand, epidermal closure driven by a pursestring mechanism such as we have suggested

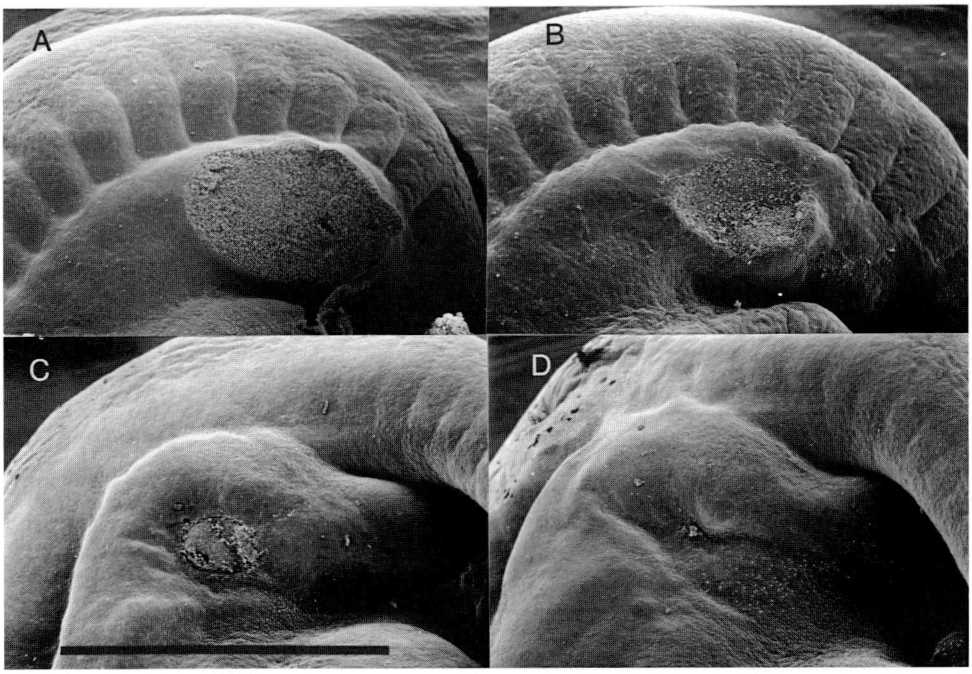

Figure 18.10 The normal course of healing in mouse embryos grown in culture after amputation of the hindlimb bud at 11.5 days of gestation. **A.** 0 hours. **B.** 6 hours. **C.** 12 hours. **D.** 24 hours; note the small pimple at the focal site of wound closure. (Scale bar = 1 mm.)

above should be independent of cell-matrix adhesion and therefore insensitive to GRGDS peptides.

We have therefore tried the effect of adding GRGDS peptide to our mouse culture medium at a concentration of 500 μg/ml; this is ten times the concentration that Donaldson et al.[46] found sufficient to inhibit migration of newt epidermal cells over a fibronectin-coated substratum. At 12 hours of healing the GRGDS treated wounds are only slightly delayed—they are 62 ± 6% closed (mean ± SD, n = 5), as compared with 75 ± 6% (mean ± SD, n = 7) for control untreated wounds at 12 hours. Such a negative result cannot be conclusive, but it strongly suggests that integrin-RGD interactions have at most a small role in healing of the embryonic epidermis. This argues against lamellipodial crawling but is consistent with our proposed pursestring model for epidermal movement.

BASIC FIBROBLAST GROWTH FACTOR ACCELERATES HEALING IN THE MOUSE EMBRYO

There are many reports that growth factors can enhance the healing of adult wounds.[27] Brown et al.[47] have shown that topically applied EGF will accelerate the healing of burn wounds on piglet backs; similar results have been seen for another related growth factor, TGFα.[48] TGFβ, which in tissue culture triggers fibroblasts to lay down matrix and to make protease inhibitors, has been shown to potentiate adult wound healing or at least to increase the strength of healing wounds[49–51]; PDGF has similar effects on healing.[52,53] The capacity of bFGF to enhance wound healing has been demonstrated on adult corneal lesions; here the

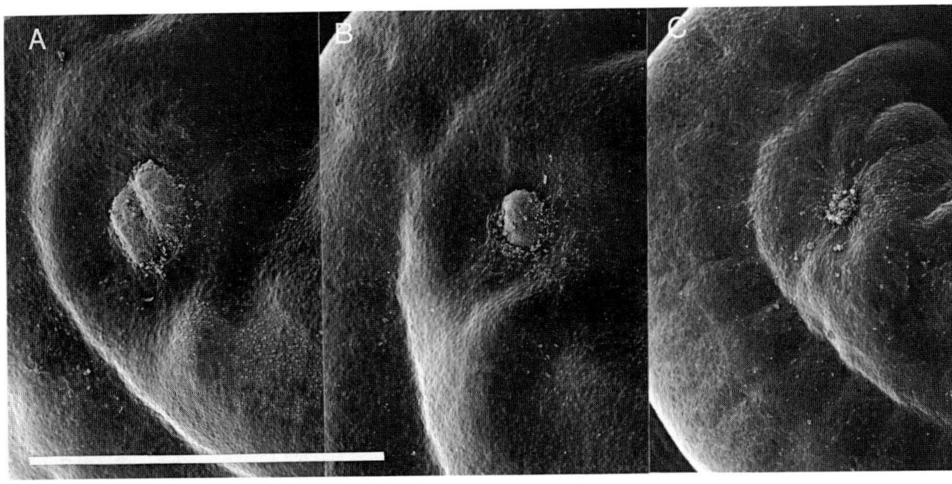

Figure 18.11 The effects of bFGF on rate of healing in mouse embryos. All three embryos have had a hindlimb amputated at 11.5 days of gestation and have then been left to heal in culture for 12 hours. **A.** In normal control culture medium. **B.** In medium with 100 ng/ml of bFGF. **C.** In medium with 1 μg/ml of bFGF; with this dosage of bFGF the wound is completely closed. (Scale bar = 1 mm.)

effect may depend on a stimulation of proliferation of the corneal epithelial cells.[54–56]

We were curious to see whether growth factors could speed up the already rapid healing of embryonic wounds. One might guess that the answer would be no, and that even in the absence of exogenous factors these wounds close as fast as their cellular machinery allows. However, when we added recombinant bFGF (Xenopus-derived, a gift from H. Isaacs & J. Thompson, ICRF, Oxford) to the culture medium we discovered a marked dose-dependent enhancement of wound closure (Fig. 18.11). The highest dose of FGF we tried—1 μg/ml—usually resulted in embryonic lesions closing completely within 12 hours, by which time without the addition of exogenous FGF they are usually only 75% closed.

We are currently repeating this experiment using other growth factors and also looking at the endogenous expression patterns of various growth factor genes during wound healing in embryos.

SUMMARY

Our data from wounds on the chick limb bud tell us that embryonic wound healing involves a forward movement of the epidermis over the mesenchyme, and probably also a certain amount of mesenchymal wound contraction. The epidermis does not appear to move by the conventional mechanism of lamellipodial crawling; rather, it seems to be drawn in by a pursestring mechanism—a tension exerted circumferentially around the margin of the wound. Pursestring contraction drags the epidermal margins together. Our observations suggest that the structural basis for the pursestring is a cable of actin which assembles within minutes of wounding in the front line of basal epidermal cells at the wound margin. The mouse embryo in culture allows us to manipulate the embryonic wound environment biochemically. In support of our view that embryonic wound epidermis does not move forward by lamellipodial crawling, we find that a high dose of GRGDS peptide, which should block cell:matrix adhesions necessary for such crawling, has only a small effect on wound closure. The mouse embryo in culture appears to be an ideal system for assaying the effects of growth factors on the rate of embryonic wound healing; our data show that bFGF significantly speeds up the healing process.

REFERENCES

1. Stanisstreet M, Smedley MJ, Veltkamp CJ: Effects of calcium antagonists and calcium-buffered salines on wound healing in Xenopus early embryos. Cytobios 1986;46:25–35.
2. Stanisstreet M, Wakely J, England MA: Scanning electron microscopy of wound healing in Xenopus and chicken embryos. J Embryol Exp Morphol 1980;59:341–353.
3. Stanisstreet M, Panayi M: Effects of colchicine, cytochalasin-B and papaverine on wound healing in Xenopus early embryos. Experientia 1980;36:1110–1112.
4. Stanisstreet M: Calcium and wound healing in Xenopus early embryos. J Embryol Exp Morphol 1982;67:195–205.
5. Radice GP: Locomotion and cell-substratum contacts of Xenopus epidermal cells in vitro and in situ. J Cell Sci 1980;44:201–223.
6. Radice GP: The spreading of epithelial cells during wound closure in Xenopus larvae. Dev Biol 1980;76:26–46.
7. Rajnicek AM, Stump RF, Robinson KR: An endogenous sodium current may mediate wound healing in Xenopus neurulae. Dev Biol 1988;128:290–299.
8. Thévenet A: Cicatrisation de la peau d'embryon de poulet de 7 jours cultivée in vitro. Arch Anat Microsc Morphol Exp 1983;72:23–46.
9. Thévenet A: Wound healing of the integument in the 5-day chick embryo. Arch Anat Microsc Morphol Exp 1981;70:227–244.
10. Thévenet A: Prolifération cellulaire au cours de la cicatrisation du tégument d'embryon de poulet de 5 jours. Arch Anat Microsc Morphol Exp 1984;73:121–132.
11. Thévenet A: Prolifération cellulaire au cours de la cicatrisation de la peau d'embryon de poulet de 7 jours cultivée in vitro. Arch Anat Microsc Morphol Exp 1985;74:121–132.
12. Weiss PA, Matoltsy AG: Wound healing in chick embryos in vivo and in vitro. Dev Biol 1959;1:302–326.
13. England MA, Cowper SV: Wound healing in the early chick embryo studied by scanning electron microscopy. Anat Embryol (Berl) 1977;152:1–14.
14. Takeuchi S: Wound healing in the cornea of the chick embryo. IV. Promotion of the migratory activity of isolated corneal epithelium in culture by the application of tension. Dev Biol 1979;70:232–240.
15. Takeuchi S: Wound healing in the cornea of the chick embryo. V. An observation and quantitative assessment of the cell shapes in the isolated corneal epithelium during spreading in vitro. Cell Tissue Res 1983;229:109–127.
16. Smedley MJ, Stanisstreet M: Scanning electron microscopy of wound healing in rat embryos. J Embryol Exp Morphol 1984;83:109–117.
17. Martin P: Tissue patterning in the developing mouse limb. Int J Dev Biol 1990;34:323–336.
18. Caplan AI, Koutroupas S: The control of muscle and cartilage development in the chick limb: the role of differential vascularization. J Embryol Exp Morphol 1973;29:571–583.
19. Feinberg RN, Beebe DC: Hyaluronate in vasculogenesis. Science 1983;220:1171–1179.
20. Martin P, Khan A, Lewis J: Cutaneous nerves of the embryonic chick wing do not develop in regions denuded of ectoderm. Development 1989;106:335–346.
21. Bard J: Morphogenesis: The Cellular and Molecular Processes of Developmental Anatomy. Cambridge: Cambridge University Press, 1990.
22. Trinkaus JP: Cells into Organs: the Forces that Shape the Embryo (2nd ed ed.). New Jersey: Prentice-Hall, 1984.
23. Vaughan RB, Trinkaus JP: Movements of epithelial cell sheets in vitro. J Cell Sci 1966;1:407–413.
24. DiPasquale A: Locomotion of epithelial cells. Factors involved in extension of the leading edge. Exp Cell Res 1975;95:425–439.

25. DiPasquale A: Locomotory activity of epithelial cells in culture. Exp Cell Res 1975;94:191–215.
26. Bereiter-Hahn J: Epidermal cell migration and wound repair. In: Bereiter-Hahn J, Matoltsy AG, Richards KS ed. Biology of the Integument. New York: Springer, 1986: 443–471.
27. Clark RAF, Henson PM: The Molecular and Cellular Biology of Wound Repair. New York: Plenum, 1988.
28. Darby I, Skalli O, Gabbiani G: Alpha-smooth muscle actin is transiently expressed by myofibroblasts during experimental wound healing. Lab Invest 1990;63:21–29.
29. Gabbiani G: Reparative processes in mammalian wound healing: the role of contractile phenomena. Int Rev Cytol 1977;48:187–219.
30. Stopak D, Harris AK: Connective tissue morphogenesis by fibroblast traction I. Tissue culture observations. Dev Biol 1982;90:383–398.
31. Martin P, Lewis J: Normal development of the skeleton in chick limb buds devoid of dorsal ectoderm. Dev Biol 1986;118:233–246.
32. Martin PB: Tissue Interactions during Embryonic Development of the Chick Wing. Ph.D. Thesis, University of London, 1988.
33. Leigh IM, Purkis PE, Navsaria HA, Phillips TJ: Treatment of chronic venous ulcers with sheets of cultured allogenic keratinocytes. Br J Dermatol 1987;117:591–597.
34. Faulstich E, Trischmann H, Mayer D: Preparation of trimethylrhodaminyl-phalloidin and uptake of the toxin into short-term cultured hepatocytes by endocytosis. Exp Cell Res 1983;144:73–82.
35. Wulf E, Deboben A, Bautz FA, Faulstich H, Wieland T: Fluorescent phallotoxin, a tool for the visualization of cellular actin. Proc Natl Acad Sci USA 1979;76:4498–4502.
36. Martin P, Lewis J: Embryonic wound healing: Actin cables and epidermal movement. Submitted, 1991.
37. Midwinter K, Lewis J, Martin P: Healing of incisional lesions to the embryonic chick wing bud. In preparation, 1991.
38. Wang Y-L: Reorganization of actin filament bundles in living fibroblasts. J Cell Biol 1984;99:1478–1485.
39. Wang Y-L: Mobility of filamentous actin in living cytoplasm. J Cell Biol 1987;105:2811–2816.
40. Schroeder TE: The contractile ring. II. Determining its brief existence, volumetric changes, and vital role in cleaving Arbacia eggs. J Cell Biol 1972;53:419–434.
41. Kolega J: Effects of mechanical tension on protrusive activity and microfilament and intermediate filament organization in an epidermal epithelium moving in culture. J Cell Biol 1986;102:1400–1411.
42. Cockroft DL: Development in culture of rat foetuses explanted at 12.5 and 13.5 days of gestation. J Embryol Exp Morphol 1973;29:473–483.
43. Clark RAF: Wound repair. Curr Opin Cell Biol 1989;1:1000–1008.
44. Grinnell F, Toda K, Takashima A: Activation of keratinocyte fibronectin receptor function during cutaneous wound healing. J Cell Sci Suppl 1987;8:199–209.
45. Ruoslahti E, Pierschbacher M: New perspectives in cell adhesion: RGD and integrins. Science 1987;238:491–497.
46. Donaldson DJ, Mahan JT, Smith GNJ: Newt epidermal cell migration over collagen and fibronectin involves different mechanisms. J Cell Sci 1988;90:
47. Brown GL, Curtsinger L3, Brightwell JR, et al.: Enhancement of epidermal regeneration by biosynthetic epidermal growth factor. J Exp Med 1986;163:1319–1324.
48. Schultz GS, White M, Mitchell R, et al.: Epithelial wound healing enhanced by transforming growth factor-alpha and vaccinia growth factor. Science 1987;235:350–352.
49. Mustoe TA, Pierce GF, Thomason A, Gramates P, Sporn MB, Deuel TF: Accelerated healing of incisional wounds in rats induced by transforming growth factor-beta. Science 1987;237:1333–1336.
50. Ammann AJ, Beck LS, DeGuzman L, et al.: Transforming growth factor-beta. Effect on soft tissue repair. Ann N Y Acad Sci 1990;593:124–134.
51. Curtsinger LJ, Pietsch JD, Brown GL, et al.: Reversal of Adriamycin-impaired wound healing by transforming growth factor-beta. Surg Gynecol Obstet 1989;168:517–522.
52. Pierce GF, Mustoe TA, Lingelbach J, et al.: Platelet-derived growth factor and transforming growth factor-beta enhance tissue repair activities by unique mechanisms. J Cell Biol 1989; 109:429–440.
53. Pierce GF, Mustoe TA, Senior RM, et al.: In vivo incisional wound healing augmented by platelet-

derived growth factor and recombinant c-sis gene homodimeric proteins. J Exp Med 1988;167:974–987.

54. Assouline M, Hutchinson C, Morton K, et al.: In vivo binding of topically applied human bFGF on rabbit corneal epithelial wound. Growth Factors 1989;1:251–261.
55. Fredj-Reygrobellet D, Plouet J, Delayre T, Baudouin C, Bourret F, Lapalus P: Effects of aFGF and bFGF on wound healing in rat corneas. Curr Eye Res 1987;6:1205–1209.
56. Fredj-Reygrobellet D, Elena PP, Moenner M, et al.: Pharmacokinetic and autoradiographic studies of basic fibroblast growth factor on deepithelialized and intact rabbit eye. Curr Eye Res 1989;8:1141–1152.

CHAPTER **19**

Fibronectin Expression During Cutaneous Wound Healing

Livingston Van De Water
Charles ffrench-Constant
Lawrence Brown

INTRODUCTION

Wound healing consists of a succession of overlapping "stages" comprising inflammation, tissue formation, and tissue remodeling. In each of these stages the host response to injury employs patterns of cellular behaviors that bear a strong resemblance to processes essential to normal embryonic development. Thus cell-cell contact, diffusible signals between more distant cells and complex interactions between epithelial and mesenchymal cells and the stromal extracellular matrix are prominent features of both the generative and regenerative processes, and studies of normal embryonic development are likely to give valuable insights into the mechanisms of wound repair.

It has become increasingly clear over the past two decades that the extracellular matrix (ECM), far from being the passive "filler" envisaged by many earlier workers, has an important instructive role in the control of cell behavior during development. One prominent matrix component that appears to be important is fibronectin (FN), a protein known to promote cellular processes in vitro such as cell adhesion and migration, extracellular matrix organization, chemotaxis, and phagocytosis. In embryogenesis, FN is localized in matrices surrounding migrating cells during gastrulation and at many later stages of specific tissue formation. Studies of migration during embryonic development have provided evidence that FN is not only present, but stimulates and possibly guides cell migrations during embryogenesis. Similarly, FN is implicated in the control of cell differentiation later in development and it seems likely that other instructive roles for FN will be found as our knowledge about the ECM increases.

Given this evidence for a role of FN in development attention has focused on the part played by FN during repair. This work has shown FN to be involved in many different aspects of healing, including platelet aggregation, clot formation, epidermal cell migration, collagen matrix assembly, and wound contraction. The purpose of this chapter is to review these roles of FN in wound healing. We shall start by describing the molecular biology of FN and its interaction with the cell. We shall then consider the mechanisms by which FN is produced in the wound and examine its role in the control of the behavior of the different cell types involved in repair. A major theme that will emerge is that the FN within the wound is derived from a number of different sources, and that these sources may each produce a form of FN that differs from the others as a result of alternative splicing of the primary gene transcript. Some of these FNs, which are not synthesized in undamaged skin, are identical to a form of FN found in the early embryo at a time of active cell migration and proliferation. This observation suggests that the reappearance of embryonic FN is an important part of the wound healing response and emphasizes the links between development and repair.

FIBRONECTINS

Structure and Biosynthesis

FNs are dimeric glycoproteins present in fluids and tissue matrices throughout the body.[1–3] Each subunit has a molecular mass of approximately 250 kilodaltons (kDa) and the two subunits are joined by C-terminal disulfide bonds (Fig. 19.1). Each subunit is comprised of a series of homologous amino acid sequences of three types, termed Types I, II, and III repeats. The fibrin binding domains, at the N- and C-termini, are examples of type I repeats (~45 amino acids) having a pair of conserved intrachain disulfide loops at their ends. The collagen site includes two type II repeats (~60 residues) which also contain intrachain disulfide bonds. Type III repeats (~90 amino acids) which are present in the central 70% of the molecule contain no disulfide bonds.

Aside from elucidating the modular structure of FN, molecular cloning evidence has demonstrated that FN exists in multiple molecular forms; these arise by transcription of a single gene to produce RNAs which can be alternatively spliced in three regions, two type III repeats, termed EIIIA (also termed ED-A) and EIIIB (or ED-B) and one nonhomologous region termed V (or IIICS). EIIIA and EIIIB can either be included (A+ or B+) or excluded (A− or B−), while the V region is subdivided in rats (3 forms of V), human (5 forms) and chicken (2 forms). At least one of these regions, V, contains a cell binding site suggesting that splicing will produce functionally different forms of FN. Taking into account all possible combinations of these three domains, at least 12 different forms are

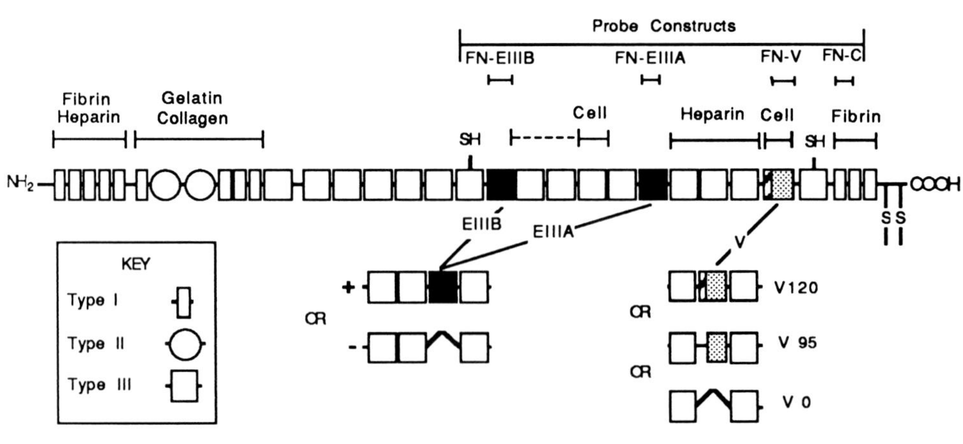

Figure 19.1 A diagrammatic representation of rat FN showing the three regions of alternative splicing and illustrating the potential heterogeneity that can be generated by this mechanism. Binding sites are denoted by bars along the length of the molecule. The four probes used for in situ hybridization are shown in the upper right: note that the V95 probe cannot distinguish the V95 and V120 forms of FN. Modified with permission from ref.[69]

potentially present in the rat (Figure 19.1) and 20 in the human as a result of alternative splicing. In addition, because two-dimensional gels resolve more proteins than predicted, there appears to be even further variation in FN forms beyond that which can be accounted for by alternative splicing.[4]

Alternative splicing of FN occurs in a cell-type specific pattern. Liver hepatocytes, for example, produce pFN which is missing the EIIIB and EIIIA domains but contains one V region per two chains; soluble plasma fibronectin (pFN) is therefore B −/−, A −/−, V +/−.[5–8] Different patterns are observed in other cell types; a developmental study in chick embryos found all four possible combinations of EIIIA and EIIIB in different cell types.[9] Taken together these studies show EIIIA, EIIIB and V to be spliced independently and suggest that many of the possible variants of FN will be present in the ECM. The mechanisms regulating this splicing are unclear. Growth factors are one obvious candidate. Recent data suggest that the inclusion of EIIIB and EIIIA domains by fibroblastic cells may be regulated by TGF-β,[10,11] while endothelial cells incubated with TGF-β give rise to forms of FN which preferentially include a region of V known to contain a cell binding site termed V25.[12]

Binding Sites

The adhesion of cells and ECM components to FN is an important part of the wound healing response. Cell binding to FN is mediated by at least three regions of the molecule. Most attention has focused on a hexapeptide in the central portion of the molecule (III-10) which contains the sequence Gly-Arg-Gly-Asp-Ser-Pro (GRGDSP) and which is sufficient for cell binding.[13–15] The critical sequence within this peptide is RGD which by itself is inactive in cell binding but is active when synthesized as a tetrapeptide, with a variety of residues in the C-terminal position. Peptides containing RGDX sequences also function as cell binding sites in other adhesive proteins.[16] The apparent affinity of cells for the RGDS site in FN is rather low, but is increased in longer fragments of FN.[17] Experiments using fusion proteins containing the RGDS sequence and peptide sequences N-terminal to it indicate that adjacent domains III-8 or III-9 contribute to an increased affinity of cell binding to the RGDS sequence and promote microfilament assembly.[18] However, this region alone cannot substitute for intact FN; even larger fragments are required to promote cell migration.[19,20] Moreover, it appears that the C-terminal heparin binding sites discussed below may be essential in addition to the RGDS region for focal contact assembly.[21,22]

The two other sites lie C-terminal to the RGDS region, one within the heparin binding site and the other within the adjacent V region of FN. The former site is one of several binding sites for glycosaminoglycans and proteoglycans. It is specific for heparin and promotes binding of certain cells[23,24] presumably through cell-surface heparin sulfate proteoglycans.[24–26] The latter site lies C-terminal to this heparin-binding site within the V region. Part of this region, containing an Arg-Glu-Asp-Val (REDV) sequence in human FN at the C-terminal end of the V region, expresses some binding activity for mouse melanoma cells.[27,28] However, the amino acid sequence within this site is not present in rat or chicken FN suggesting that it may not function in all species.[29] Another part, within the N-terminal 25 amino acids of the V region (V25, CS-1), binds melanoma cells efficiently but not some other cell types which do bind via the RGD sequences.[28] This region is well conserved in chicken, rat, and human, suggesting that it represents a genuine cell binding site. At present, therefore, there appear to be three and possibly four cell binding sites in FN: an RGDS site in the central region, a C-terminal proteoglycan site, and one definite and one possible site within the V region.

What are the cellular surface receptors that bind FN? Recent work defines a family of heterodimeric proteins, termed integrins, which range in mass from 115 kD to 165 kD.[30–33] These cell surface proteins are integral membrane proteins composed of two chains, termed α and β. They form a family of molecules that bind to a wide range of ECM ligands, with a limited number of β chains being covalently linked to one of a larger number of different α chains that apparently confer different binding specificities (Table 19.1). There are several integrins which are known to bind FN, including $\alpha_3\beta_1$, $\alpha_4\beta_1$, $\alpha_5\beta 1$, $\alpha_v\beta_1$, $\alpha_{IIb}\beta_3$ and $\alpha_v\beta_5$ integrins, and the expression of these on individual cells may determine which cells migrate, spread or become immobile on FN. The $\alpha_5\beta_1$, $\alpha_{IIb}\beta_3$ integrins bind to the GRGDS sequence within FN[34] while $\alpha_4\beta_1$ binds to the V25 (CS-1) portion of FN[35,36] and both $\alpha_v\beta_1$ and $\alpha_3\beta_1$ appear to bind to the RGD within FN.[37,38] The mechanism by which $\alpha_v\beta_3$ and $\alpha_v\beta_5$ exert FN receptor activity are presently unknown, although recent data suggests that the $\alpha_v\beta_3$ may serve as a cofactor for $\alpha_5\beta_1$ function for certain cells.[39] A number of cells express $\alpha_5\beta_1$, including platelets, monocytes, fibroblasts, endothelial cells and keratinocytes.[30–33] The $\alpha_4\beta_1$ integrin is found on lymphocytes and monocytes, while $\alpha_{IIb}\beta_3$ is expressed by platelets. The distribution of $\alpha_3\beta_1$, $\alpha_v\beta_3$, $\alpha_v\beta_5$ on cells have not yet been elucidated.

In addition to cells, a number of ECM ligands important to wound healing bind at discrete regions within the FN subunit.[1–3] These regions include two binding sites for fibrin and fibrinogen, one at the N-terminal 25–30 kD which can be cross-linked to factor XIIIa, and one at the C-terminus which is not cross-linked. Collagen (Types I–IV and possibly V) bind to a 40–45 kD region of FN near the N-terminus. The affinity of FN for denatured collagens appears higher than that for native collagen and this binding site on FN provides one basis for affinity puri-

TABLE 19.1 The Integrin Receptor Family

Sub-families		α Subunits	Ligands
β_1	α_1	= VLA-1 (CD49a)	LM (COL)
	α_2	= VLA-2 (CD49b) platelet GP Ia	COL (LM)
	α_3	= VLA-3 (CD49c)	FN, LM, COL
	α_4	= VLA-4 (CD49d)	FN (IIICS, V25) V-CAM
	α_5	= VLA-5 (CD49e) platelet GP Ic	FN
	α_6	= VLA-6 (CD49f) platelet GP Ic	LM
	α_v	= CD51	FN
β_2	α_L	= LFA-1 (CD 11a)	I-CAM
	α_M	= MAC-1 (CD 11b)	C3bi, FB
	α_x	= α chain o fp150,95 (CD11c)	C3bi?
β_3	α_{IIb}	= platelet GPIIb (CD41)	FB, FN, VN, VWF
	α_v	= vitronectin receptor (CD51)	VN, FB, VWF, TSP
β_4	α_6	= (CD49f/CD?) [on epithelial cells]	LM?
$\beta_5 = \beta_x = \beta_s$	α_v	= (CD51/CD?) [on epithelial cells and some carcinomas]	VN, FN
β_p	α_4	= VLA-4 L-PAM-1	Peyers Patch HEV

Abbreviations: LM, laminin; COL, collagen; FN, fibronectin; FB, fibrinogen; VN, vitronectin; VWF, von Willebrand's factor; TSP, thrombospondin.

fication.[40] Plasma FN is reported to bind to dermatan sulfate proteoglycans at least in part through the protein core[41] and this binding may be at the C-terminal site within FN. These interactions of FN with proteoglycans are potentially important in tissue repair as recent data indicates that the pattern of proteoglycan expression changes during wound healing.[42] Interactions between FN and cell surface proteoglycans provide an additional mechanism by which cells adhere to extracellular matrices.[24,25,43,44]

Sources of FN in Wound Healing

Plasma FN

One of the first events after wounding is the establishment of a provisional matrix of fibrin-FN.[45] This results from clotting of blood plasma proteins which spill from damaged vessels and also from undamaged vessels rendered leaky by the action of factors promoting permeability.[46,47] An extensive meshwork of fibrin-FN is assembled throughout the bed of the wound which, because it is assembled from pFN, is largely missing the EIIIB and EIIIA domains (pFN is B−/−, A−/−, V+/−). The fibrin within the clot is cross-linked to itself and to pFN by the action of factor XIIIa.[48] Factor XIIIa is produced by the liver as a heterotetramer, a_2b_2, which circulates in blood plasma and is also produced by monocytes/macrophages in culture as the a_2 homodimer.[49,50] Most of the fibrin isolated from the provisional matrix within wounds is cross-linked.[51] However, approximately 50% of FN is cross-linked to fibrin gels in vitro,[48] suggesting that there is an appreciable amount of soluble pFN within the gel. This matrix provided by factor XIIIa-dependent FN cross-linking to fibrin appears to be especially good at promoting the adhesion of fibroblasts.[52] FN may also have activities within the clot other than cell adhesion, such as modulation of the structure of the fibrin gel.[53]

Platelet FN

Platelets, also present in the fibrin gel, contain several adhesive glycoproteins within their alpha granules including FN, thrombospondin, fibrinogen, and von Willebrand factor (vWF).[54] FN is present in platelets at a level of 3 $\mu g/10^9$ cells[55,56] and has been localized to the alpha granules by immunoelectron microscopy[57]; no detectable FN is found on the surfaces of unactivated platelets.[58,59] Several integrins are found on the surfaces of these cells, including glycoprotein IIb/IIIa ($\alpha_{IIb}\beta_3$) at the level of 50,000 to 120,000 sites per cell, with much smaller numbers (few thousand per cell) of $\alpha_2\beta_1$, $\alpha_5\beta_1$, $\alpha_6\beta_1$.[60–66] These latter three integrins bind collagen, FN, laminin, respectively.[32,33] It is by these receptors and by ternary interactions between the granule proteins and plasma glycoproteins that platelets adhere to extravascular fibrin gels and to sub-endothelial basement membrane components to develop a thrombus.

On activation the platelets release their granule contents and express "activated" glycoprotein IIb/IIIa which then is capable of binding fibrin, FN, thrombospondin and vWF, including those within the granule contents. The FN within the platelet alpha granules is not identical to the pFN found within the clot, but includes the EIIIA domain (67). The platelet contributes its own EIIIA+ FN to the clot in amounts which are about 1% of those contributed by pFN within plasma.[54–56] In this way, platelets activated by thrombin during coagulation express glycoprotein IIb/IIIa, bind pFN, and probably bind their own EIIIA+ FN which may in turn promote other platelet functions such as aggregation, adhesion, and spreading. Moreover, these platelets release growth factors such as PDGF and TGF-β which have profound effects on the mitogenic and synthetic function of stromal cells in the wound.

Local Expression of FN During Wound Healing

Against the background of FN synthesized at some distance from the cutaneous wound (e.g., liver, megakaryocytes) and carried to the wound by blood plasma and platelets, FN is also synthesized locally in the wound. This was established by the ingenious transplantation experiments of Clark and colleagues using a model system of rat skin grafted onto the flank of a mouse.[68] Once the graft was well healed the rat skin was wounded and species-specific antibodies used to determine the source of the FN in the wound. As early as 4 days after wounding rat FN predominated, showing that local synthesis makes the dominant contribution to the FN in the wound by this stage. Our own in situ hybridization experiments also emphasize the degree to which local synthesis contributes to the FN in the wound.[69] Normal rat skin produces a low level of FN mRNA (Fig. 19.2). However, two days after wounding, a marked increase is observed in the total amount of FN mRNA (Fig. 19.3). Labeling was seen in cells in the wound bed immediately beneath the clot as well as in a well-defined band of labeling that was observed along the margins of wound. In addition, many more labeled cells

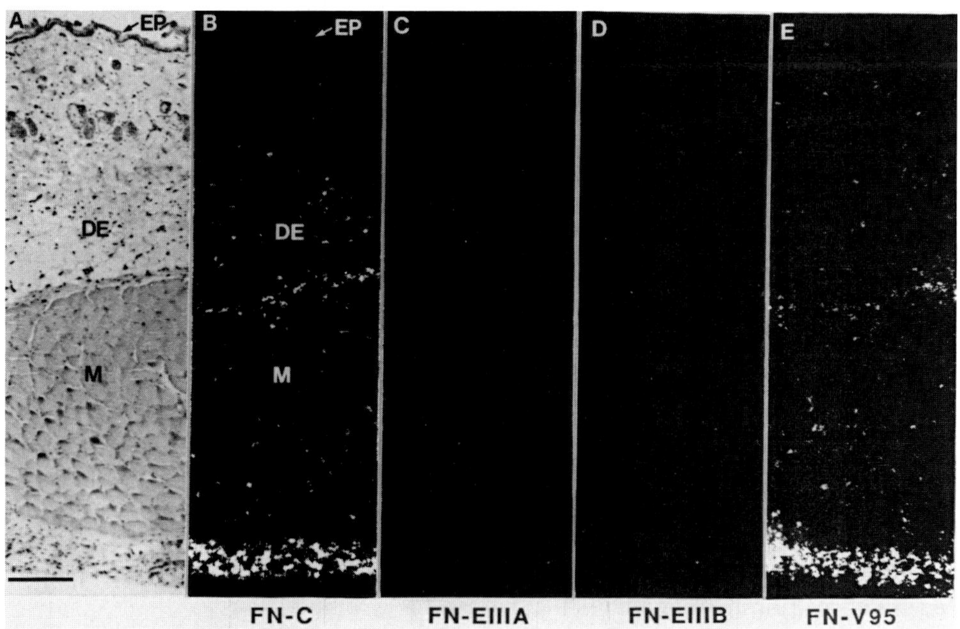

Figure 19.2 Four closely adjacent sections of normal adult rat skin hybridized with the FN-C, FN-EIIIA, FN-EIIIB, and FN-V probes as indicated, and then viewed with darkfield optics (B-E). A representative section viewed with brightfield optics is shown (A). Scattered labeling with FN-C is seen in the reticular dermis (DE), whereas the epidermis (EP) is unlabeled. Labeling is also seen on either side of the striated muscle layer (M) below the dermis, and occasionally within the muscle itself. The segment-specific probes show an identical pattern of labeling with FN-V, but no labeling with FN-EIIIA or FN-IIIB, suggesting that the FN mRNA in normal rat skin is A−B−V+. Bar, 200 μm. With permission from ref.[69]

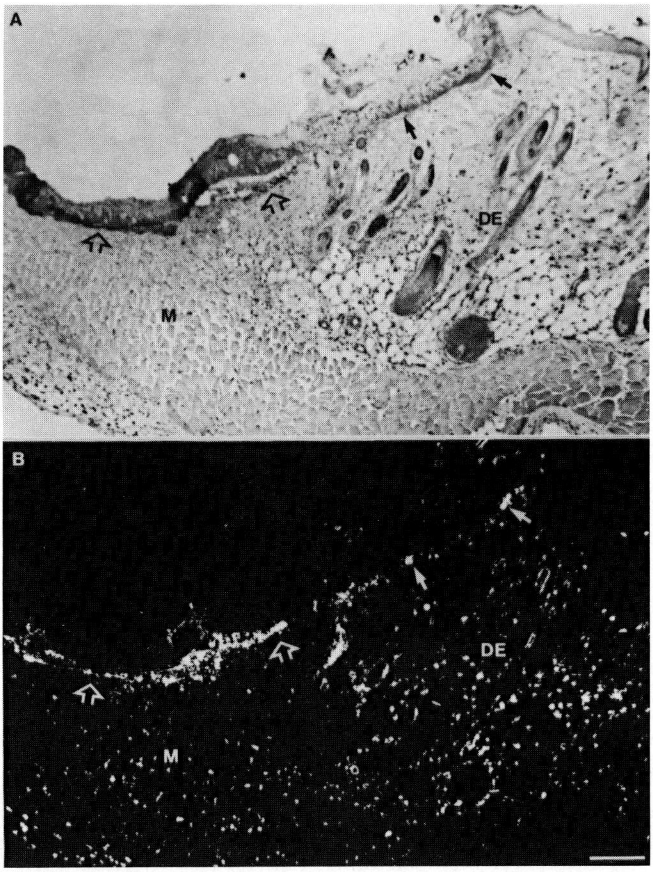

Figure 19.3 A section through one edge of a 2-day wound, hybridized with FN-C and viewed with brightfield (A) and darkfield (B) optics. Extensive scattered labeling is seen in the dermis (DE) and muscle (M). Labeling is also seen at the base (hollow arrow) and edge (arrows) of the wound as well as in the uninjured dermis lateral to the wound (DE). Note that the epidermal cells (EP) have not yet started to migrate centrally. They will migrate down the edge and over the base of the wound during healing. Bar, 200 μm. With permission from ref.[69]

were seen in the neighboring dermis and subadjacent striated muscle than had been observed in the normal skin.

Re-expression of Embryonic Forms of FN During Cutaneous Wound Repair

The FN expressed at high levels in healing wounds is therefore derived from pFN, from platelets, and from local synthesis. Our recent studies suggest that these FNs have important differences generated as a result of different patterns of alternative RNA splicing. As described earlier, different forms of FN can be produced by alternative splicing of the primary gene transcript in three regions: EIIIA, EIIIB, and V. The pFN deposited in the wound is synthesized in the liver and this form of FN has been shown to lack EIIIA and EIIIB, while the platelet FN includes EIIIA.[6,67,70–72] In contrast to both these forms at least some of the FN synthesized in the region of the wound appears to include these exons. The evidence for this comes from in situ hybridization studies using segment-specific probes for the EIIIB, EIIIA and V95 regions of FN (Figure 19.1 and ref. 69). In normal rat skin no hybridization was observed with probes spanning the EIIIB and EIIIA regions, but approximately equivalent labeling was observed with a probe to all forms of FN (FN-C) and to the V95 region (Figure 19.2). The FN mRNA in normal undamaged skin therefore appears to be A–B–V95+. Following wounding a greatly increased level of this pattern of FN mRNA was seen in the dermis adjacent to the wound (Figure 19.3). Additionally, however, FN mRNA including EIIIA and EIIIB was seen in the granulation tissue at the base of the wound and in the cells of the superficial dermis at the edge of the wound over which epidermal cell migration occurs (Fig. 19.4). This labeling by the EIIIA and EIIIB probes was maximal between four and seven days but was also observed at much reduced levels in one to two day wounds, suggesting that this pattern of FN mRNA splicing is an early response to injury. Taken together with cell culture studies showing that the pattern of FN protein reflects that of FN mRNA,[73] these observations show that locally synthesized FNs containing EIIIA and EIIIB will be present in the wound alongside both the A−B− forms derived from local synthesis and from exudation of pFN and relatively minor amounts of A+ forms derived from platelets.

As well as demonstrating heterogeneity of FNs in the healing wound these studies have also allowed the determination of the cell types responsible for the production of FNs containing EIIIA and EIIIB. The macrophages that increase in prominence during the first 4 days after wounding in the region of the base of the wound express FN mRNA containing EIIIA and EIIIB, while those more distant from the wound in the underlying muscle and connective tissue also express FN mRNA in which little if any EIIIB or EIIIA is present (Fig. 19.5, and ref. 74). Later at four to seven days the fibroblasts becoming abundant within granulation tissue also express B+ and A+ FN mRNAs while neutrophils, in contrast, do not synthesize detectable FN mRNA at any stage.[74] These results

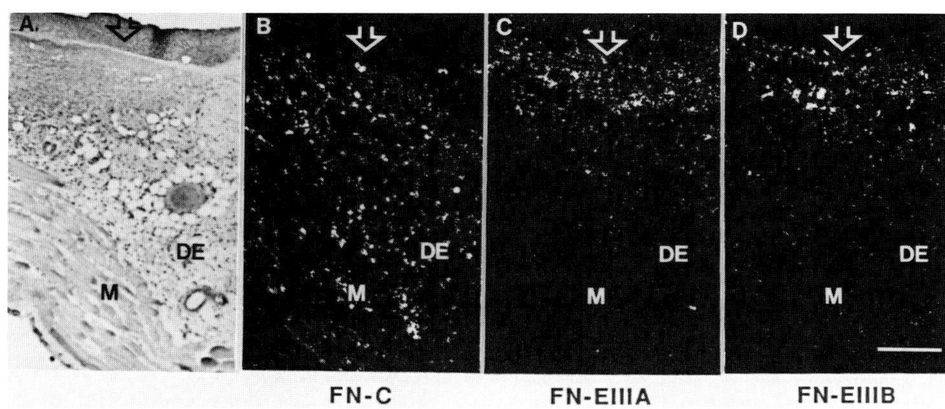

Figure 19.4 Three closely adjacent sections through the base of a 4-day wound hybridized with FN-C, FN-EIIIA, and FN-EIIIB, exposed for 1, 2, and 7 d, respectively, and then viewed with dark-field optics (B-D). A representative section is shown in brightfield optics (A). As explained in the text, the absence of labeling in the dermis (DE) and muscle (M) with FN-EIIIA and FN-EIIIB in the presence of more intense labeling in the base of the wound (hollow arrow) with these probes than with the FN-C probe shows that the restricted expression of EIIIA and EIIIB after wounding reflects a difference in RNA splicing between the two regions. Bar, 300 μm. With permission from ref.[69]

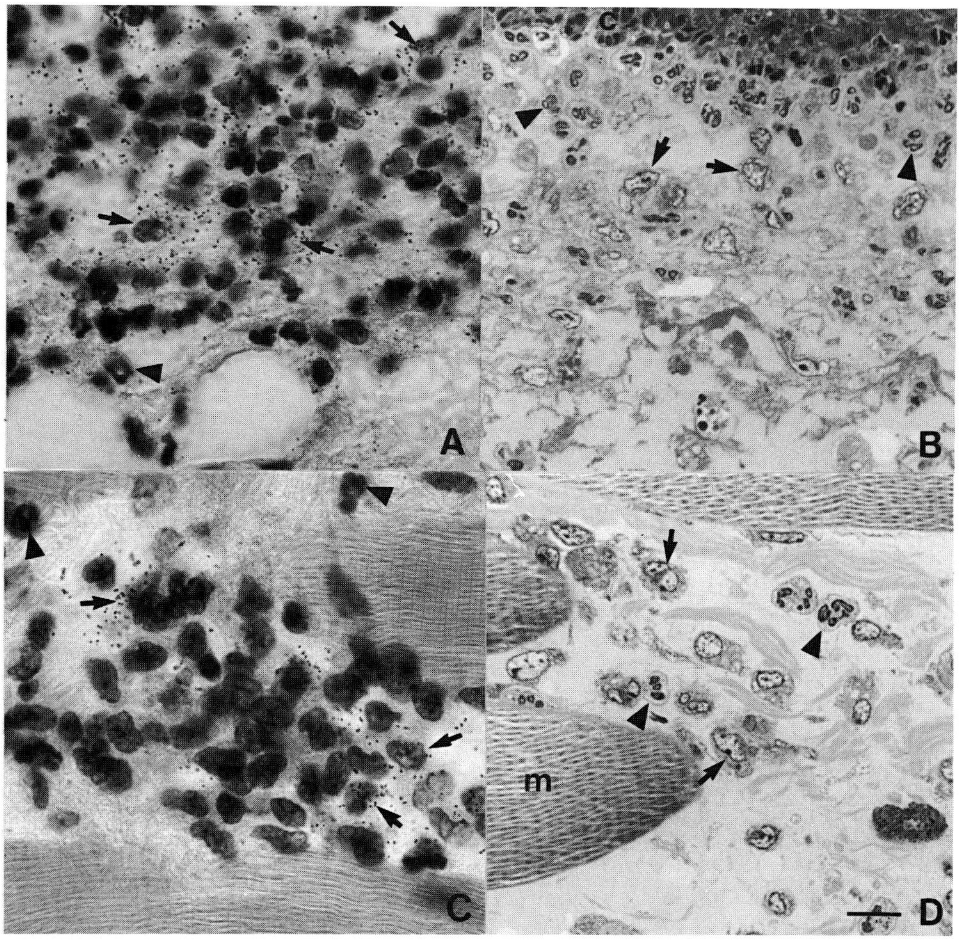

Figure 19.5 Paraffin sections from 2 day wounds (panels A, C) hybridized with FN-C and illustrating expression of FN mRNA by macrophages just beneath the blood clot (panel A) or within the subjacent muscle layer (panel C). These are regions within the wound in which cells are known to express FN mRNAs containing or lacking EIIIB and EIIIA regions, respectively (see Figure 19.4). One micron Epon sections (panels B, D) illustrate the presence of granulocytes (arrowhead), macrophages (arrow) and other inflammatory cells (e.g., lymphocytes, mast cells) just beneath the blood clot (c, panel B) and within subjacent muscle fibers (m, panel D). Bar, 5 μm.

suggest that the production of FNs containing EIIIA and EIIIB is shared by macrophages and fibroblasts, with macrophages predominating early in repair during events such as the migration of epidermal cells through the provisional matrix, while fibroblasts produce the same forms of FN later during activities such as the endothelial migration during angiogenesis or fibroblast-mediated contraction of the wound.

The appearance of EIIIA and EIIIB during wound repair is interesting. Developmental studies have shown that EIIIA+ EIIIB+ FN mRNAs form the great majority of the FN mRNA present in the early embryo at a time when cell migration and proliferation are underway.[9] Later in development as growth is completed, forms of FN mRNA lacking EIIIA and/or EIIIB are seen in cell-type specific patterns within different tissues.[75] Although we do not know the functions of EIIIA and EIIIB these results suggest that A+B+ forms of FN might be functionally the most appropriate for cell migration and proliferation, with other forms being more appropriate for the maintenance of a differentiated structure. Cell migration and proliferation of keratinocytes, macrophages and fibroblasts are essential components of the wound healing response and the reappearance of this early embryonic pattern of FN splicing may therefore be an essential part of this response.

The in situ hybridization analysis also suggested that the two forms of A−B− FN, derived from local synthesis and from exudation of pFN, might differ in their inclusion of the V region. This third region of FN mRNA splicing is known to be excluded in 50% of the FN mRNA encoding pFN.[67,76,77] In wounds, however, the approximately equivalent labeling with FN-C and V95 suggests that most, if not all, FN mRNA includes this region. Healing wounds therefore contain at least four distinct FN mRNAs, with A−B− V95−, A−B−V95+/− and A+B−V? forms in addition to the A+B+V95+ form described above. The functional significance of this added heterogeneity within the V region is, however, unclear. The region of V known to contain a cell binding site, V25 in the rat, is spliced independently of V95 and the probes used in our studies will not distinguish between V25 + and − forms. Studies using specific probes are underway to determine the temporal and spatial distribution of V25. Until these are completed, the attractive hypothesis that splicing of this region contributes to the production of functionally distinct forms of FN in different regions of the wound remains unproven.

Role of FNs in the Cellular Response to Injury

Neutrophils

Neutrophils appear in the cutaneous wound within hours of the initial injury and are the principal elements that sterilize the wound both by phagocytosis and the release of oxygen free radicals.[78] While circulating in the blood, these cells contain small amounts of intracellular FN, very little FN mRNA and no surface bound FN.[79,80] The type of FN within neutrophilic granules is unknown. The amounts of FN expressed by these cells are greatly increased in synovial fluids from patients with rheumatoid arthritis.[80] In contrast, neutrophils within rat cutaneous wounds express no detectable FN mRNA, raising the possibility that FN production by these cells is very specific to the type of inflammatory response.[74]

Adhesion to FN of neutrophils activated by chemotactic agents promotes cellular functions such as complement-mediated phagocytosis (e.g., f-Met-Leu-Phe[81]). Neutrophils do express integrins within the β_3 group which may function as transducers of this cellular activation and certain integrins are shuttled from the granules to the cell surface upon activation.[82] The dense granules also contain neutral proteases which are capable of degrading FN and other extracellular matrix proteins and are likely to be important in the generation of fragments of FN within the fibrin gel.[78] Fragments of FN containing RGD sequences have been shown to be chemotactic for monocytes and thus may have a promotional role in the immigration of monocytes into the wound.[83]

Macrophages

Uninjured skin contains very few macrophages. During an inflammatory reaction such as wounding, however, the number of cells increases dramatically and in adult cutaneous wound healing macrophages are quite evident by two days. Kinetic studies using ^{3}H-thymidine labeling indices demonstrated that some 99% of the macrophages appearing in the wound are derived from the circulation.[84] While early studies put forth the idea that macrophages were primarily phagocytic cells, it has become increasingly clear that these cells are essential for a smooth transition from the inflammatory reaction to the reparative processes. Administration of hydrocortisone systemically, which decreases the number of macrophages that appear in cutaneous wounds, also causes a decrease in the appearance of fibroblasts and the subsequent deposition of scar tissue.[85] It is now quite clear that macrophages elaborate a large variety of cytokines, growth factors and adhesive proteins, a topic presented in Chapter 3 and the subject of recent reviews.[86,87] These mediators are clearly important in this transition to tissue repair.

Peripheral blood monocytes do not secrete FN when freshly explanted, nor do they contain detectable FN mRNA.[73,88] After a period of 5–10 days in culture, these cells acquire properties of macrophages and begin to synthesize FN. The amount of FN mRNA and the secreted protein rise concomitantly during this induction period suggesting that there is a linear relationship between the amount of mRNA and protein secreted.[73] Macrophages explanted from the peritoneum or alveoli are also capable of synthesizing and secreting FN but do not assemble it into their own extracellular matrix.[89–91] Such FN synthesis appears to be a feature of the macrophage response to injury. FN mRNA expression rises in macrophages derived from patients with idiopathic pulmonary fibrosis, a disorder associated with exaggerated amounts of FN in the lower respiratory tract.[91] During the first two days following cutaneous injury in the rat, FN mRNA is also expressed by macrophages; no detectable FN mRNA was observed in neutrophils or other granulocytes observed within the wound.[74] In healing cutaneous wounds it appears that macrophages are the first cells entering the wound to produce FN mRNA and they express it in regions along which epidermal cell migration occurs. This finding suggests that macrophage FN production may be critical to the early closure of the cutaneous wound.

FN promotes certain macrophage functions. Monocytes are chemotactic toward fragments of FN containing the RGDS cell binding domain.[83,92] Given the large amount ($\sim$300 μg/ml) of pFN in the provisional matrix, of which some 50% is uncrosslinked,[48] as well as the significant potential for neutral proteases elaborated by neutrophils to degrade FN, it seems likely that large amounts of diffusible fragments are generated and may play a role, with other chemotactic factors (e.g., C5a, see review 93), in recruiting blood monocytes to the wound area. On the other hand, under certain conditions, FN may modulate migration. When macrophages encounter the fibrin-FN cross-linked gel, macrophage migration is decreased.[94]

FN has direct effects on macrophage phagocytosis. The observation that FN binds to gram-negative and gram-positive bacteria, spirochetes, and to yeast, encouraged the notion that FN might serve as an opsonin for microorganisms.[95–99] However, there is no convincing evidence for this role of FN.[97] FN does promote the uptake of particles coated with denatured collagen and fibrin suggesting that it may play a role in the task of tissue remodeling by macrophages.[89,100–103] Bacterial adhesion to host tissue is promoted by FN, indicating that FN is a host protein used to the advantage of the microorganism.[104]

FN also appears to promote macrophage phagocytosis indirectly. Peripheral blood monocytes express receptors for particles opsonized with C3b and iC3b;

however, these receptors exhibit little activity until the cells are activated by extracellular conditions including adhesion to substrata coated with FN,[105–107] laminin,[108] serum amyloid P,[107] or vitronectin.[109] Activation is dependent upon the presence of an RGD sequence in FN,[110] does not require any increase in the numbers of receptors or in protein synthesis and appears to involve activation of protein kinase C.[106,107,111] Monocytes and macrophages express FN receptors; however, the mechanism by which these receptors may function to activate cells is unclear.[112–115] Phagocytosis is not the only cell function increased by adherence to FN, as monocytes and macrophages also express increased PDGF mRNA.[116]

Epidermal Cells

An early and essential event in healing skin wounds is the inward migration of epidermal cells from the wound edges to cover the injured surface. This re-epithelialization is crucial to successful cutaneous wound healing as it provides increased tensile strength and, by closing the wound, prevents further infection and dessication. Immunohistochemical staining for FN indicates that these migrating cells are underlaid by an irregular band of fibrin and FN,[46,47,68] while in normal, uninjured skin the epidermal basal lamina contains little or no fibrin or FN.[117] However, when in situ hybridization is carried out, neither migrating nor normal epidermal cells appear to express significant amounts of FN mRNA.[69] Instead, the cells beneath the migrating epidermis appear responsible for the synthesis of FN. Without competition by endogenous FN, receptors on epidermal cells may then be maximally responsive to FN encountered in the pathway. Although a number of reports demonstrate that epidermal cells express FN when explanted into culture,[118–123] it is not clear how this data applies to wound healing. However, the fact that these cells, while in culture, express the capacity for FN synthesis suggests that under certain conditions they may produce FN in situ.

How do these cells employ FN to migrate? Both biochemical data from cells in culture and immunohistochemical data on healing wounds indicate that epidermal cells express integrins in the β_1 sub-family.[124–127] Low levels of β_1 is expressed on normal, uninjured epidermis and is found on the basolateral surface.[124] Conversely, migrating epidermis expresses elevated levels of the β_1 integrins. Biochemical data demonstrate that epidermal cells express $\alpha_2\beta_1$, $\alpha_3\beta_1$, and $\alpha_5\beta_1$ on their surfaces and as these cells differentiate into involucrin-positive cells the activity of the $\alpha_5\beta_1$ receptor diminishes, followed by a loss of all three β_1 receptors from the cell surface.[127] Taken together this data suggests a model of epidermal function in which adhesion to the FN-fibrin provisional matrix is essential for prompt migration and closure of healing wounds. Progressive loss of adhesion to FN by integrins is accompanied by maturation of the basal cells and progression to terminally differentiated cells.[127]

Fibroblasts

Among the diverse cell types present in normal dermis, fibroblasts constitute a large potential reservoir for FN production. When explanted into culture, fibroblasts from a variety of tissues secrete relatively large amounts (on order of μgs/day/10^6 cells) of FN (reviewed in 3). Moreover, these cells produce all combinations of alternatively spliced FNs indicating that they have the potential for production of these forms in situ.[8] Supplementation of the growth medium with TGF-β results in increased secretion and deposition of FN[128–131] and in some instances may increase the ratios of B+/B−[10] and A+/A−[11] forms produced. By contrast, in situ hybridization data indicates that normal dermal fibroblasts produce little FN mRNA (Figure 19.2). However, by four to seven days following wounding, these cells contain large amounts of FN mRNA and appear to be the major cell type producing FN in granulation tissue.[74] Wounding must therefore stimulate a cascade of events starting with macrophage FN expression and culminating in the increased production of appropriate forms of FN by fibroblasts in forming granulation tissue.

What then might be the functions of the fibroblast-derived FN in granulation tissue? This FN may be instructive, guiding the orderly deposition of collagen within the granulation tissue. At the tissue level fibroblasts, and fibrils of FN and collagen[124,132] appear to orient themselves in a direction parallel to the overlying epidermis. Ultrastructural analysis reveals associations between the FN and collagen fibrils in forming granulation tissue.[133] Biochemical evidence demonstrates that all FNs bind to native (Types I–IV) and more avidly to denatured (Types I–IV, especially Type III) collagens.[134–136] Moreover, FN appears first in granulation tissue followed by Types III and I collagen.[47,137] This is confirmed by the sequential appearance of FN and Type I collagen mRNA in forming granulation tissue when analyzed by in situ hybridization (Van De Water and Brown, unpublished). In culture, fibroblasts assemble FN into fibrils which also contain Types I and III collagen.[133] This is not a passive process, but requires the involvement of cells which express cell assembly "sites."[138–140] Collagenase digestion removes collagen but not FN from these matrices, while trypsin or thrombin treatments that digest FN remove both.[141–143] Moreover, treatment of cultures with antibody to the gelatin-binding site perturb collagen deposition in these cultures.[144] Taken together these observations indicate that FN provides important structural information for assembly of a collagen-containing matrix in culture and in maturing granulation tissue.

Consideration of the role of such a matrix brings us to a second important possible function, wound contraction. This is a process essential to successful cutaneous wound remodeling, but one that can be deleterious resulting in the impaired function of affected organs.[145] Wound contraction occurs by the concerted function of collagen-rich fibrils outside the cells and the actomyosin contractile system within cells.[146] That FN functions as one link in such a system was demonstrated by immunolocalization studies on tissue culture fibroblasts in which FN fibrils outside of cells were observed to be oriented in a colinear fashion with intracellular actin filaments.[147,148] These seem to terminate at a structure at the plasma membrane, termed the fibronexus,[149] which contains receptors for FN and cytoskeletal proteins.[3,150] Fibronexi have also been observed on fibroblasts in situ in granulation tissue five to seven days after wounding.[132,151] Tissue collagens were observed to associate with immunoreactive FN which in turn co-aligns with intracellular actin microfilament bundles. Moreover, FN receptor expression, microfilament bundle formation and extensive cell-matrix links occur concomitantly and temporally precede measurable wound contraction.[132] Taken together these data are consistent with a model in which FN is an important link between collagen and fibroblasts which generate the force needed for wound contraction.

Endothelial Cells

Angiogenesis is an essential component of granulation tissue formation in which new vessels form by budding of endothelial cells from existing vessels.[152] Endothelial cells migrating away from the parent vessel are followed closely by a population of dividing cells.[153] FN is found in the vessel basement membrane near cutaneous wounds and reaches a peak of expression at approximately the same time as the peak in cell division, suggesting a role for FN in endothelial cell migration.[154] That this FN is locally produced is demonstrated by skin transplant experiments in which cells from donor skin deposited FN in vessel basement membranes.[68] FN promotes endothelial attachment and migration in tissue culture and these cultivated cells synthesize FN and produce an FN-rich matrix in culture (reviewed in Chapter 3). Recent evidence indicates that endothelial cells produce EIIIA+ forms[155] and assemble FNs on the basolateral surface.[156] This data implicates FN but does not prove a role for it in the establishment of new vessels during embryogenesis and during the tissue regeneration that accompanies tissue repair. Although FN is made by endothelial cells in culture, it is not clear that these cells make it during wound healing. Experiments done with in situ hybridization for FN on healing adult wounds suggests that endothelial cells in new vessels make very little FN mRNA during granulation tissue formation (Van De Water and Brown, unpublished data). Instead the FN mRNA may be produced by accessory cells (fibroblasts) or the "pioneering" endothelial cells suggested by McAuslan et al.[157,158]

In summary, a succession of cells are important in the sequence of events in wound healing. Of these, most, if not all, of the above-mentioned cells either store FN in intracellular granules or have been found to produce FN in culture. However, it appears that not all of these cells may produce FN mRNA during wound healing. In situ hybridization data indicates that monocytes/macrophages are the earliest cells appearing in the wound which produce FN locally. This FN may be involved in epidermal cell migration, differentiation or division. The process of synthesis initiated by macrophages is gradually replaced by fibroblasts which are major producers of FN in forming granulation tissue; this FN may serve important roles in the contraction of the wound. It is evident that endothelial cells bind FN which may have important roles in angiogenesis; however, the source of this FN is unclear.

An obvious question raised by our work on the splicing of FN during wounding is how the various cell types respond to the different FNs in the wound. Answers to this question are clearly essential before one can understand how the different FNs are utilized during wound healing. Until recently it has not been possible to address this issue as the FN purified from sources such as cultured cells contains an unknown mixture of EIIIA and EIIIB. The availability of purified recombinant FNs of any desired splicing pattern should enable this obstacle to be overcome in the near future.[159]

CONCLUSIONS AND LESSONS FOR FETAL WOUNDING

The central point that emerges from the work described in this chapter is that FN is not a single molecule but rather a family of molecules produced by alternative splicing that may each have different functions. This splicing is precisely regulated; in situ hybridization demonstrates first, that only certain cells in embryos or in healing wounds express FN mRNA and second, that there is spatial segregation of FN splicing. The mechanisms controlling this splicing remain unclear although growth factors such as TGF-β are obvious candidates.

The observation that adult wound healing is associated with a reappearance of an embryonic FN may explain some of the unique features of fetal wound healing, namely that it takes place in the absence of large numbers of inflammatory cells, proceeds with rapid re-epithelialization of the defect and produces little scar. It is possible that the functionally appropriate forms of FN produced during morphogenesis and organogenesis will still remain in the tissues and will hasten repair by circumventing the need for production of these FNs by the infiltrating macrophages and fibroblasts so prominent in adult wound healing. Analysis of FN synthesis and alternative splicing patterns during fetal wound healing may support this hypothesis and may guide future efforts to promote re-epithelialization or limit scarring in adult tissue repair.

REFERENCES

1. McDonagh J: Plasma Fibronectin: Structure and Function; Marcel Dekker, New York, 1985.
2. Mosher DF: Fibronectin. Academic Press, New York, 1989.
3. Hynes R: Fibronectins. Springer-Verlag, New York, 1990.
4. Paul J, Hynes RO: Multiple fibronectin subunits and their post-translational modifications. J Biol Chem. 259:13477–13487, 1984.
5. Gutman A, Kornblihtt AR: Identification of a third region of cell-specific alternative splicing in human fibronectin mRNA. Proc Natl Acad Sci USA 84:7179–7182, 1987.
6. Kornblihtt AR, Vibe-Pedersen K, Baralle FE: Human fibronectin: cell specific alternative mRNA splicing generates polypeptide chains differing in the number of internal repeats. Nuc Acid Res 12:5853–5868, 1984.
7. Norton PA, Hynes RO: Alternative splicing of chicken fibronectin in embryos and in normal and transformed cells. Mol Cell Biol 7:4297–4307, 1987.
8. Schwarzbauer JE, Patel RS, Fonda D, Hynes RO: Multiple sites of alternative splicing of the rat fibronectin gene transcript. EMBO Journal 6:2573–2580, 1987.
9. ffrench-Constant C, Hynes RO: Patterns of fibronectin gene expression and splicing during cell migration in chicken embryos. Development 104:369–382, 1988.
10. Balza E, Borsi L, Allemanni G, Zardi L: Transforming growth factor β regulates the levels of different fibronectin isoforms in normal human cultured fibroblasts. FEBS Lett 228:42–44, 1988.
11. Borsi L, Castellani P, Risso A, Leprini A, Zardi L: Transforming growth factor-β regulates the splicing pattern of fibronectin messenger RNA precursor. FEBS Lett 261:175–178, 1990.
12. Kocher O, Kennedy S, Madri J: Alternative splicing of endothelial cell fibronectin mRNA in the IIICS region. Am J Pathol 137:1509–1524, 1990.
13. Pierschbacher MD, Hayman EG, Ruoslahti E: Location of the cell-attachment site in fibronectin with monoclonal antibodies and proteolytic fragments of the molecule. Cell 26:259–267, 1981.
14. Pierschbacher MD, Hayman EG, Ruoslahti E: Synthetic peptide with cell attachment activity of fibronectin. Proc Natl Acad Sci USA 80:1224–1227, 1983.
15. Pierschbacher MD, Ruoslahti E: Cell attachment activity of fibronectin can be duplicated by small synthetic fragments of the molecule. Nature 309:30–33, 1984.
16. Pierschbacher MD, Ruoslahti E: Influence of stereochemistry of the sequence Arg-Gly-Asp-Xaa on binding specificity in cell adhesion. J Biol Chem 262:17294–17298, 1987.
17. Akiyama SK, Yamada KM: The interaction of plasma fibronectin with fibroblastic cells in suspension. J Biol Chem 260:4492–4500, 1985.
18. Obara M, Kang MS, Yamada KM: Site-directed mutagenesis of the cell-binding domain of human fibronectin: separable, synergistic sites mediate adhesive function. Cell 53:649–657, 1988.
19. McCarthy JB, Hagen ST, Furcht LT: Human fibronectin contains distinct adhesion- and motility-promoting domains for metastatic melanoma cells. J Cell Biol 102:179–188, 1986.
20. Dufour S, Duband J-L, Kornblihtt AR, Thiery JP: The role of fibronectins in embryonic cell migration. Trends Genet 4:198–203, 1988.
21. Izzard C, Radinsky R, Culp L: Substratum contacts and cytoskeletal reorganization of Balb/c

3T3 cells on a cell-binding fragment and heparin binding fragments of plasma fibronectin. Exp Cell Res 165:320–336, 1986.

22. Woods A, Couchman J, Johansson S, Hook M: Adhesion and cytoskeletal organization of fibroblasts in response to fibronectin fragments. EMBO J 5:665–670, 1986.
23. Rogers S, Letourneau PC, Peterson BA, Furcht LT, McCarthy JB: Selective interaction of peripheral and central nervous system cells with two distinct cell-binding domains of fibronectin. J Cell Biol 105:1435–1442, 1987.
24. Saunders S, Bernfield M: Cell surface proteoglycan binds mouse mammary epithelial cells to fibronectin and behaves as a receptor for interstitial matrix. J Cell Biol 106:423–430, 1988.
25. LeBaron R, Esko J, Woods A, Johansson S, Hook M: Adhesion of glycosaminoglycan-deficient chinese hamster ovary cell mutants to fibronectin substrate. J Cell Biol 106:945–952, 1988.
26. McCarthy JB, Chelberg MK, Mickelson DJ, Furcht LT: Localization and chemical synthesis of fibronectin peptides with melanoma adhesion and heparin binding activities. Biochemistry 27:1380–1388, 1988.
27. Humphries M, Akiyama S, Komoriya A, Olden K, Yamada K: Identification of an alternatively spliced site in human plasma fibronectin that mediates cell type-specific adhesion. J Cell Biol 103:2637–2647, 1986.
28. Humphries M, Komoriya A, Akiyama S, Olden K, Yamada K: Identification of two distinct regions of the type III connecting segment of human plasma fibronectin that promote cell type-specific adhesion. J Biol Chem 262:6886–6892, 1987.
29. Norton P, Hynes R: Alternative splicing of chicken fibronectin in embryos and in normal and transformed cells. Mol Cell Biol 7:4297–4307, 1987.
30. Hynes RO: Integrins: a family of cell surface receptors. Cell 48:549–554, 1987.
31. Ruoslahti E: Fibronectin and its receptors. Ann Rev Biochem 57:375–413, 1988.
32. Albeda S, Buck C: Integrins and other cell adhesion molecules. FASEB J 4:2868–2880, 1990.
33. Hemler ME: VLA proteins in the integrin family: structures, functions, and their role on leukocytes. Ann Rev Immunol 8:365–400, 1990.
34. Ruoslahti E, Pierschbacher MD: New perspectives in cell adhesion: RGD and integrins. Science 238:491–497, 1987.
35. Wayner E, Garcia-Pardo A, Humphries M, McDonald J, Carter W: Identification and characterization of the T lymphocyte adhesion receptor for an alternative cell attachment domain (CS-1) in plasma fibronectin. J Cell Biol 109:1321–1330, 1989.
36. Guan J, Hynes R: Lymphoid cells recognize an alternatively spliced segment of fibronectin via the integrin receptor $\alpha_4\beta_1$. Cell 60:53–61, 1990.
37. Vogel B, Tarone G, Giancotti F, Gailit J, Ruoslahti E: A novel fibronectin receptor with an unexpected subunit composition ($\alpha_v\beta 1$). J Biol Chem 265:5934–5937, 1990.
38. Elices M, Urry L, Hemler M: Receptor functions for the integrin VLA-3: Fibronectin, collagen and laminin binding are differentially influenced by Arg-Gly-Asp peptide and by divalent cations. J Cell Biol 112:169–181, 1991.
39. Charo I, Nannizzi L, Smith J, Cheresh D: The vitronectin receptor $\alpha v\beta 3$ binds fibronectin and acts in concert with $\alpha 5\beta 1$ in promoting cellular attachment and spreading on fibronectin. J Cell Biol 111:2795–2800, 1990.
40. Engvall E, Ruoslahti E: Binding of soluble form of fibroblast surface protein, fibronectin, to collagen. Int J Cancer 20:1–5, 1977.
41. Schmidt G, Robenek H, Harrach B, et al.: Interactions of small dermatan sulfate proteoglycan from fibroblasts with fibronectin. J Cell Biol 104:1683–1691, 1987.
42. Yeo T-K, Brown L, Dvorak H: Alterations in proteoglycan synthesis common to healing wounds and tumors. Am J Pathol. 138:1437–1450, 1991.
43. Laterra J, Silbert JE, Culp LA: Cell surface heparan sulfate mediates some adhesive responses to glycosaminoglycan-binding matrices, including fibronectin. J Cell Biol 96:112–123, 1983.
44. McCarthy JB, Skubitz AP, Qi Z, et al.: RGD-independent cell adhesion to the carboxy-terminal heparin-binding fragment of fibronectin involves heparin-dependent and -independent activities. J Cell Biol 110:777–787, 1990.
45. Clark RAF, Henson PM: The Molecular and Cellular Biology of Wound Repair. Plenum Press, New York, 1988, pp 597.
46. Clark RA, Lanigan JM, DellaPelle P, Manseau E, Dvorak HF, Colvin RB: Fibronectin and fibrin provide a provisional matrix for epidermal cell migration during wound reepithelialization. J Invest Dermatol 79:264–269, 1982.
47. Dvorak HF, Form DM, Manseau EJ. Smith BD: Pathogenesis of desmoplasia. I. Immunoflu-

orescence identification and localization of some structural proteins of line 1 and line 10 guinea pig tumors and of healing wounds. J Natl Cancer Inst 73:1195–1205, 1984.

48. Mosher DF: Action of fibrin-stabilizing factor on cold-insoluble globulin and alpha2-macroglobulin in clotting plasma. J Biol Chem 251:1639–1645, 1976.
49. Yorifuji H, Anderson K, Lynch GW, Van De Water L, McDonagh J: B protein of factor XIII: differentiation between free B and complexed B. Blood 72:1645–1650, 1988.
50. Kradin RL, Lynch GW, Kurnick JT, Erikson M, Colvin RB, McDonagh J: Factor XIII A is synthesized and expressed on the surface of U937 cells and alveolar macrophages. Blood 69:778–785, 1987.
51. Brown LF, Van De Water L, Harvey VS, Dvorak HF: Fibrinogen influx and accumulation of cross-linked fibrin in healing wounds and in tumor stroma. Am J Pathol 130:455–465, 1988.
52. Grinnell F, Feld M, Minter D: Fibroblast adhesion to fibrinogen and fibrin substrata: requirement for cold-insoluble globulin (plasma fibronectin). Cell 19:517–525, 1980.
53. Carr MJ, Gabriel DA, McDonagh J: Influence of factor XIII and fibronectin on fiber size and density in thrombin-induced fibrin gels. J Lab Clin Med 110:747–752, 1987.
54. Ginsberg M, Plow E: Fibronectin: A contender in platelet adhesive function. In Mosher D (ed): Fibronectin; Academic Press, New York, 1989, pp 474.
55. Plow E, Birdwell C, Ginsberg M. Identification and quantitation of platelet associated fibronectin antigen. J Clin Invest 63:540–543, 1979.
56. Zucker M, Mosesson M, Broekman M, Kaplan K: Release of platelet fibronectin (cold-insoluble globulin) from alpha granules induced by thrombin or collagen: Lack of requirement for plasma fibronectin in ADP-induced platelet aggregation. 54:8–11, 1979.
57. Wencel-Drake J, Painter R, Zimmerman T, Ginsberg M: Ultrastructural localization of human platelet thrombospondin, fibrinogen, fibronectin and von Willebrand factor in frozen thin sections. Blood 65:929–938, 1985.
58. Hynes R, Ali I, Destree A, et al.: A large glycoprotein lost from the surfaces of transformed cells. NY Acad Sci 312:317–342, 1978.
59. Ginsberg M, Plow EJ: Supramol. Struct. 17:91–98, 1981.
60. Gardner J, Hynes R: Interaction of fibronectin with its receptor on platelets. Cell 42:439–448, 1985.
61. Parise L, Phillips D: Platelet membrane glycoprotein IIb-IIIa complex incorporated into phospholipid vesicles: Preparation and morphology. J Biol Chem 260:1750–1756, 1985.
62. Plow E, Pierschbacher M, Ruoslahti E, Marguerie G, Ginsberg M: The effect of arg-gly-asp-containing peptides on fibrinogen and von Willebrand factor binding to platelets. Proc Natl Acad Sci 82:8057–8061, 1985.
63. Pytela R, Pierschbacher M, Ginsberg M, Plow E, Ruoslahti E: Platelet membrane glycoprotein IIb/IIIa: Members of a family of arg-gly-asp-specific adhesion receptors. Science 231:1559–1562, 1986.
64. Kunicki T, Nugent D, Staats S, Orchekowski R, Wayner E, Carter W: The human fibroblast class II extracellular matrix receptor mediates platelet adhesion to collagen and is identical to the platelet glycoprotein Ia-IIa complex. J Biol Chem 263:4516–4519, 1988.
65. Hemler M, Crouse C, Takada Y, Sonnenberg A: Multiple very late antigen (VLA) heterodimers on platelets: evidence for distinct VLA-2, VLA-5 (fibronectin receptor) and VLA-6 structures. J Biol Chem 263:7660–7665, 1988.
66. Pischel K, Bluestone H, Woods V: Platelet glycoproteins Ia, Ic and IIa are physiochemically indistinguishable from the very late activation antigens adhesion-related proteins of lymphocytes and other cell types. J Clin Invest 81:505–508, 1988.
67. Paul J, Schwarzbauer J, Tamkun J, Hynes R: Cell-type-specific fibronectin subunits generated by alternative splicing. J Biol Chem 261:12258–12265, 1986.
68. Clark RA, Winn HJ, Dvorak HF, Colvin RB: Fibronectin beneath reepithelializing epidermis in vivo: sources and significance. J Invest Dermatol 26s–30s, 1983.
69. ffrench-Constant C, Van De Water L, Dvorak HF, Hynes RO: Reappearance of an embryonic pattern of fibronectin splicing during wound healing in the adult rat. J Cell Biol 109:903–914, 1989.
70. Borsi L, Carnemolla B, Castellani P, et al.: Monoclonal antibodies in the analysis of fibronectin isoforms generated by alternative splicing of mRNA precursors in normal and transformed human cells. J Cell Biol 104:595–600, 1987.
71. Peters JH, Ginsberg MH, Bohl BP, Sklar LA, Cochrane C: Intravascular release of intact cellular fibronectin during oxidant-induced injury of the in vitro perfused rabbit lung. J Clin Invest 78:1596–1603, 1986.

72. Schwarzbauer J, Patel R, Fonda D, Hynes R: Multiple sites of alternative splicing of the rat fibronectin gene transcript. EMBO Journal 6:2573–2580, 1987.
73. Yamauchi K, Martinet Y, Crystal R: Modulation of fibronectin gene expression in human mononuclear phagocytes. J Clin Invest 80:1720–1727, 1987.
74. Van De Water L, Brown L, Dubin D, Lavigne L, Murphy T: Macrophages regulate their fibronectin splicing pattern during wound healing. Submitted, 1991.
75. ffrench-Constant C, Hynes RO: Alternative splicing of fibronectin is temporally and spatially regulated in the chicken embryo. Development 375–388, 1989.
76. Schwarzbauer JE, Paul JI, Hynes RO: On the origin of species of fibronectin. Proc Natl Acad Sci USA 82:1424–1428, 1985.
77. Hershberger R, Culp L: Cell-type-specific expression of alternatively spliced human fibronectin IIICS mRNAs. Mol Cel Biol 662–671, 1990.
78. Tonnesen M, Worthen G, Johnston R: Neutrophil emigration, activation and tissue damage. In Clark RAF and Henson PM, (eds): The Molecular and Cellular Biology of Wound Repair. Plenum Press, New York, 1988, pp 149–183.
79. Beaulieu T, Audette M, Menard C, Parent C, Duval M: Studies on fibronectin in inflammatory vs non-inflammatory polymorphonuclear leukocytes of patients with rheumatoid arthritis. I. Immunofluorescent and flow cytometric analysis. Clin Exp Immunol 60:339–346, 1985.
80. La Fleur M, Beaulieu AD, Kreis C, Poubelle P: Fibronectin gene expression in polymorphonuclear leukocytes: accumulation of mRNA in inflammatory cells. J Biol Chem 262:2111–2115, 1987.
81. Pommier CG, O'Shea J, Chused T, et al.: Studies on the fibronectin receptors of human peripheral blood leukocytes: morphological and functional characterization. J Exp Med 159:137–151, 1984.
82. Singer II, Scott S, Kawka DW, Kazazis DM: Adhesomes: specific granules containing receptors for laminin, C3bi/fibrinogen, fibronectin, and vitronectin in human polymorphonuclear leukocytes and monocytes. J Cell Biol 3169–3182, 1989.
83. Clark RAF, Wilkner N, Doherty D, Norris D: Cryptic chemotactic activity of fibronectin for human monocytes resides in the 120-kDa fibroblastic cell-binding fragment. J. Biol. Chem. 263:12115–12123, 1988.
84. van Furth R, Diesselhoff-den Dulk M, Sluiter W, van Dissel J: New perspectives on the kinetics of mononuclear phagocytes. In van Furth R, (eds): Mononuclear Phagocytes: Characteristics, Physiology and Function; Martinus Nijhoff, Dordrecht, Holland, 1985, pp 201–208.
85. Leibovich S, Ross R: The role of the macrophage in wound repair. A study with hydrocortisone and antimacrophage serum. Am J Pathol 78:71–100, 1975.
86. Nathan C: Secretory products of macrophages. J Clin Invest 79:319–326, 1987.
87. Rappolee D, Werb Z: Secretory products of phagocytes. Curr. Opin. in Immunol. 1:47–55, 1988.
88. Alitalo K, Hovi T, Vaheri A: Fibronectin is produced by human macrophages. J Exp Med 151:602–613, 1980.
89. Van De Water L, Schroeder S, Crenshaw E, Hynes RO: Phagocytosis of gelatin-latex particles by a murine macrophage line is dependent on fibronectin and heparin. J Cell Biol 90:32–39, 1981.
90. Villiger B, Kelley D, Engleman W, Kuhn C, McDonald J: Human alveolar macrophage fibronectin; Synthesis, secretion, and ultrastructural localization during gelatin-coated latex particle binding. J. Cell Biol 90:711–720, 1981.
91. Rennard S, Hunninhake G, Bitterman P, Crystal R: Production of fibronectin by the human alveolar macrophage: Mechanism for the recruitment of fibroblasts to sites of tissue injury in interstitial lung diseases. Proc Natl Acad Sci 78:7147–7151, 1981.
92. Norris DA, Clark RAF, Swigart LM, Huff JC, Weston WL, Howell SE: Fibronectin fragment(s) are chemotactic for human peripheral blood monocytes. J Immunol 129:1612–1618, 1982.
93. Riches D: The multiple roles of macrophages in wound healing. In Clark RAF and Henson PM, (eds): The Molecular and Cellular Biology of Wound Repair. Plenum Press, New York, 1988, pp 213–242.
94. Lanir N, Ciano PS, Van De Water L, McDonagh J, Dvorak AM, Dvorak HF: Macrophage migration in fibrin gel matrices. II. Effects of clotting factor XIII, fibronectin, and glycosaminoglycan content on cell migration. J Immunol 140:2340–2349, 1988.
95. Kuusela P: Fibronectin binds to Staphylococcus aureus. Nature 276:718–720, 1978.
96. Proctor R, Mosher D, Olbrantz P: Fibronectin binding to Staphylococcus aureus. J Biol Chem 257:14788–14794, 1982.
97. Van De Water L, Destree A, Hynes R: Fibronectin binds to some bacteria but does not promote their uptake by phagocytic cells. Science 220:201–204, 1983.

98. Van De Water L. Phagocytosis. In McDonagh J, (ed): Plasma Fibronectin. Dekker, New York, 1985, pp 175–196.
99. Ryden C, Rubin K, Speziale P, Hook M, Lindberg M, Wadstrom T: Fibronectin receptors from Staphylococcus aureus. J Biol Chem 258:3396–3401, 1983.
100. Hormann H, Jelinic V: Fibronectin VII. Binding of cold-insoluble globulin and of denatured collagen by macrophages. Hoppe Seylers Z Physiol Chem 361:379–387, 1980.
101. Gudewicz P, Molnar J, Lai M, et al.: Fibronectin-mediated uptake of gelatin-coated latex particles by peritoneal macrophages. J Cell Biol 87:427–433, 1980.
102. Doran J, Mansberger A, Reese A: Cold-insoluble globulin-enhanced phagocytosis of gelatinized targets by macrophage monolayers: A model system. J Reticuloendothel Soc 27:471–483, 1980.
103. Marquette D, Molnar J, Yamada K, Schlesinger D, Darby S, Van Alten P: Phagocytosis-promoting activity of avian plasma and fibroblastic cell surface fibronectins. Mol Cell Biochem 36:147–155, 1981.
104. Hook M, Switalski L, Wadstrom T, Lindberg M: Interactions of pathogenic microorganisms with fibronectin. In Mosher D, (ed): Fibronectin. Academic Press, New York, 1989, pp 295–308.
105. Bevilacqua M, Amrani D, Mosesson M, Bianco C: Receptors for cold-insoluble globulin (plasma fibronectin) on human monocytes. J Exp Med 153:42–60, 1981.
106. Pommier CG, Inada S, Fries LF, Takahashi T, Frank MM, Brown EJ: Plasma fibronectin enhances phagocytosis of opsonized particles by human peripheral blood monocytes. J Exp Med 157:1844–1854, 1983.
107. Wright SD, Craigmyle LS, Silverstein SC: Fibronectin and serum amyloid P component stimulate C3b- and C3bi-mediated phagocytosis in cultured human monocytes. J Exp Med 158:1338–1343, 1983.
108. Bohnsack JF, Kleinman HK, Takahashi T, O'Shea JJ, Brown EJ: Connective tissue proteins and phagocytic cell function. Laminin enhances complement and Fc-mediated phagocytosis by cultured human macrophages. J Exp Med 161:912–923, 1985.
109. Parker C, Frame R, Elstad M: Vitronectin (S protein) augments the functional activity of monocyte receptors for IgG and complement. Blood 71:86–93, 1988.
110. Wright SD, Meyer BC: Fibronectin receptor of human macrophages recognizes the sequence Arg-Gly-Asp-Ser. J. Exp Med 162:762–767, 1985.
111. Wright SD, Licht MR, Craigmyle LS, Silverstein SC: Communication between receptors for different ligands on a single cell: Ligation of fibronectin receptors induces a reversible alteration in the function of complement receptors on cultured human monocytes. J. Cell Biol. 99:336–339, 1984.
112. Brown E, Goodwin J: Fibronectin receptors of phagocytes: characterization of the Arg-Gly-Asp binding proteins of monocytes and polymorphonuclear leukocytes. J Exp Med 167:777–793, 1988.
113. Brown D, Phillips D, Damsky C, Charo I: Synthesis and expression of the fibroblast fibronectin receptor in human monocytes. J Clin Invest 84:336–370, 1989.
114. Garcia-Pardo A, Ferreira O, Valinsky J, Bianco C: Fibronectin receptors of mononuclear phagocytes: binding characteristics and biochemical isolation. Exp Cell Res 181:420–431, 1989.
115. Van De Water L, Aronson D, Braman V: Alteration of fibronectin receptors (integrins) in phorbol ester-treated human promonocytic leukemia cells. Cancer Res 48:5730–5737, 1988.
116. Thorens B, Mermod J-J, Vassalli P: Phagocytosis and inflammatory stimuli induce GM-CSF mRNA in macrophages through posttranscriptional regulation. Cell 48:671–679, 1987.
117. Couchman JR, Gibson WT, Thom D, Weaver AC, Rees DA, Parish WE: Fibronectin distribution in epithelial and associated tissues in the rat. Arch Dermatol Rev 266:295–310, 1979.
118. Clark RA, Nielsen LD, Howell SE, Folkvord JM: Human keratinocytes that have not terminally differentiated synthesize laminin and fibronectin but deposit only fibronectin in the pericellular matrix. J Cell Biochem 28:127–141, 1985.
119. Kubo M, Kan M, Isemura M, Yamane I, Tagami H: Effects of extracellular matrices on human keratinocyte adhesion and growth and on its secretion and deposition of fibronectin in culture. J Invest Dermatol 88:594–601, 1987.
120. Kariniemi A-L, Lehto V-P, Vartio T, Virtanen I: Cytoskelton and pericellular matrix organization of pure adult human keratinocyte cultured from suction-blister roof epidermis. J Cell Sci 58:49–61, 1982.
121. O'Keefe E, Woodley D, Castillo G, Russell N, Payne R: Production of soluble and cell-associated fibronectin by cultured keratinocytes. J. Inv. Dermatol. 82:150–155, 1984.
122. O'Keefe EJ, Woodley DT, Falk RJ, Gammon WR, Briggaman RA: Production of fibronectin by epithelium in a skin equivalent. J Invest Dermatol 88:634–639, 1987.

123. Alitalo K, Kuismanen E, Myllyla R, Kiistala V, Asko-Seljavaana S, Vaheri A: Extracellular matrix proteins of human epidermal keratinocytes and feeder 3T3 cells. J Cell Biol 94:497–505, 1982.
124. Clark RA: Fibronectin matrix deposition and fibronectin receptor expression in healing and normal skin. J Invest Dermatol 128S–134S, 1990.
125. Larjava H, Peltonen J, Akiyama SK, et al.: Novel function for β1 integrins in keratinocyte cell-cell interactions. J Cell Biol 110:803–815, 1990.
126. Toda K, Grinnell F: Activation of human keratinocyte receptor function in relation to other ligand-receptor interactions. J Invest Dermatol 88:412–417, 1987.
127. Adams J, Watt F: Changes in keratinocyte adhesion during terminal differentiation: Reduction in fibronectin binding precedes $\alpha_5\beta_1$ integrin loss from the cell surface. Cell 63:425–435, 1990.
128. Roberts A, Sporn M, Assoian R, et al.: Transforming growth factor type β: Rapid induction of fibrosis and angiogenesis in vitro and stimulation of collagen formation in vitro. Proc Natl Acad Sci 83:4167–4171, 1986.
129. Raghow R, Postlethwaite A, Keski-Oja J, Moses H, Kang A: Transforming growth factor-β increases steady state levels of Type I procollagen and fibronectin messenger RNAs postranscriptionally in cultured human dermal fibroblasts. J Clin Invest 79:1285–1288, 1987.
130. Ignotz RA, Massague J: Cell adhesion protein receptors as targets for transforming growth factor-β. J Cell Biol 262:6443–6446, 1987.
131. Ignotz R, Endo T, Massague J: Regulation of fibronectin and type I collagen mRNA levels by transforming growth factor-β. J Biol Chem 262:6443–6446, 1987.
132. Welch MP, Odland GF, Clark RA: Temporal relationships of F-actin bundle formation, collagen and fibronectin matrix assembly, and fibronectin receptor expression to wound contraction. J Cell Biol 110:133–145, 1990.
133. Furcht L, Wendelschafer-Crabb G, Mosher D, Foidart J: Ascorbate-induced fibroblast cell matrix: Reaction of antibodies to procollagen I and III and fibronectin in an axial periodic fashion. Prog Clin Biol Res 41:829–843, 1980.
134. Engvall E, Ruoslahti E, Miller EJ: Affinity of fibronectin to collagens of different genetic types and to fibrinogen. J Exp Med 147:1584–1595, 1978.
135. Jilek F, Hormann H: Cold-insoluble globulin (fibronectin), IV affinity to soluble collagen of various types. Hoppe-Seyler's Z Physiol Chem 359:247–250, 1978.
136. Ingham K, Landwehr R, Engel J: Interaction of fibronectin with Clq and collagen. Effects of ionic strength and denaturation of the collagenous component. Eur J Biochem 148:219–224, 1985.
137. Kurkinen M, Vaheri A, Roberts PJ, Stenman S: Sequential appearance of fibronectin and collagen in experimental granulation tissue. Lab Invest 43:47–51, 1980.
138. Fogerty FJ, Akiyama SK, Yamada KM, Mosher DF: Inhibition of binding of fibronectin to matrix assembly sites by anti-integrin ($\alpha_5\beta_1$) antibodies. J Cell Biol 111:699–708, 1990.
139. McKeown-Longo P, Mosher D: Mechanism of formation of disulfide-bonded multimers of plasma fibronectin in cell layers of cultured human fibroblasts. J Biol Chem 12210–12215, 1984.
140. McKeown-Longo P, Mosher D: Interaction of the 70 kilodalton amino-terminal fragment of fibronectin with the matrix-assembly receptor of fibroblasts. J Cell Biol 100:364–374, 1985.
141. Carter WG, Hakomori S: A new cell surface, detergent-insoluble glycoprotein matrix of human and hamster fibroblasts. The role of disulfide bonds in stabilization of the matrix. J Biol Chem 256:6953–6960, 1981.
142. Hedman K, Kurkinene M, Alitalo K, Vaheri A, Johansson S, Hook M: Isolation of the pericellular matrix of human fibroblast cultures. J Cell Biol 81:83–91, 1979.
143. Vaheri A, Kukinen M, Lehto V, Lindner E, Timpl R: Codistribution of pericellular matrix proteins in cultured fibroblasts and loss in transformation: Fibronectin and procollagen. Proc Natl Acad Sci 75:4944–4948, 1978.
144. McDonald J, Kelley D, Broekelmann T: Role of fibronectin in collagen deposition: Fab' to the gelatin-binding domain of fibronectin inhibits both fibronectin and collagen organization in fibroblast extracellular matrix. J Cell Biol 92:485–492, 1982.
145. Peacock E, Van Winkle W: Surgery and Biology of Wound Repair. WB Saunders, Philadelphia, 1970, pp 356.
146. Skalli O, Gabbiani G: The biology of the myofibroblast relationship to wound contraction and fibrocontractive diseases. In Clark RAF and Henson PM, (eds): The Molecular and Cellular Biology of Wound Repair. Plenum Press, New York, 1988, pp 373–402.
147. Hynes RO, Destree AT: Relationships between fibronectin (LETS protein) and actin. Cell 15:875–886, 1978.

148. Heggeness M, Ash J, Singer S: Transmembrane linkage of fibronectin to intracellular actin-containing filaments in cultured human fibroblasts. Ann NY Acad Sci 312:414–417, 1978.
149. Singer II: The fibronexus: a transmembrane association of fibronectin-containing fibers and bundles of 5 nm microfilaments in hamster and human fibroblasts. Cell 16:675–685, 1979.
150. Singer II, Scott S, Kawka DW, Kazazis DM, Gailit J, Ruoslahti E: Cell surface distribution of fibronectin and vitronectin receptors depends on substrate composition and extracellular matrix accumulation. J Cell Biol 106:2171–2182, 1988.
151. Singer II, Kawka DW, Kazazis DM, Clark RA: In vivo co-distribution of fibronectin and actin fibers in granulation tissue: immunofluorescence and electron microscope studies of the fibronexus at the myofibroblast surface. J Cell Biol 98:2091–2106, 1984.
152. Madri J, Pratt B: Angiogenesis. In Clark RAF and Henson PM, (eds): The Molecular and Cellular Biology of Wound Healing. Plenum Press, New York, 1988, pp 337–358.
153. Ausprunk D, Folkman J: Migration and proliferation of endothelial cells in preformed and newly formed blood vessels during tumor angiogenesis. Microvasc Res 14:53–65, 1977.
154. Clark RA, DellaPelle P, Manseau E, Lanigan JM, Dvorak HF, Colvin RB: Blood vessel fibronectin increases in conjunction with endothelial cell proliferation and capillary ingrowth during wound healing. J Invest Dermatol 79:269–276, 1982.
155. Peters JH, Sporn LA, Ginsberg MH, Wagner DD: Human endothelial cells synthesize, process, and secrete fibronectin molecules bearing an alternatively spliced type III homology (ED1). Blood 75:1801–1808, 1990.
156. Kowalczyk AP, Tulloh RH, McKeown-Longo PJ: Polarized fibronectin secretion and localized matrix assembly sites correlate with subendothelial matrix formation. Blood 75:2335–2342, 1990.
157. McAuslan B, Hannan G, Reilly W, Stewart F: Variant endothelial cells: Fibronectin as a transducer of signals for migration and neovascularization. J Cell Physiol 104:177–186, 1980.
158. McAuslan B, Hannan G, Reilly W: Signals causing change in morphological phenotype, growth mode, and gene expression of vascular endothelial cells. J Cell Physiol 112:96–106, 1982.
159. Guan J-L, Trevitnick JE, Hynes RO: Retroviral expression of alternatively spliced forms of rat fibronectin. J Cell Biol 110:833–847, 1990.

CHAPTER **20**

Regulation of Prolyl Hydroxylase Activity in Fetal and Adult Fibroblasts

Brian W. Duncan
Jing Qian
Xuan Liu
Rajendra S. Bhatnagar

INTRODUCTION

Tissue repair in the fetus differs markedly from adult repair. Injured fetal tissues undergo repair without acute inflammation and scarring,[1–4] whereas inflammation is an essential part of adult tissue repair.[5] These observations suggest that fundamental biochemical differences may exist in repair mechanisms between fetal and adult tissues. Fetal tissues exist in a highly dynamic state and exhibit higher rates of macromolecular turnover than adult tissues. The biochemical processes that regulate differentiation and macromolecular turnover are down-regulated in normal adult tissues due to the decreased need for tissue reorganization and growth. These mechanisms must be re-initiated following injury to accommodate the increased turnover required for the restoration and remodeling of tissue. Therefore, repair processes in the adult are at least partially reminiscent of tissue ontogeny.

The differences between fetal and adult repair may arise from the superimposition of the considerably slower adult biosynthetic rates on tissue remodeling initiated by injury. In order to delineate the differences between fetal and adult repair processes, it is necessary to understand the mechanisms that modulate crucial biochemical pathways in fetal and adult cells.

The objective of repair is to restore form and function to the injured tissue. While studies on fetal wound repair have been initiated quite recently, wound repair in the adult has been the subject of long-term investigation (see Chapter 2). Whereas the stages of acute inflammation and granulation tissue deposition do not play prominent roles in fetal wound healing, the rapid restoration and remodeling of the extracellular matrix (ECM) is crucial. The modulation of ECM turnover is elicited by the cells in repair tissues via the action of a Pandora's box of growth factors and other biologically active molecules that immigrate or are produced in situ. In addition, exogenous factors such as ascorbate and oxygen are important in regulating extracellular matrix turnover. Free radicals also accumulate in tissues during inflammation and can induce growth factor production.

Recent studies in developmental biology suggest that growth factors are important in the control of gene expression as well as in morphological organization. The growth factors involved in development and in repair act by both paracrine and autocrine mechanisms. For instance, transforming growth factor β (TGF-β) is present during the earliest stages of development and is a major regulator of cell proliferation, cell differentiation, and ECM turnover.[6,7] Elucidation of the regulatory role of various factors during wound repair is an area of intense investigation. It is particularly interesting to delineate the disparate mechanisms that regulate repair in fetal and adult tissues.

COLLAGEN SYNTHESIS IN INJURED ADULT AND FETAL TISSUES

Collagen synthesis is crucial for wound repair because collagen: 1) modulates cell behavior including proliferation, migration, and specific gene expression, 2) is a major determinant of tissue biomechanical properties,[8] 3) is important in the wound contraction process,[9] and 4) promotes re-epithelialization by constituting the substratum, along with fibrin and fibronectin, for the migration of epidermal cells.[10]

During dermal wound healing, elevated rates of collagen synthesis are seen, with much greater type III collagen expression than in normal skin.[11] The highest rates of type III collagen synthesis are seen during the initial 10 hours after wounding, but normal ratios of type I to type III collagen expression are seen within 24 hours.[12] Type III collagen accounts for nearly 20% of the total collagen production at this time. Prolyl hydroxylase catalyzes a major post-translational step in collagen synthesis, and enzyme activity is increased two to five fold in healing wounds compared to uninjured skin in the adult humans and in rats.[13,14]

These observations are particularly interesting when considered along with the effect of age on collagen synthesis. The highest rates of collagen synthesis are observed in fetal skin and decrease with age, up to about 30–40 years.[15] The activities of enzymes involved in the post-translational modification of collagen, i.e., prolyl hydroxylase, lysyl hydroxylase, collagen galactosyl transferase and collagen glucosyl transferase, are also similarly decreased in aging human skin.[16–18] The parameters of collagen synthesis are decreased to one-fourth or less during aging from fetus to adult. Adult tissue injury may elevate both collagen synthesis and related enzyme activities close to fetal levels, consistent with the suggestion that a healing wound in the adult may replay the ontogeny of the tissue.

In contrast to observations in adult wounds, there is some disagreement as to the levels of collagen synthesis and deposition in fetal wound tissue. It has been suggested that fetal wound healing may not involve collagen synthesis and may instead depend on the deposition of a proteoglycan-rich matrix as a template for subsequent tissue reconstruction.[19,20] Other workers suggest that small amounts of collagen may be synthesized in fetal wounds.[21] Adzick and coworkers have shown that fetal wound healing proceeds with both mesenchymal cell proliferation and collagen deposition.[2] Both collagen synthesis and cell proliferation are more rapid in fetal wounds than in wound tissue in neonatal or adult animals.

It is not clear whether the decreasing ability of tissues to repair as a function of age[22] is related to decreasing collagen synthesis. Data presented in Chapter 11 reveals that the fetus appears to heal by regeneration rather than scar formation until late in gestation, yet collagen deposition is abundant in scarless fetal lamb wound healing. Granulomas from older animals were found to have lower biomechanical strength compared to granulomas in younger animals.[23] These differences may arise from decreased cross-linking of newly synthesized collagen in the granulomas in older animals although biochemical evidence for this is not available.

REGULATION OF COLLAGEN SYNTHESIS IN THE WOUND ENVIRONMENT

The differences in adult and fetal repair may arise from differences in the mechanisms which modulate collagen synthesis. Collagen synthesis is subject to regulation by a variety of endogenous and exogenous factors in the wound environment. Since inflammation contributes to increased collagen synthesis in adult tissues, it has been suggested that processes related to inflammation may be essential for repair.[8] In fact, inflammation and subsequent granulation processes bring into the wound environment a large number of biologically active molecules which directly or indirectly contribute to increased turnover of collagen. Although chemical signals arising from inflammation and from its attendant cells affect many aspects of repair, we will discuss only those factors that influence collagen synthesis. The species present in the wound environment that can affect collagen synthesis may be classified into three categories (Table 20.1). In the first category are oxygen free radicals, starting with superoxide. Superoxide is a product of the metabolism of oxygen, is present in all cells,[24] and is produced in large quantities by phagocytosing cells.[25] The mechanism of action of superoxide and other free radicals is discussed in a later section.

A number of biologically active peptide growth factors comprise the second category. Growth factors play a major role in wound healing. Among growth factors known to affect collagen synthesis directly are platelet derived growth factor,[26] epidermal growth factor,[27] fibroblast growth factor,[28] and TGF-β.[29] Growth factors are known to be produced by cells of the inflammatory response in adult wounds. Since fetal wounds repair without acute inflammation, the pres-

TABLE 20.1 Factors in the Wound Environment that Modulate Collagen Synthesis

Metabolic Factors	
Superoxide	Product of oxygen metabolism Product of phagocytic cells, e.g. PMNs
Lactate	Metabolism
Growth Factors	
Platelet derived growth factor	
Epidermal growth factor	
Fibroblast growth factor	
Transforming growth factor β	
External Factors	
Oxygen	Oxygen delivery
Ascorbate	Nutrient

ence and source of growth factors in the fetal wound are unknown. Epidermal growth factor may elevate collagen synthesis by promoting fibroblast proliferation rather than by increasing the expression of collagen.[30] The effect of epidermal growth factor is modulated by the extracellular matrix.[31] TGF-β is present in fetal and embryonic tissues in the earliest stages of development and it plays a crucial role in differentiation and phenotypic expression.[6,7] TGF-β1 stimulates collagen synthesis in fibroblast cultures, although the proportion of collagen to total protein is not altered.[29] TGF-β1 alone has no enhancing effect on type III collagen synthesis in cultures of dermal fibroblasts, but acts synergistically with ascorbate to enhance types I and III collagen synthesis and to maintain steady state levels of mRNAs for these collagens.[32] Wound implants containing TGF-β1 elicited an adult-like response characterized by inflammation and fibrosis in fetal rabbits.[33] Since fibrosis and scarring are not seen in fetal healing, it is not clear what role members of the TGF-β family may play in fetal repair.

The third category of factors that influence collagen synthesis in the wound environment are oxygen and ascorbic acid. In addition to its importance for cellular metabolism, oxygen is a substrate for post-translational hydroxylation of proline and lysine in collagen.[34] Collagen synthesis is enhanced in the presence of elevated levels of oxygen.[34] Fetal tissues, however, are relatively hypoxic[1] but are efficiently able to repair. Ascorbate is an essential nutrient for primates and one of its principal roles is the synthesis and maintenance of connective tissues. Ascorbate is a co-factor in the hydroxylation of proline and lysine during collagen synthesis.[34] It also modulates the synthesis of collagen at the level of gene expression.[36,37]

REGULATION OF COLLAGEN SYNTHESIS AT THE EPIGENETIC LEVEL BY POLYADP-RIBOSYLATION

Our aim is to determine a central point in the cellular pathways that may serve as the regulatory site for collagen synthesis. Elucidation of this site may provide the means to control collagen synthesis during repair. Since the production of collagen is an important aspect of cell differentiation, epigenetic mechanisms operating at the level of gene expression are crucial in determining both the types and amounts of collagen to be synthesized. One such mechanism is the polyADP-ribosylation of chromatin proteins.[38,39] The modification of chromatin proteins by polyADP-ribosylation is an important role for cell differentiation, cellular transformation, sister chromatid exchange, nucleic acid metabolism and DNA repair.[38–41] This modification alters the conformation of chromatin resulting in the transcription of specific genes.[42] PolyADP-ribosylation of chromatin is subject to alteration with age.[43] PolyADP-ribosylation is related to the so-called "pro-oxidant" state and is initiated as a result of interaction of oxygen free radicals with DNA.[44]

In adult tissues, increased generation of oxygen free radicals by neutrophils and other cells that infiltrate the injured tissue as components of inflammation[45] may elicit increased polyADP-ribosylation that is needed for mediating specific gene expression and cell differentiation as part of repair. Our studies suggest that the activity of prolyl hydroxylase may be modulated at the epigenetic level by polyADP-ribosyl synthetase. PolyADP-ribosyl synthetase activity is increased in the presence of many unrelated stimulants of collagen synthesis and prolyl hydroxylase. The marked decrease in the activity of prolyl hydroxylase by inhibitors of polyADP-ribosyl synthetase suggests a central locus for the regulation of collagen synthesis and it may explain the differences in the collagen synthesis in fibroblasts derived from fetal and adult tissues.

It can be expected that the modulation of collagen synthesis by processes related to aging may play an important role in differentiating between fetal and adult tissue repair. Relative collagen synthesis is greater in fetal fibroblasts than in adult fibroblasts.[46] The enzyme prolyl hydroxylase catalyzes the hydroxylation of proline in collagen sequences and is a key post-translational step in collagen synthesis. The activity of prolyl hydroxylase is an index of the rate of collagen synthesis. We have examined the activity of prolyl hydroxylase in fibroblasts derived from fetal human dermis from various gestational ages and from adult dermis, as a measure of the cellular capacity to synthesize collagen at different stages in development. In other studies in our laboratory,[47] we have observed marked reduction in the ascorbate stimulated collagen polypeptide synthesis in the presence of inhibitors of polyADP-ribosyl synthetase.

PROLYL HYDROXYLASE ACTIVITY IN FIBROBLAST CULTURES IS UNDER THE CONTROL OF POLYADP-RIBOSE SYNTHETASE

Our previous studies showed concomitant increases in collagen synthesis, prolyl hydroxylase activity and polyADP-ribose synthetase in cells and tissues exposed to the fibrogenic agents ozone and Bleomycin.[48,49] If polyADP-ribose synthetase is a part of the regulatory pathway for collagen and prolyl hydroxylase, its activity should be modulated by other agents that increase collagen synthesis. Ascorbate is known to increase collagen synthesis and prolyl hydroxylase activity in fibroblast cultures.[35,36] We examined the effect of ascorbate on polyADP-ribose synthetase activity in cultures of neonatal human (foreskin) fibroblasts. As seen in Figure 20.1, polyADP-ribose synthetase activity was increased by 50% within 30 minutes after exposure to 50 μg/ml ascorbate. The enzyme activity doubled after 120 min exposure.

The effect of ascorbate on prolyl hydroxylase activity was examined in neonatal human dermal fibroblasts (foreskin), IMR-90 cells (an established line of diploid fibroblasts derived from fetal human lung), and in dermal fibroblasts from a 78-year-old male. As seen in Table 20.2, prolyl hydroxylase activity increased in the

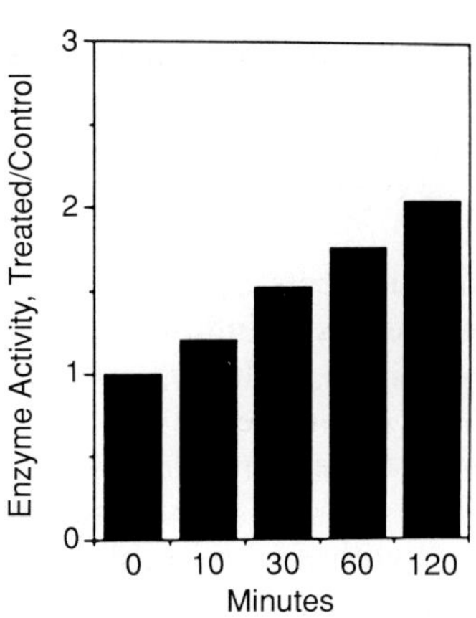

Figure 20.1 Ascorbate-mediated increase in polyADP-ribose synthetase (PADPRS). These experiments were carried out using cultures of neonatal human dermal (foreskin) fibroblasts in passage 8. Ascorbate (50 μg/ml) was added to confluent cultures and the cells were harvested at the indicated times. PolyADP-ribose synthetase activity was assayed by a previously published method[48,49] by monitoring the incorporation of ^{14}C-NAD into an acid insoluble product and was related to cellular DNA content.[64]

TABLE 20.2 Inhibitors of PolyADP-ribose Synthetase Abolish the Ascorbate-Induced Increase in Prolyl Hydroxylase Activity.

Cell Type and Experiment	Enzyme Activity dpm ^3H/mg Protein × 10^{-3}	Treated/ Control	Inhibitor/ Ascorbate
Fetal dermal fibroblasts (22 weeks)			
Control	3.14		
+ Ascorbate	6.00	1.91	
+ Ascorbate + 3-aminobenzamide	3.60	1.15	0.60
+ Ascorbate + 6-aminonicotinamide	2.97	0.96	0.50
Neonatal dermal fibroblasts (foreskin)			
Control	3.08		
+ Ascorbate	5.59	1.81	
+ Ascorbate + 3-aminobenzamide	3.41	1.11	0.61
+ Ascorbate + 6-aminonicotinamide	3.22	1.05	0.58
IMR-90 fibroblasts			
Control	1.68		
+ Ascorbate	3.44	2.05	
+ Ascorbate + 3-aminobenzamide	1.76	1.05	0.51
+ Ascorbate + 6-aminonicotinamide	1.64	0.98	0.48
Adult dermal fibroblasts (78 years)			
Control	2.83		
+ Ascorbate	3.43	1.21	
+ Ascorbate + 3-aminobenzamide	3.13	1.11	0.91
+ Ascorbate + 6-aminonicotinamide	2.72	0.96	0.80

All cells were used between 5th and 10th passage. Ascorbate (3.5 mM) and/or 3-aminobenzamide (2 mM) or 6-aminonicotinamide (2 mM) were added at confluence. The cells were harvested 24 h after the addition of ascorbate and/or inhibitors of polyADP-ribose synthetase. Prolyl hydroxylase activity was determined as described in the legend to Fig. 20.2.

presence of ascorbate in all cells. In order to determine if the ascorbate-induced increase in polyADP-ribose synthetase is involved in the regulation of prolyl hydroxylase, we examined the effect of inhibiting polyADP-ribose synthetase on the ascorbate-induced increase in prolyl hydroxylase. Table 20.2 also shows that the ascorbate-induced increase in prolyl hydroxylase was abolished by 3-aminobenzamide and 6-aminonicotinamide, inhibitors of polyADP-ribose synthetase. The concentrations of these compounds used are similar to those used in other studies[50] and the compounds are not toxic at this level. The inhibitors of polyADP-ribose synthetase did not have any significant effect on its activity in cells not treated with ascorbate. Control experiments showed that these compounds did not inhibit prolyl hydroxylase in vitro.

REGULATION OF COLLAGEN SYNTHESIS IN HUMAN FETAL FIBROBLASTS

Our studies suggest that elevated levels of polyADP-ribose synthetase correlate with elevation of collagen synthesis and prolyl hydroxylase. Since fetal fibroblasts display a higher rate of relative collagen synthesis,[46] it was of interest to examine if polyADP-ribose synthetase is involved. We did not measure the activity of polyADP-ribose synthetase in fibroblasts, but examined the effect of inhibitors of this enzyme on both unstimulated and ascorbate-stimulated production of prolyl hydroxylase in human fetal dermal fibroblasts derived from gestational ages 11,

13, 16, 17, 18, 19, 20, 21, 24, and 28 weeks respectively. Fetal skin was obtained from therapeutic abortion material after obtaining signed consent for the use of this tissue for research purposes under an approved human subjects research protocol at the University of California, San Francisco.

The constitutive levels of prolyl hydroxylase observed in cells below 20 weeks gestation in the absence of ascorbate were significantly higher than those in fibroblasts from post-20 week gestation or in postnatal cells, even in the presence of ascorbate.[51] We examined the effect of inhibiting polyADP-ribose synthetase both in the presence and absence of ascorbate in these cells.

Treatment of fetal fibroblasts with 6-aminonicotinamide, an inhibitor of polyADP-ribose synthetase, resulted in marked decrease in prolyl hydroxylase activity (Fig. 20.2). The effect was greatest on cells from fetuses 20 weeks or less in gestation, resulting in more than 50% decrease in enzyme activity. The decrease was much less in fibroblasts from longer gestation (26 weeks) or in neonatal fibroblasts.

As seen in Figure 20.3, the addition of ascorbate had a paradoxical effect on the activity of prolyl hydroxylase in fibroblasts derived from fetal dermal skin from less than 20 weeks gestation. The activity of prolyl hydroxylase was not increased after the addition of ascorbate, and in each case a small but significant decrease was observed. In contrast, fibroblasts from 20 weeks or longer gestation

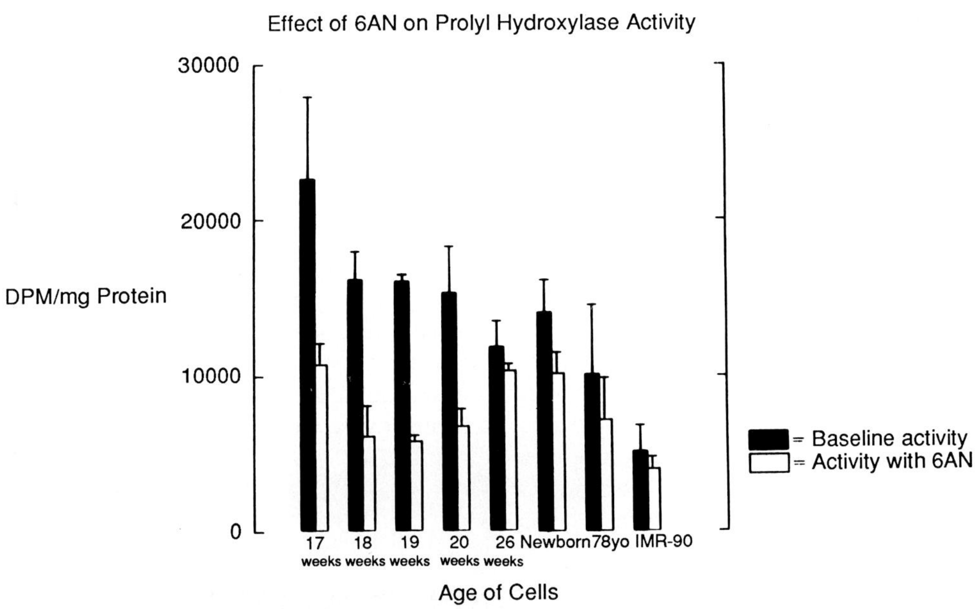

Figure 20.2 Prolyl hydroxylase activity as a function of age of fibroblast source. Dermal fibroblast cultures were prepared from tissues explanted from fetal skin of various gestational ages, or from neonatal (foreskin) or adult skin (78 y). Prolyl hydroxylase levels were determined in confluent cultures. In cultures to examine the role of polyADP-ribose synthetase, 6-aminonicotinamide (an inhibitor of the enzyme) was added at a concentration of 2 mM, 24 h prior to harvesting the cells. Prolyl hydroxylase activity was determined as described previously[65] using ^{3}H-proline labeled unhydroxylated collagen as a substrate. Total protein content in the cell homogenates was determined by a standard procedure.[63] The enzyme activity, measured as the radioactivity in ^{3}H released as a result of hydroxylation of ^{3}H-proline, was related to cellular protein content and was expressed as a specific activity term, d.p.m. ^{3}H released/mg cellular protein.

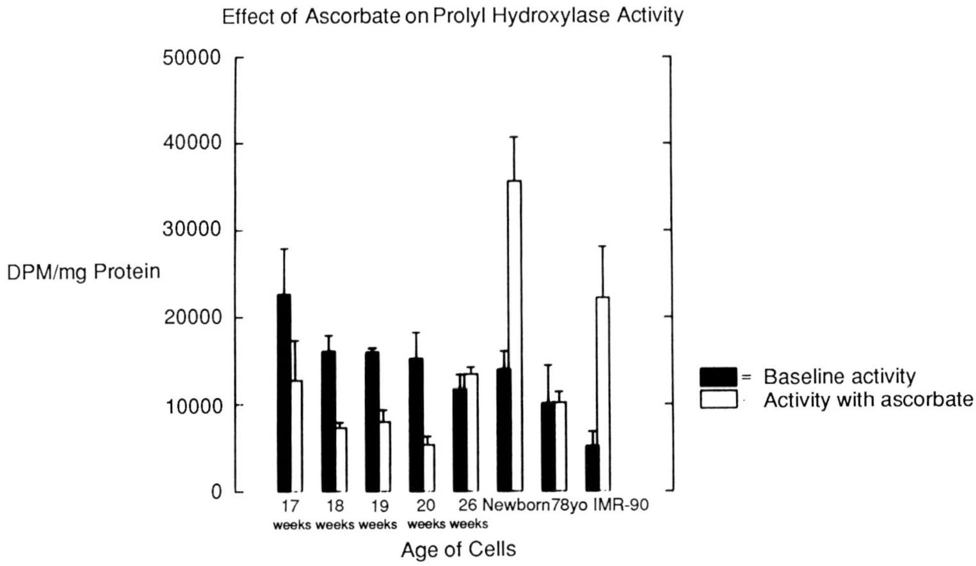

Figure 20.3 Effect of ascorbate on fibroblast prolyl hydroxylase activity. Ascorbate (50μg/ml) was added 24 h prior to harvesting the cells. All measurements were made in confluent cultures, using the procedures described in the legends to Figures 1 and 2.

gestation fetal skin exhibited marked increase in enzyme activity in the presence of ascorbate. Inhibiting polyADP-ribose synthetase with 3-aminobenzamide resulted in reversal of the effect of ascorbate in all cells (Fig. 20.4). In fibroblasts from tissues at less than 20-week gestation, there was a slight increase in prolyl hydroxylase activity, reversing the decrease induced in the presence of ascorbate. In contrast, there was a marked decrease in the ascorbate-stimulated levels of prolyl hydroxylase activity in cells from 20 weeks and older fetuses.

Our observations supported the involvement of polyADP-ribose synthetase in

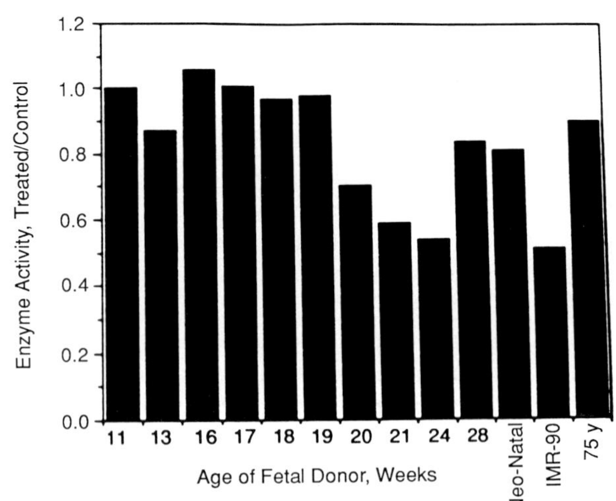

Figure 20.4 The effect of 3-aminobenzamide, an inhibitor of polyADP-ribose synthetase, on the stimulation of prolyl hydroxylase by ascorbate. Experimental conditions and procedures are described in legends to Figures 20.1–20.3. 3-aminobenzamide was added at a concentration of 2mM along with ascorbate.

TABLE 20.3 Agents that Increase PolyADP-ribose Synthetase Increase Fibroblast Prolyl Hydroxylase Activity

Experiment	Enzyme Activity dpm ^{3}H/mg Protein × 10^{-3}	Treated/ Control	Inhibitor/ Stimulant
Control	2.62		
+ Phorbol ester (50 ng/ml)	3.79	1.45	
+ 3-aminobenzamide (2 mM)	2.73	1.04	0.72
+ Cholera toxin, 10 ng/ml	3.48	1.33	
+ 3-aminobenzamide (2 mM)	2.71	1.03	0.78
+ Dihydroxyfumarate (35 μM)	3.69	1.41	
+ 3-aminobenzamide (2 mM)	2.47	0.94	0.67

These experiments were carried out with neo-natal (foreskin) human dermal fibroblasts in the 8th passage. All additives were added at confluence and the cells were harvested after 24 h with the reagents. Dihydroxyfumarate was added as a generator of superoxide. Prolyl hydroxylase activity was determined as described in the legend to Fig. 20.2.

the regulation of prolyl hydroxylase activity. We further confirmed this by exposing neonatal fibroblast cultures to other agents that are known to elevate levels of polyADP-ribose synthetase (Table 20.3). Cells exposed to cholera toxin, an inducer of polyADP-ribosylation,[52] showed elevated levels of prolyl hydroxylase. The increase was abolished by 3-aminobenzamide. Increased polyADP-ribose synthetase activity is induced on exposure to oxygen free radicals such as superoxide.[53] Exposure of fibroblasts to dihydroxyfumarate,[53] a generator of superoxide, also caused a marked increase in prolyl hydroxylase activity and this increase was also abolished by 3-aminobenzamide. The activity of prolyl hydroxylase was also elevated in cells exposed to phorbol ester (12-O-tetradecanoylphorbol-13-acetate) and this increase was abolished by 3-aminobenzamide. Phorbol ester is a tumor promotor whose effects are mediated by polyADP-ribosylation.[54]

DIFFERENCES IN THE REGULATION OF COLLAGEN SYNTHESIS WITH AGING

Our studies support the concept that fibroblast prolyl hydroxylase activity is subject to regulation at the epigenetic level by polyADP-ribose synthetase. Our studies show that constitutive levels of prolyl hydroxylase are quite high in early gestation fetal fibroblasts. These levels may reflect the maximal potential of fibroblasts to synthesize collagen. The decrease in enzyme activity after 20 weeks gestation suggests that mechanisms related to aging in the context of collagen synthesis and wound healing may be initiated during gestation. The sharp break in the properties of fibroblasts related to collagen synthesis at the 20-week gestation landmark represents a remarkable change in cell behavior and may represent the transition point from fetal to adult-type healing in humans.

These experiments clearly show that before 20 weeks gestation, the cells do not require ascorbate to activate collagen synthesis. This is in marked contrast to the observation that postnatal tissues and cells appear to have a marked requirement for ascorbate in order to induce increased collagen synthesis.[35,36] A possible explanation for this seeming paradox is based on our observations that the effect of ascorbate may be mediated by polyADP-ribose synthetase.

The activity of polyADP-ribose synthetase is elevated in tissues undergoing development and differentiation.[40–44] The enzyme itself is subject to down-regulation as a function of age.[43] It is likely that early gestation fetal cells closely reflect the properties characteristic of the early developmental stage of the tissues from which they are derived. These properties would include elevated levels of polyADP-ribose synthetase, necessary for the increased rates of gene expression and other differentiation-related events. The decrease in prolyl hydroxylase caused by inhibitors of polyADP-ribose synthetase in these cells supports this concept further.

Why is ascorbate needed to induce collagen synthesis in cells from "older" tissues? With advancing development and "aging," the levels of polyADP-ribose synthetase are decreased. In order to stimulate collagen synthesis, polyADP-ribose synthetase activity must be increased by other means. Ascorbate is a well-known generator of oxygen free radicals including superoxide.[55] We have previously reported the induction of increased oxygen synthesis by superoxide in fibroblasts[56] and in hepatocytes.[57] These experiments showed that the stimulatory effect of ascorbate on collagen synthesis is abolished by superoxide dismutase and that ascorbate may be replaced by increased cellular levels of superoxide generated by dihydroxyfumarate, xanthine, xanthine oxidase, or paraquat.[57,58] We have shown that the stimulatory effect of ozone and Bleomycin on collagen synthesis is accompanied by increased activity of polyADP-ribose synthetase.[48,49] These agents are known to act through oxygen-free radicals. The increase in collagen synthesis seen in inflamed tissues is not known to be related to increased concentrations of ascorbate, but is likely to be caused by the increased production of superoxide. Finally, the effect of ascorbate appears to be abolished by inhibitors of polyADP-ribose synthetase. We have made similar observations with respect to collagen synthesis.[47]

A MODEL FOR THE REGULATION OF COLLAGEN SYNTHESIS

A model for the regulation of collagen synthesis is described in Figure 20.5. Fibroblasts are committed to synthesizing collagen, and therefore are able to express collagen genes as necessary. During early development, the turnover of collagen

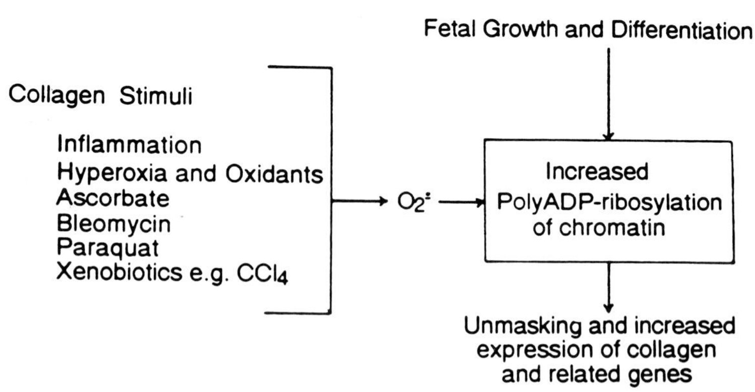

Figure 20.5 Relationship between polyADP-ribose synthetase and collagen synthesis.

proceeds at elevated rates. During this stage, the levels of polyADP-ribose synthetase are elevated to accommodate the increased synthesis not only of collagen, but presumably of many other proteins necessary for rapid tissue development and remodeling. As proposed in the "pro-oxidant state" hypothesis, increased cellular metabolic activity provides the needed stimulus in the form of oxygen-free radicals.[44] It is interesting to note in this context that the levels of superoxide dismutase, the enzyme that would neutralize superoxide, are very low in early development and then increase as a function of age.[58] Increased superoxide dismutase would curtail the availability of superoxide which appears to be a stimulus for collagen synthesis acting through the induction of polyADP-ribose synthetase. We have shown that the inhibition of intracellular superoxide dismutase results in a marked stimulation of collagen synthesis and increased prolyl hydroxylase activity.[57] This situation is further complicated by the down-regulation of polyADP-ribose synthetase itself as a function of age. Thus, increased superoxide production and inflammation are not necessary for collagen synthesis and repair in fetal tissues, whereas older tissues need this additional help to activate this essential component of repair. Our studies suggest that it may be possible to develop strategies based on either the induction or inhibition of polyADP-ribose synthetase to manipulate repair, to increase collagen, or to decrease scarring.

REFERENCES

1. Burrington JD: Wound healing in the fetal lamb. J Pediatr Surg 6:523–528, 1971.
2. Adzick NS, Harrison MR, Glick PL, et al.: Comparison of fetal, newborn, and adult wound healing by histologic, enzyme-histochemical and hydroxyproline determinations. J Pediatr Surg 20:315–319, 1985.
3. Hallock GG, Rice DC, Merkel JR, DiPaolo BR: Analysis of collagen content in the fetal wound. Ann Plast Surg 21:310–315, 1988.
4. Krummel TM, Nelson JM, Diegelmann RF, et al.: Fetal response to injury in the rabbit. J Pediatr Surg 22:640–644, 1987.
5. Chavapil M, Koopman CF: Scar formation: Physiology and pathological states. Otolaryngol Clin North Amer 17:265–272, 1984.
6. Hay ED: in Role of Extracellular Matrix in Development, Trelstad RL (ed). Alan R. Liss, New York, 1984, pp 1–33.
7. Ehrlich HP: The role of connective tissue matrix in wound healing. In Barbul A, Pines E, Caldwell M, and Hunt TK (eds): Growth Factors and Other Aspects of Wound Healing: Biological and Clinical Implications; Alan R. Liss, New York, 1987, pp 243–258.
8. Hunt TK, Halliday B: Inflammation in wound healing: From laudable pus to primary repair and beyond. In TK Hunt (ed): Wound Healing and Wound Infection. Theory and Surgical Practice. Appleton Century Crofts, New York, 1980, pp 281–293.
9. Ehrlich HP: The role of connective tissue matrix in hypertrophic wound contracture. In Hunt TK, Heppenstall RB, Pines E, and Rovee D (eds): Soft and Hard Tissue Repair. Praeger, New York, 1984, pp 533–553.
10. Clark RAF, Lanigan BS, Dellapille P, et al.: Fibronectin and fibrin provide a provisional matrix for epidermal cell migration during wound epithelialization. J Invest Dermatol 79:264–269, 1982.
11. Bailey AJ, Boyin S, Sims TJ, et al.: Characterization of the collagen of human hypertrophic and normal scars. Biochim Biophys Acta 405:412–421, 1975.
12. Clore JN, Cohen IK, Diegelmann RF: Quantitation of collagen types I and III during wound healing in the rat. Proc Soc Exp Biol Med 160:458–462, 1979.
13. Stein HD, Keiser HR, Sjoerdsma A: Collagen synthesis in granulating wounds in rats and man. Surg Forum 20:63–65, 1969.
14. Stein HD, Kaiser HR: Collagen metabolism in granulating wounds. J Surg Res 11:277–283, 1971.
15. Uitto J: Connective tissue biochemistry of the aging dermis: Age-related alterations in collagen and elastin. Dermatol Clin 4:433–446, 1986.
16. Anttinen Oikarinen A, Kivirikko KI: Age-related changes in human skin collagen galactosyl transferase and collagen-glucosyl transferase activities. Clin Chim Acta 76:95–101, 1977.

17. Anttinen H, Orava S, Ryhanen L, Kivirikko KI: Assay of protocollagen lysyl hydroxylase in the skin of human subjects and changes in the activity with age. Clin Chim Acta 47:289–294, 1973.
18. Uitto J, Halme J, Hannuksela M, et al.: Protocollagen proline hydroxylase activity in the skin of normal human subjects and patients with scleroderma. Scand J Clin Lab Invest 23:241–244, 1976.
19. DePalma RL, Krummel TM, Nelson JM, et al.: Fetal wound matrix is composed of proteoglycan rather than collagen. Surg Forum 38:626–628, 1987.
20. Krummel TM, Nelson JM, Diegelmann RF, et al.: Wound healing in the fetal and neonatal rabbit. Surg Forum 37:595–596, 1986.
21. Hallock GG, Rice DC, Merkel JR, DiPaolo BR: Analysis of collagen content in the fetal wound. Ann Plast Surg 21:310–315, 1988.
22. Eaglestein WH: Wound healing and aging. Dermatol Clin 4:481–484, 1986.
23. Holm-Pederson P, Zenderfeldt B: Granulation tissue formation in subcutaneously implanted cellulose sponges in young and old rats. Scand J Plast Reconstr Surg 5:13–16, 1971.
24. Fridovich I: Superoxide dismutases. Adv Enzymol 58:61–97, 1986.
25. Weiss SJ: Oxidative stress. Acta Physiol Scand Suppl 548:9–37, 1986.
26. Grotendorst GR, Martin GR, Pancev D, et al.: Stimulation of granulomatous tissue formation by platelet-derived growth factor in normal and diabetic rats. J Clin Invest 76:2323–2329, 1985.
27. Lawrence WT, Norton JA, Sporn MB, et al.: The effect of chemoattractants and growth factors on wound healing in a wound chamber model in adriamycin-treated rats. Ann Surg 203:142–147, 1986.
28. Davidson J, Buckley A, Woodward S, et al.: Mechanisms of accelerated wound repair using epidermal growth factor and basic fibroblast growth factor. Progr Clin Biol Res 266:63–75, 197.
29. Narayanan AS, Page RC, Swanson J: Collagen synthesis by human fibroblasts. Regulation by transforming growth factor β in the presence of other inflammatory mediators. Biochem J 260:463–469, 1989.
30. Laato M, Kahari VM, Niinikoski J, Vuorio E: Epidermal growth factor increases collagen production in granulation tissue by stimulation of fibroblast proliferation and not by activation of procollagen genes. Biochem J 247:385–388, 1987.
31. Colige A, Nusgens B, Lapiere CM: Effect of EGF on human fibroblasts is mediated by the extracellular matrix. Arch Dermatol Res 280(Suppl):S42–46, 1988.
32. Appling WD, O'Brien WR, Johnson DA, Duvic M: Synergistic enhancement of type I and III collagen production in cultured fibroblasts by transforming growth factor β and ascorbate. FEBS Letts 250:541–544, 1989.
33. Krummel TM, Michna BA, Thomas BL, et al.: Transforming growth factor β (TGFβ) induces fibrosis in a fetal wound model. J Pediatr Surg 23:647–652, 1988.
34. Prockop DJ, Berg RA, Kivirikko KI, Uitto J: Intracellular steps in biosynthesis of collagen. In Ramachandran GN and Redde AH (eds): Biochemistry of Collagen. Plenum Press, New York, 1976, pp 163–253.
35. Hunt TK, Pai MP: The effect of varying ambient oxygen tensions on wound metabolism and collagen synthesis. Surg Gynecol Obstet 135:561–567, 1972.
36. Sandell LJ, Daniel JC: Effects of ascorbic acid on collagen MRNA levels in short term chondrocyte cultures. Connective Tissue Res 17:11–22, 1988.
37. Pinnell SR: Regulation of collagen synthesis by ascorbic acid: A review. Yale J Biol Med 58:553–559, 1985.
38. Gall JC, Pearson CK: Covalent modification of proteins by ADP-ribosylation. Trends in Biochem Sci 11:171–175, 1986.
39. Thakur MK, Prasad S: ADP-ribosylation of HMG proteins and its modulation by different effectors in the liver of aging rats. Mech Aging Dev 53:91–100, 1990.
40. Ueda K, Hayaishi O: ADP-ribosylation. Ann Rev Biochem 54:79–100, 1985.
41. Shall S: ADP-ribosylation as a cellular control mechanism. In Althaus FR, Hilz H, and Shall S (eds): ADP-Ribosylation of Proteins; Spinger-Verlag, Berlin, 1985, pp 9–29.
42. Aubin RJ, Frechette A, de Murcia G, et al.: Correlation between endogenous nucleosomal hyper(ADP)ribosylation of histone H1 and induction of chromatin relaxation. EMBO J 2:1685–1693, 1983.
43. Shambaugh GE III, Koehler RR, Radosevich JA: Developmental pattern of poly(ADP-ribose) synthetase and NAD glycohydrolase in the brain of the fetal and neonatal rat. Neurochem Res 13:973–981, 1988.
44. Cerutti P: Pro-oxidant states and tumor production. Science 227:375–381, 1985.
45. Tonnensen MG, Worthen GS, Johnston RB Jr: Neutrophil emigration, activation, and tissue dam-

age. In Clark RAF and Henson PM (eds): The Molecular and Cellular Biology of Wound Repair. Plenum Press, New York, 1988, pp 149–183.
46. Thomas BL, Krummel TM, Melany M, et al.: Collagen synthesis and type expression by fetal fibroblasts in vitro. Surg Forum 39:642–644, 1987.
47. Blaisdell RJ, Qian JJ, Bhatnagar RS: Molecular mechanism of modulation of collagen synthesis by ascorbate: Inhibition of increased polyADP-ribosylation in the presence of ascorbate blocks increase in collagen synthesis. Submitted for publication (1991).
48. Hussain MZ, Mustafa MG, Ghani QP, Bhatnagar RS: Stimulation of poly (ADP-ribose) synthetase activity in the lungs of mice exposed to low level of ozone. Arch Biochem Biophys 241:477–485, 1985.
49. Hussain MZ, Giri SN, Bhatnagar RS: Poly(ADP-ribose) synthetase activity during Bleomycin induced lung fibrosis in hamsters. Exptl Mol Pathol 43:162–176, 1985.
50. Brac T, Ebisuzaki K: PolyADP ribosylation and Friend erythroleukemic-cell differentiation: Action of poly(ADP-ribose) polymerase inhibitors. Differentiation 34:139–143, 1987.
51. Duncan BW, Liu X, Qian JJ, et al.: Fetal prolyl hydroxylase is under the control of PADPR synthetase. Submitted for publication (1991).
52. Qian JJ, Liu X, Zha J, Bhatnagar RS: Inducers of poly(ADP-ribose) synthetase elevate prolyl hydroxylase activity in fibroblasts. Submitted for publication (1991).
53. Bhatnagar RS, Hussain MZ, Lee SD: The role of collagen as a primary molecular site of environmental injury. In Bhatnagar RS (ed): The Molecular Basis of Environmental Toxicity. Ann Arbor Science, Ann Arbor, MI, 1980, pp 531–558.
54. Ludwig A, Dietel M, Schafer G, et al.: Nicotinamide and nicotinamide analogues as anti-tumor promoters in mouse skin. Cancer Res 50:2470–2475, 1990.
55. Shinar E, Navok T, Chevion M: The analogous mechanism of enzymatic inactivation induced by ascorbate and superoxide in the presence of copper. J Biol Chem 258:14778–14783, 1983.
56. Bhatnagar RS: Role of superoxide in oxidant induced pulmonary fibrosis. In Lee SD (ed): Biochemical Effects of Environmental Pollutants. Ann Arbor Science, Ann Arbor, MI, 1977, pp 47–58.
57. Hussain MZ, Watson JA, Bhatnagar RS: Increased prolyl hydroxylase activity and collagen synthesis in hepatocyte cultures exposed to superoxide. Hepatology 7:502–507, 1987.
58. Allen RG, Balin AK: Developmental changes in the superoxide dismutase activity of human skin fibroblasts are maintained in vitro and are not caused by oxygen. J Clin Invest 82:731–734, 1988.
59. Bradford M: A rapid sensitive method for the quantitation of microgram quantities of protein utilizing the principle of dye binding. Anal Biochem 72:248–254, 1976.
60. Shatkin AJ: Colorimetric reactions for DNA, RNA, and protein determinations. In Habel K and Salzman NP (eds): Fundamental Techniques in Virology. Academic Press, New York, 1969, pp 231–237.
61. Hutton JJ Jr, Tappel AL, Udenfriend S: A rapid assay for collagen prolyl hydroxylase. Anal Biochem 16:348–394, 1966.

CHAPTER **21**

Scarless Fetal Healing: Therapeutic Implications

N. Scott Adzick
Michael T. Longaker

The purpose of this chapter is to call attention to the fetal wound healing process as a paradigm for ideal tissue repair. The therapeutic goal is to apply the lessons that the fetus is teaching us about wound healing to control the quality of healing. This lodestar may provide the tools for the surgeon to regulate each step of the adult wound healing process: re-epithelialization, inflammation, angiogenesis, contraction, and extracellular matrix synthesis, deposition, and remodeling. Pare's humble statement from over four hundred years ago that "I dressed the wound, and God healed it" may finally be outdated.

The emerging field of "wound pharmacology" is replete with papers that focus on the effect of vulnerary agents, such as growth factors, on wound healing acceleration.[1,2] Peacock points out that this approach is far too confining: "To limit our interest in healing to the speed of its various reactions is almost as restrictive as it would be to continue embryological investigation in the hope that a baby can be produced in less than 9 months."[3] With the exception of chronic nonhealing wounds and bone repair, the time required to reestablish tissue continuity and tensile strength after injury is usually not the major clinical issue. Of far greater importance is the restoration of normal tissue structure and function without scar formation.

THE CONSEQUENCES OF SCAR FORMATION

Scarring and fibrosis dominate some diseases in virtually every branch of medicine and surgery (Table 21.1). For example, the surgeon confronts the consequences of excessive scar formation daily. Skin incisions heal with scar, and sometimes pathologic processes such as keloids and hypertrophic scars are the unanticipated sequelae. Abdominal surgery invariably leads to intraperitoneal fibrous adhesions, and repeated bouts of mechanical intestinal obstruction can result. Strictures occur at anastomotic sites, whether of the bowel, blood vessel, trachea, ureter, or bile duct. The pediatric surgeon is frustrated with the tragic problem of biliary atresia in babies—a progressive, fibrotic obliteration of the hepatobiliary tree. Other examples include esophageal stricture after caustic ingestion, post-traumatic urethral stricture, tendon adhesions after hand surgery, and transmission loss after peripheral nerve injury.

TABLE 21.1 Consequences of Scar Formation

SKIN:	Keloid	**LUNG:**	Interstitial fibrosis
	Hypertrophic scar		Bronchopulmonary dysplasia
	Burn contracture	**HEART:**	Rheumatic HD
	Scleroderma		LV Aneurysm
GI:	Stricture	**EYE:**	Retrolental fibroplasia
	Adhesions		Diabetic retinopathy
	Chronic pancreatitis	**NERVE:**	Transmission loss
LIVER:	Cirrhosis	**BONE:**	Ankylosis
	Biliary atresia		Osteoarthritis
			Glomerulonephritis

Pathologic scarring and fibrosis also frequently occur in non-surgical specialties. The ophthalmologist observes retrolental fibroplasia in premature infants as well as a similar fibrotic retinopathy in diabetics. The gastroenterologist attempts to mollify the bleeding, liver failure, and encephalopathic complications of hepatic cirrhosis. The pulmonologist detects bronchopulmonary dysplasia in the tiny premature baby and diagnoses pulmonary fibrosis in the aging cigarette smoker. The radiotherapist worries about radiation-induced fibrosis. The cardiologist wishes to ameliorate the fibrotic endpoints of rheumatic heart disease—shortened, distorted chordae and scarred valve leaflets. The dermatologist deals with scleroderma. And this is only a partial list.

All of these problems are notoriously difficult to prevent or treat. The clinician's therapeutic role is largely to "hope for the best," much as physicians did in the past when confronted with what were then unsolved problems: appendicitis until 100 years ago, bacterial infections until 50 years ago, and organ replacement until recently. An understanding of fetal wound healing may lead to therapeutic strategies to help avert scarring and fibrosis. Healing without scar would have a tremendous impact on both medical and surgical practice.

DIFFERENCES IN THE FETAL AND ADULT WOUND ENVIRONMENT

The mechanisms that underlie scarless fetal tissue repair are unknown but may be unique to fetal cells, the fetal wound environment, or a combination of both. The fetal wound environment is quite different from the wound environment after adult tissue injury. The fetus is profoundly hypoxemic with an arterial pO_2 of 20 mm Hg.[4,5] There is only a minimal inflammatory response to fetal injury, since polymorphonuclear leukocytes and immunoglobulins are not present in the fetal wound matrix.[6,7] Finally, fetal skin wounds are continually bathed in warm, sterile amniotic fluid known to be rich in growth factors that are crucial for development.[8]

The lower fetal oxygen tension, the absence of acute inflammation, and the amniotic fluid environment might each dramatically influence wound healing. But the contribution of these differences to tissue repair may be partially discounted by recent results from fetal animal studies. Fetal tissue oxygenation remains consistently low throughout gestation, yet there is a spectrum to fetal wound healing as a function of gestational age: skin wound healing in the rat or the lamb fetus becomes adult-like with scar formation late in gestation.[9–11] Although the absence of polymorphonuclear leukocytes in the fetal wound matrix suggests that some of the characteristic inflammatory mediators of adult wound healing may be absent in fetal wounds, Simpson and Ross have shown that elimination of neutrophils in guinea pig wounds does not diminish scar formation.[12] Several lines of evidence suggest that amniotic fluid exposure is not crucial for scarless tissue repair. At birth, the opossum is physiologically and anatomically a fetus, and remains attached to the mother's nipple for 4–5 weeks before weaning. Although the "fetal" development of the marsupial continues in the non-sterile environment of the pouch/nipple and in the absence of an amniotic fluid milieu, scarless skin healing still occurs.[13] Fetal lamb studies have shown that exclusion of wounds from amniotic fluid by a silastic patch does not obviate scarless repair,[14] and that adult skin transplanted to the fetus heals with scar formation despite exposure to the fluid intrauterine environment.[15]

THE FETAL WOUND EXTRACELLULAR MATRIX

Scarless fetal wound healing may be attributed to the organization of a unique extracellular matrix (ECM). The fetal ECM has an entirely different profile of macromolecular structural constituents compared to the adult ECM. In particular, the early appearance and prolonged maintenance of an environment rich in hyaluronic acid (HA) facilitates cell mobility, cell proliferation, and regeneration in fetal wounds.[16,17] Hyaluronidase-treated polyvinyl alcohol sponges that are implanted into fetal rabbits show a significant reduction in HA content with concomitant striking fibroblast infiltration and collagen deposition.[18] Fetal serum, amniotic fluid, wound fluid and a number of fetal tissues contain a glycoprotein called hyaluronic acid stimulating activity (HASA).[19–21] This factor is present in the fetal wound for a prolonged period of time, which results in a prolonged HA-rich response in fetal wounds, a mechanism entirely absent in the adult wound.

Studies in our laboratory have examined the mechanisms by which HA is deposited in such abundance in the fetal wound, delineated the nature of fetal wound collagen deposition, and compared these processes with adult wound healing. Based on these studies, a theoretical model of HA deposition in wounds can be proposed. In the adult wound, the early deposition of HA by the platelet plug and the fibrin clot obviates the need for an exogenous mechanism for stimulating local HA production.[22] Following the initial deposition of HA, hyaluronidase is produced, HA is removed, sulfated glycosaminoglycans are then deposited, and finally collagen is laid down in a scar pattern. In contrast, fetal wounds are characterized by a persistent presence of HASA which underlies the prolonged presence of HA. Thus, the mechanism for eliciting the early HA-rich response in adult wounds is entirely different from the prolonged HA-rich response in fetal wounds.

Although the precise mechanisms of action of HA in fetal wound healing are unknown, an HA-rich ECM may provide a permissive environment for the orderly deposition of collagen.[6] The deposition of collagen without scarring in the fetal lamb model has been firmly established using histologic, immunohistochemical, biophysical, and biochemical techniques.[23] Siebert has postulated that HA influences the reorganization of wound collagen by acting as a carrier for biologically active proteins.[24,25] In addition, several proteins have been recently isolated from the ECM and found to be able to bind HA; they appear to be involved in the structuring of the ECM.[26,27]

MODULATION OF ADULT TISSUE REPAIR

What is the evidence that adult wounds can be modulated by HA to heal in a fetal-like manner? Historically, it is intriguing that reports from over 50 years ago documented that application of "embryonic tissue juices" enhanced wound repair.[28] Raedelli investigated the effect of HA on wound healing in rats and found that treated wounds develop greater wound breaking strength than untreated controls.[29] This finding was attributed to an early deposition of organized collagen fibers. Hellstrom and Laurent studied the healing of experimental tympanic membrane perforations in rats treated with topical HA.[30] Membranes treated with HA not only close faster than the untreated controls, but also show much less scar tissue with a discernible organized collagen fiber layer. The healing rate and degree of scar tissue were dependent on the concentration of HA, not on the molecular weight of HA. Abatangelo reported that topical HA enhances epithelial migration in wounded diabetic rats.[31] Balasz postulated that hyaluronate gels are ideally suitable as viscosurgical implants to prevent postoperative adhesions and to control scar formation.[32] Other experimental studies confirm the impression that HA is associated with healing that results in less scarring.[33,34] The efficacy of applying agents to maintain an HA-rich wound environment by either stimulating the deposition of HA or retarding HA breakdown must be tested.[19,35]

Immunocytochemistry, in situ hybridization, and wound fluid analysis should help elucidate the unique growth factor and ECM molecular profile of fetal tissue repair. For example, the deposition of fibronectin and tenascin occurs early in the fetal wound matrix and these phenomena may underlie rapid re-epithelialization in fetal wounds.[36,37] Recent documentation of the predominance of an embryonic pattern of fibronectin splicing during wound healing in the adult rat suggests that this fibronectin type is functionally more appropriate for the cell migration and proliferation associated with tissue repair.[38] When applied topically, fibronectin expedites wound healing in rats[39] and promotes healing of human corneal ulcers.[40] While there has been a considerable rush to document the therapeutic efficacy of various peptide growth factors on adult tissue repair, the characteristics of the normal growth environment in adult wound healing have been largely ignored. Preliminary studies examining the profile of peptide growth factors in fetal versus adult sheep wound fluid have already shown dramatic differences in insulin-like growth factor II and TGF-β isoform levels.[41]

Fetal wound healing research may also permit control of wound contraction. Wound contraction is the process by which the surrounding uninjured tissue is pulled over an open wound defect. When the cicatrization process continues after completion of wound closure, pathologic scar contracture results. Scar contracture can compromise tissue architecture and anatomic function—burn wound contracture and anastomotic stricture are two clinical examples. In vitro studies on fetal wound contraction have shown that amniotic fluid can inhibit (rabbit or human)[42,43] or stimulate (lamb)[44] fibroblast populated collagen lattice (FPCL) contraction. Additional studies in vivo are needed to confirm that adult wound contraction can be modulated when exposed to amniotic fluid. Recently, a protein has been identified in sheep amniotic fluid that specifically stimulates human FPCL contraction.[45] Development of blocking antibodies against this protein or isolation of a contraction inhibitor from human amniotic fluid may have substantial clinical utility in preventing scar contracture.

THE FETAL CLEFT LIP DILEMMA

Recently there have been several articles and editorials advocating surgical correction of cleft lip in utero.[46–49] Anticipated benefits of this form of surgery would be: 1) restoration of normal lip form without visible scarring, 2) normal mid-facial growth unrestricted by scar formation, and 3) prevention of secondary nasal deformities associated with cleft lip. But if fetal surgery is to be effective, the optimal time during gestation when surgery should be performed must be determined. In the fetal lamb model there is a change to a more adult type of healing with scar formation during the third trimester.[9] In humans, the precise time at which this transition from fetal to adult type repair occurs is unknown. In addition, human embryos show evidence of secondary deformities associated with clefting beginning at 10 weeks gestation.[50] Repair later in gestation may partially correct these deformities but repair during the first trimester may be necessary to provide complete correction.

Advances in prenatal diagnosis, particularly ultrasound, have led to fetal surgery becoming a reality. Diagnosing cleft lip and palate ultrasonographically is not difficult, but there is evidence that the rate of severe defects associated with cleft lip and palate is much higher in clefts diagnosed in utero compared to those diagnosed at birth.[51] Thus, the prenatal assessment must also ensure that the fetus found to have a cleft does not have other significant anatomic or chromosomal anomalies.

Fetal surgery for cleft lip and palate carries the same fetal and maternal risks as does surgery for life-threatening fetal anomalies, while the benefits, although potentially substantial and attractive, are unproven. Further experimental studies on fetal wound healing and new developments in fetoscopic surgery may eventually allow in utero repair of cleft lip and palate. At present, performance of fetal surgery for human clefts is inappropriate.

SUMMARY

Using the fetal wound healing "blueprint," novel guidelines for scarless tissue repair may be defined. Adult wound healing is a complex process involving a variety of cell types, serum components, and cell products. The constituents of fetal wound healing require analysis in order to understand the control mechanisms that endow the fetus with unique healing abilities. The ultimate aim is to understand the biology of fetal tissue repair, then apply these lessons to prevent fibrosis and contracture in children and adults.

REFERENCES

1. Barbul A, Pines E, Caldwell M, Hunt TK, eds: Growth factors and other aspects of wound healing: Biological and clinical implications. Progress in Clinical and Biological Research. Vol. 266. New York: Alan R. Liss, 1988.
2. Mustoe TA, Pierce GF, Thomason A, et al.: Accelerated healing of incisional wounds in rats induced by transforming growth factor-B. Science 237:1333–1335, 1987.
3. Peacock EE: Wound Repair. WB Saunders, Philadelphia: 1986, p.ix.
4. Nelson NM: Respiration and circulation before birth, in Smith CA, Nelson NM (eds): The Physiology of the Newborn Infant, 4th Ed. Thomas, Springfield, Illinois, 1976.
5. Hock RJ: The physiology of high altitude. Sci Amer 22:52–59, 1970.

6. Longaker MT, Whitby DJ, Adzick NS, et al.: Studies in fetal wound healing: VI. Second and early third trimester fetal wounds demonstrate rapid collagen deposition without scar formation. J Pediatr Surg 25:63–69, 1990.
7. Adzick NS, Harrison MR, Glick PL, et al.: Comparison of fetal, newborn and adult wound healing by histologic, enzyme-histochemical, and hydroxyproline determination. J Pediatr Surg 20:315–320, 1985.
8. Mulvihill SJ, Stone MM, Fonkalsrud EW: Trophic effects of amniotic fluid on fetal gastrointestinal development. J Surg Res 40:291–296, 1986.
9. Dixon JB: Inflammation in the foetal and neonatal rat: The local reactions to skin burns. J Path Bact 80:73–78, 1960.
10. Ihara S, Motobayashi Y, Nagao E, et al.: Ontogenetic transition of wound healing pattern in rat skin occurring at the fetal stage. Development 110:671–680, 1990.
11. Longaker MT, Adzick NS: The biology of fetal wound healing: A review. Plastic Reconstr Surg 87:788–798, 1990.
12. Simpson DM, Ross R: The neutrophilic leukocyte in wound repair. A study with antineutrophil serum. J Clin Invest 51:2009–2020, 1972.
13. Howarth G, Ferguson MWJ: A comparison of wound healing in adult and pouch young of Monodelphis Domestica. Presented at the British Society of Cell Biology meeting. Manchester, England, April 1990.
14. Longaker MT, Burd DAR, Yen TSB, et al.: Midgestation fetal lamb excisional wounds contract in utero. J Pediatr Surg (in press).
15. Longaker MT, Whitby DJ, Jennings RW, et al.: Adult skin in the fetal environment heals with scar formation. Surgical Forum 41:639–641, 1990.
16. DePalma RL, Krummel TM, Durham LA III, et al.: Characterization and quantitation of wound matrix in the fetal rabbit. Matrix 9:224–230, 1989.
17. Longaker MT, Chiu ES, Adzick NS, et al.: Studies in fetal wound healing: V. A prolonged presence of hyaluronic acid characterizes fetal wound fluid. Ann Surg 213:292–296, 1991.
18. Mast BA, Haynes JH, Schatzki PF, et al.: Hyaluronic acid regulates the cellular response in fetal wound healing. Presented at the 35th Annual Meeting of the Plastic Surgery Research Council, Washington, DC, 1990.
19. Longaker MT, Chiu ES, Harrison MR, et al.: Studies in fetal wound healing: IV. Hyaluronic acid stimulating activity distinguishes fetal wound fluid from adult wound fluid. Ann Surg 210:667–672, 1989.
20. Longaker MT, Adzick NS, Crombleholme TM, et al.: Studies in fetal wound healing. VII: Fetal wound healing may be modulated by elevated hyaluronic acid stimulating activity in amniotic fluid. J Pediatr Surg 25:430–433, 1990.
21. Decker M, Chiu ES, Dollbaum C, et al.: Hyaluronic acid stimulating factor in serum from the bovine fetus and from breast cancer patients. Canc Res 49:3499–4004, 1989.
22. Weigel PH, Fuller GM, LeBoeuf RD: A model for the role of hyaluronic acid and fibrin in the early events during the inflammatory response and wound healing. J Theor Biol 119:219–226, 1986.
23. Burd DAR, Longaker MT, Adzick NS, et al.: Fetal wound healing in a large animal model: The deposition of collagen is confirmed. Brit J Plast Surg 43:571–577, 1990.
24. Siebert JW, Burd DAR, McCarthy JG, et al.: Fetal wound healing: A biochemical study of scarless healing. Plast Reconstr Surg 85:495–499, 1990.
25. Burd DAR, Siebert JW, Ehrlich HP, et al.: Human skin and post-burn hyaluronan: Demonstration of the association with collagen and other proteins. Matrix 9:322–328, 1989.
26. Turley EA, Brassel P, Moore D, et al.: A hyaluronan-binding protein shows a partial and temporally regulated codistribution with actin on locomoting chick heart fibroblasts. Exp Cell Res 187:243–248, 1990.
27. Yoneda M, Suzuki S, Kimata K: Hyaluronic acid associated with the surfaces of cultured fibroblasts is linked to a serum-derived 85-kD protein. J Biol Chem 265:5247–5252, 1990.
28. Arey LB: Wound healing. Physiol Reviews 16:327, 1936.
29. Radaelli E, Piazzini A, Marrazzi M, et al.: Role of hyaluronic acid in wound healing. Ultrastructural observations. International Symposium on Cutaneous Development, Aging, and Repair, University of Padova, 1982, p.42.
30. Hellstrom S, Laurent C: Hyaluronan and healing of tympanic membrane perforations. An experimental study. Acta Otolaryngology Suppl 442:54–61, 1987.
31. Abatangelo G, Marrelli M, Vecchia RP: Healing of hyaluronic acid-enriched wounds: Histological observations. J Surg Res 35:410–416, 1983.

32. Balasz EA, Denlinger JL: Clinical uses of hyaluronan. In: Evered D, Whelan J (eds). The Biology of Hyaluronan. J. Wiley & Sons, 1989, p. 265.
33. Chung JH, Fagerholm P, Lindstrom B: Hyaluronate in healing of corneal alkali wounds in the rabbit. Exp Eye Res 48:569–576, 1989.
34. Wiig ME, Amiel D, Van de Berg J, et al.: The early effects of high molecular weight hyaluronan (Hyaluronic Acid) on anterior cruciate ligament healing: An experimental study in rabbits. J Orthoped Res 8:425–434, 1990.
35. Decker M, Chiu ES, Dollbaum C, et al.: Hyaluronic acid stimulating factor in serum from the bovine fetus and from breast cancer patients. Can Res 49:3499, 1989.
36. Longaker MT, Whitby DJ, Crombleholme TM, et al.: Studies in fetal wound healing: III. Early deposition of adhesion molecules distinguishes fetal from adult wounds. J Pediatr Surg 24:799, 1989.
37. Whitby DJ, Longaker MT, Adzick NS, et al.: Rapid epithelialization of fetal wounds is associated with the early deposition of tenascin. J Cell Science (in press).
38. ffrench-Constant C, Van De Water L, Dvorak HF, et al.: Reappearance of an embryonic pattern of fibronectin splicing during wound healing in the adult rat. J Cell Biol 109:903, 1989.
39. Cheng CY, Martin DE, Legget CG, et al.: Fibronectin enhances healing of excised wounds in rats. Arch Dermatol 124:221, 1988.
40. Kono I, Matsumoto Y, Kano K, et al.: Beneficial effect of topical fibronectin in patients with keratoconjunctivitis sicca of Sjogren's syndrome. J Rheumatol 12:487, 1985.
41. Longaker MT, Adzick NS: Unpublished data.
42. Krummel TM, Ehrlich HP, Nelson JM, et al.: Fetal wounds do not contract in utero. Surg Forum 40:613, 1989.
43. Chang B, Siebert JW, Longaker MT, et al.: Do human fetal wounds contract? Presented at the 35th Annual Meeting of The Plastic Surgery Research Council, Washington, DC April 1990.
44. Burd DAR, Longaker MT, Rittenberg T, et al.: In vitro fetal wound contraction: The effect of amniotic fluid. Brit J Plast Surg 44:302–305, 1991.
45. Rittenberg T, Longaker MT, Adzick NS, et al.: Sheep amniotic fluid has a protein factor which stimulates human fibroblast populated collagen lattice contraction. J Cell Physiol (in press).
46. Christ JE: Fetal surgery: A frontier for plastic surgery. Plast Reconstr Surg 77:645, 1986.
47. Dado DV, Kernahan DA, Gianopoulos JG: Intrauterine repair of cleft lip: What's involved. Plast Reconstr Surg 85:461–465, 1990.
48. Sullivan WG: Intrauterine repair of cleft lip: What's involved (Discussion) Plast Reconstr Surg 85:466–467, 1990.
49. Hallock GG: In defense of intrauterine repair of cleft lip. Plast Reconstr Surg 85:801, 1990.
50. Akimoto N, Ikeda T, Satow Y, et al.: Craniofacial and oral malformations in an autopsy population of Japanese human fetuses and newborns. J Craniofacial Genet Develop Biol Supp 2:213–230, 1986.
51. Saltzman DH, Benacerraf BR, Frigoletto FD: Diagnosis and management of fetal facial clefts. Am J Obstet Gynecol 155:377–380, 1986.
52. Longaker MT, Whitby DJ, Adzick NS, et al.: Fetal surgery for cleft lip: A plea for caution. Plast Reconst Surg (in press).

Index

H

I